Multidrug Resistant Pediatric Infections

Multidrug Resistant Pediatric Infections

Editors

Nupur Ganguly
Associate Professor
Department of Pediatrics
Institute of Child Health, Kolkata

Ritabrata Kundu
Professor
Department of Pediatrics
Institute of Child Health, Kolkata

Tapan Kr Ghosh
Scientific Coordinator
Institute of Child Health, Kolkata

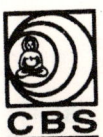

CBS

CBS Publishers & Distributors Pvt. Ltd.

New Delhi • Bangalore • Pune • Chennai • Cochin

ISBN : 978-81-239-1766-5

First Edition : 2009
Reprint : 2011

Published by Satish Kumar Jain and produced by V.K. Jain for
CBS Publishers & Distributors Pvt. Ltd.,
CBS Plaza, 4819/XI Prahlad Street, 24 Ansari Road, Daryaganj,
New Delhi - 110002, India. • Website: www.cbspd.com
e-mail: delhi@cbspd.com, cbspubs@vsnl.com, cbspubs@airtelmail.in
Ph.: 23289259, 23266861, 23266867 • Fax: 011-23243014

Branches:
• *Bengaluru:* Seema House, 2975, 17th Cross, K.R. Road,
  Bansankari 2nd Stage, Bengaluru - 560070   Ph.: +91-80-26771678/79
  Fax: +91-80-26771680 • E-mail: cbsbng@gmail.com,
  bangalore@cbspd.com
• *Pune:* Bhuruk Prestige, Sr. No. 52/12/2+1+3/2,
  Narhe, Haveli (Near Katraj-Dehu Road By-pass), Pune - 411051
  Ph.: +91-20-64704058/59, 32342277 • E-mail: pune@cbspd.com
• *Kochi:* 36/14, Kalluvilakam, Lissie Hospital Road,
  Kochi - 682018, Kerala • Ph.: +91-484-4059061-65
  Fax: +91-484-4059065 • E-mail: cochin@cbspd.com
• *Chennai:* 20, West Park Road, Shenoy Nagar, Chennai - 600030
  Ph.: +91-44-26260666, 26208620 • Fax: +91-44-42032115
  E-mail: chennai@cbspd.com

Printed at :
India Binding House, Noida (UP)

Preface

A few years back the present editors brought out an exclusive book on most common multidrug resistant infections in children for the first time, where many stalwarts in this field had contributed their chapters. This time an updated version of those issues and topics is made with broader perspective including some of the most common problems, which were not included last time. This book is completely a new venture, which has tried to specify the problems and causes behind development of antimicrobial resistance by the microorganisms and also to disseminate knowledge on these multidrug resistant infectious diseases in the pediatric age group.

Problem of antimicrobial resistance is currently a burning issue in the entire world. The first line and cheap drugs are no longer effective in the treatment of most infectious diseases making the health scenario very complicated and expensive. Even the Governments of these countries are also becoming financially hard pressed day-by-day with their fixed and limited health budgets. With the change of time the practice of empirical antimicrobial therapy on presumption is no longer recommended except in very selected cases and situations. Every effort should be made to diagnose and isolate the offending agent. By this, not only definitive treatment will be ensured but also target specific antibiotic can be administered. Previous practice of use of broad-spectrum antibiotics even for trivial infection is presently highly discouraged. It only increases the emergence of resistance strains of offending organisms and cost of therapy. In the process of hospital-based treatment the child acquires infection from the hospital setting. These bugs are more virulent and resistant to the commonly used broad-spectrum antibiotics.

Here, in addition to typhoid, tuberculosis and malaria the three most common MDR infections in children, other bacteriological infections, which are also emerging as MDR organisms have been included. Various strains of organisms like MRSA, ESBL, VRE and Pan drug-resistant organisms are discussed. The four most common steps to prevent multidrug resistance: (i) Proper establishment of the diagnosis before starting the antimicrobial treatment, (ii) choosing the narrow spectrum effective antimicrobial, (iii) avoiding the prescription of irrational combinations, and (iv) not prescribing antimicrobials in trivial and common viral infection, will definitely help in reducing this problem in community to a great extent.

Hope this book will help our readers and encourage them to work in the right direction.

Editors
Nupur Ganguly
Ritabrata Kundu
Tapan Kr Ghosh

List of Contributors

Ajay Kalra
Professor of Pediatrics,
S N Medical College, Agra
Email: drajaykalra@yahoo.com

Anju Aggarwal
Associate Professor of Pediatrics,
University College of Medical Sciences and
Guru Tegh Bahadur Hospital, New Delhi
Email: aggar_anju@yahoo.com

Ashok Kr Dutta
Director, Professor and Head of the Department of
Pediatrics(Ex), LHMC & Associated Hospital,
New Delhi. Email : drdutta@gmail.com

Ashok Kapse
Associate Professor of Pediatrics (Retd),
Surat Institute of Medical Education and Research
and Government Medical College,
Surat. Presently Consultant Pediatrician, Surat.
Email: ashok.kapse@gmail.com,
        ashokkapse@hotmail.com

Baldev Prajapati
Associate Professor of Pediatrics,
Sheth L G General Hospital,
Smt NHL Municipal Medical College, Ahmedabad.
Aakanksha Children Hospital and Neonatal Nursery,
Nava Vadaj Road, Ahmedabad-380 013.
Email: baldevprajapati55@yahoo.com

Camilla Rodrigues
Consultant Microbiologist, P D Hinduja National
Hospital, Mumbai
Email: dr_crodrigues@hindujahospital.com

Digant D Shastri
Consultant Pediatrician, Killol Children Hospital,
Surat, Email: drdigant@hotmail.com

Indu Khosla
Consultant Pediatrician, Mumbai
Email: drinduk@yahoo.com

Ira Shah
Incharge, Pediatric HIV and TB Clinic,
B.J.Wadia Hospital for Children
Editor – Pediatric Oncall
Asian Editor – Journal of Pediatric Infectious Diseases
Email: irashah@pediatriconcall.com

Jaydeep Choudhury
Assistant Professor of Pediatrics, Institute of Child
Health, Calcutta, Kolkata 700017
Email: drjaydeep_choudhury@yahoo.co.in

Joydeep Das
Assistant Professor of Pediatrics, Institute of Child
Health, Calcutta, Kolkata 700 017
Email: dr_joydeepdas@yahoo.com

M Indrasekhar Rao
Professor of Pediatrics,
Osmania Medical College, Hyderabad
Email: indramummulla@yahoo.co.in

Monjori Mitra
Assistant Professor of Pediatrics,
Institute of Child Health, Calcutta, Kolkata 700 017
Email: monjorim@vsnl.net

Nigam Prakash Narain
Associate Professor of Pediatrics,
Patna Medical College, Patna
Email: nigampn@gmail.com

Nitin K Shah
Consultant Pediatrician and Pediatric Hematologist,
PD Hinduja National Hospital, Mumbai, National
President, Indian Academy of Pediatrics (2006)
Email: drnitinshah@hotmail.com

Nupur Ganguly
Associate Professor of Pediatrics,
Institute of Child Health, Calcutta, Kolkata 700 017
Email: nupur_diya@yahoo.com

Parang N Mehta
Consultant Pediatrician,
Mehta Hospital, Surat
Email: parang@mehtachildcare.com,
        parang@iqara.net

Pratima Shah
Associate Professor of Pediatrics (Retd),
Smt NHL Municipal Medical College, Ahmedabad.

Rajal B. Prajapati
Associate Professor, Sheth V S General Hospital,
Smt NHL Municipal Medical College, Ahmedabad.

Raju C Shah
Associate Professor of Pediatrics,
Smt NHL Municipal Medical College, Ahmedabad
National President IAP (2005), President,
Pediatric Association of SAARC (2005-08),
Ankur Institute of Child Health,
Ashram Road, Ahmedabad 380 009
Email: rajucshah@rediffmail.com,
        rajucshah@lycos.com

Ritabrata Kundu
Professor of Pediatrics,
Institute of Child Health, Calcutta, Kolkata 700 017
Email: rkundu22@gmail.com

Sangeeta Sharma
Pediatrician and Head, Department of Pediatrics,
LRS Institute of Tuberculosis and Respiratory
Diseases, New Delhi
Email: sangeetasharma2000@gmail.com

Shivananda
Professor and Head of the Department of Pediatrics
(Retd), Bangalore Medical College, Superintendent,
Vani Vilas Hospital, Bangalore
Email: sssiddhi@rediffmail.com

Soumya Swaminathan
Deputy Director, Division of HIV/AIDS,
Tuberculosis Research Center, ICMR, Chennai
Email: doctorsoumya@yahoo.com

Tapan Kr Ghosh
Scientific Co-ordinator, Institute of Child Health,
Calcutta, Kolkata 700 017
Email: dr_tkghosh@rediffmail.com

Tanu Singhal
Consultant, Pediatric Infectious Diseases,
Kokilaben Ambani Hospital, Andheri, Mumbai.
Email: tanusinghal@yahoo.com

T U Sukumaran
Professor of Pediatrics, Pushpagiri Institute of Medical
Sciences, Tiruvalla, Kerala
Email: tusukumaran@hotmail.com

Vijay N Yewale
Consultant Pediatrician, Dr.Yewale Hospital and
Vashi Criticare, Navi Mumbai,
Editor-in-Chief, Pediatric Infectious Diseases
Email: vnyewale@gmail.com

Contents

Section 1: Typhoid

Section 2: Tuberculosis

Section 3: Malaria

Section 4: Other Resistant Bacterial Infections

Section 1
Typhoid

1

Epidemiology of Typhoid Fever

Ajay Kalra

Typhoid fever occurs in all parts of the world where water supply and sanitation are substandard. The disease is uncommon in developed countries where most of the cases that occur are either imported by immigrants or acquired abroad[1]. Worldwide typhoid fever affects 17 million people (range 6–33 million) with more than 5–6 lakh deaths every year[2,3]. By other estimates, in the year 2000, there were 21.6 million typhoid cases in the world with 216,000 deaths[4,5]. Ninety percent of cases and deaths are in Asia and the rest in Africa and Latin America[4].

In India, typhoid fever is endemic especially in the urban areas. One percent of children below 17 years of age suffer from typhoid fever every year[1]. It is estimated that the incidence of typhoid fever in India is 214.7 cases per one lakh population per year making it an area of high incidence[4].

Case fatality rate is 1–4% in treated patients[2,5,6]. If left untreated case fatality can climb to 10–20%[7,8]. Children 4 years or younger may have a high fatality rate, 10 times higher than older children, that is 4% as compared to 0.4%[9]. Hospitalization rates vary from 10–40%[10].

Causative Organism

Salmonella typhi, a non motile, non capsulated Gram negative bacillus is the cause of typhoid fever. Paratyphoid is caused by *Salmonella paratyphi* A, B and C. The bacilli has several antigens of which three main ones are O, H and Vi. Antibodies to O and H antigens are used in serodiagnosis. *S. typhi* has more than 80 phage types. Phage typing is a useful epidemiological tool in tracing the source of epidemics.

S. typhi and *paratyphi* together form a group of fevers referred to as enteric fever. Typhoid forms 90% of this group. The organism survives intracellularly; it grows rapidly on ordinary media and under aerobic as well as anaerobic conditions. It is rapidly killed by drying, pasteurization and common disinfectants.

Reservoir

Man is the only reservoir in the form of cases and carriers. The cases may be subclinical (missed) or clinical (mild to severe). Carriers may be temporary as seen during the stages of incubation and convalescence, or they may be chronic, in 3–5% patients, who excrete bacillus for more than one year (may be even up to 50 years).

Incubation Period

The incubation period is 10–14 days but may be as short as 3 days and as long as 3 weeks. This depends on the dose of the bacillus ingested. *S. typhi* rapidly divides in less than half hour of infection. So that, after one to two weeks, the amount of bacilli that result from even a single bacillus are tremendous. Thus, the total bacilli that result from infection with millions of organisms would be stupendous and beyond calculation. The incubation period is inversely proportional to the size of inoculum. However, the normal intestinal flora is an important defence against invasion by typhoid bacillus and not all cases who get infected would get the disease.

Spread of Infection

Poverty, inadequate sanitary facilities and questionable water supplies are conditions prevalent in developing countries and conducive to getting typhoid fever. Besides this, the possibility of inadequate facilities for processing human waste leading to heavy contamination of water supplies always prevails.

The primary sources of infection are the feces and urine of cases and carriers, while the secondary sources are contaminated water, food and dissemination by hands and flies. *S. typhi* does not multiply in water but can survive for about a week, although a majority die within 48 hours. In average, the organism can survive for weeks. The organism cannot survive in sea water as it is bactericidal. In soil irrigated with water from sewage, *S. typhi* may survive for nearly two months. The organism does not get killed in low temperature but cannot multiply below 5°C. Thus the *S. typhi* can survive for more than a month in ice and ice creams[11].

S. typhi can also grow rapidly in milk without altering its taste or appearance. Milk can get infected either by hands of a human carrier or by means of infected water used at some stage of collection or distribution. Milk products like cream, ice creams and cheese have also been known to have caused epidemics.

Vegetables grown on sewage irrigated farms may be infected with typhoid bacilli and can be a source of infection if taken raw without being washed properly or by using chlorine and potassium permanganate in the water.

Other food sources which can commonly lead to infection are meat products (when not cooked well) and untreated shellfish. The organism remains viable on external surface of houseflies for as long as 20 days[11]. These flies carry the bacillus from the feces to food and are thus an important source of infection.

Chemicals which can help on preventing the spread of infection by destroying the bacteria are phenols, mercuric chloride, formaldehyde and quaternary ammonium compounds, chlorine and potassium permanganate and gamma radiations can be used for treating food.

There are various personal, social factors and practices which are conducive for the spread of infection. These are not washing hands properly after toilets, low standard of food and kitchen hygiene, washing infected material near kitchen, defecation and urination in open spaces, illiteracy and lack of health education. The problem is further compounded by scarcity of water due to a rapidly increasing population and urbanization. Patients with parasitic infections such as roundworms or schistosomiasis are also readily infected with *S. typhi* as the organism gets adhered to the surface of the parasites with help of pili.

There are now increasing reports of outbreaks of multidrug resistant typhoid fever (MDRTF). These epidemics begin abruptly and the disease spreads to involve large areas of a whole city or even a state. High attack rates lead to clustering of cases. In India, several MDRTF outbreaks have occurred during 1989-1996[12]. Ninety percent of the resistant isolates belonged to a single phage type E1 suggesting that there could have been a common source of infection. It has been further seen that children constitute about 40–50% of these cases and of these 15–50% were below the age of 5 years. This has led to increase in the incidence of severe cases, hospitalization and mortality.

Age Distribution

It may occur at any age but is more prevalent in children and young adults. The peak incidence is in children aged 5–15 years. As the person grows older he becomes relatively immune because of the acquired immunity due to sub-infectious exposure to typhoid bacilli.

Recent reports[4,13-16] indicate that while school aged children continue to be at a particular high risk, the incidence of typhoid fever in pre-school children (even as young as 2 years old) in the high incidence areas is of the same order of magnitude as that for school children, some times even more. This has led to the need to develop a conjugate vaccine.

Gender Predeliction

Both sexes are equally susceptible but cases of typhoid fever are seen more commonly in males. The females are more prone to become chronic carriers, the incidence being nearly three folds as compared to males.

Seasonal Variation

Cases occur throughout the year but increase during the summers, the peak months being July to September[7].

Serological Profile

In endemic areas the individual titers of O (somatic) and H (flagellar) antibodies in general population is high as compared to areas or countries with better sanitation conditions. Therefore, in a Widal test, a single measurement of these antibodies indicates only a past exposure to the bacilli. To be diagnostic of typhoid fever an antibody titers of at least 1/160 against O antigen or, better still, a four fold or greater rise of these antibodies in paired serum specimens collected two weeks apart, is of significance. These antibodies reach a peak during the third week of illness and then gradually decline to reach the pre-illness level in a few months.

References

1. Park K. Typhoid fever. In Park K, ed. Park's Text. book of Preventive and Social Medicine, 16th ed. Jabalpur: Banarasidas Bhanot Publishers, 2000: 175-8.
2. Crump JA *et al*. The global burden of typhoid fever. *Bull WHO* 2004; 82,346-98.
3. World Health Organization. Background document: The diagnosis, treatment and prevention of typhoid fever. Geneva: WHO, 2003 (WHO/ V&B/03.07).
4. Ochiai RL, Acosta CJ, Danovaro Holliday MC, Baiquing D, *et al*. A study of typhoid fever in five Asian countries : Disease burden and implications for control. *Bull WHO*, 2008;86:260-8.
5. Ivanoff BN, Levine MM, Lambert PH. Vaccination against typhoid fever – present status. *Bull WHO* 1994;72:1957-76.
6. Parry CM. The treatment of multidrug-resistant and naladixic acid-resistant typhoid fever in Viet-Nam. *Trans Royal Soc Trop Med Hyg* 2004;83:413-22.
7. Levine MM, Black RE, Lanata C. Chilean Typhoid Committee. Precise estimation of the numbers of chronic carriers of *Salmonella typhi* in Santiago, Chile, an endemic area. *J Infec Dis* 1982;146:724-26.
8. Hessel L, Debois H, Fletcher M, Dumas R. Experience with *Salmonella typhi* Vi capsular polysaccharide vaccine. *Eur J Clin Microbiol Infect Dis* 1999;18:609-20.

9. Bhutta ZA. Impact of age and drug resistance on mortality in typhoid fever. *Arch Dis Child* 1996:72: 214-17.

10. Parry CM, Hien TT, Dougan G, Wite NJ, Farrar JJ. Typhoid Fever. *N Engl J Med* 2002;347:1770-82.

11. Ichhpujani RL, Bhatia R. Magnitude of problem. In: Typhoid Fever, 1st ed. Delihi: Top Publications, 1997:9-14.

12. Gupta A. Multidrug resistant typhoid fever in children: Epidemiology and therapeutic approach. *Pediatr Infect Dis.* 1994;13:134-40.

13. Sinha A, *et al.* Typhoid fever in children aged less than 5 years. *Lancet* 1999;354,734-7.

14. Saha SK, Baqui AH, *et al.* Typhoid fever in Bangladesh : Implications for vaccination policy, *Pediatr Infect Dis J* 2001;20:521-4.

15. Gupta A Swarnkar, NK, *et al.* Changing antibiotic sensitivity in enteric fever *J Tropical Pediatr* 2001;147,369-71.

16. Saha MR, *et al.* A note on incidence of typhoid fever in diverse age groups in Kolkata, India. *Japanese J Infect Dis.* 2003;56:121-2.

2

Pathogenesis of Typhoid Fever

Nigam Prakash Narain

Salmonella are a group of gram-negative bacteria belonging to the enterobacteriacea family. Typhoid fever is a systemic infection caused by *Salmonella enterica* serotype *typhi* . Salmonella are further subdivided into serovars based on the detection of 3 major antigenic determinants; the somatic lipopoly-saccharide O antigen (O9 and O12), the surface capsular polysaccharide Vi antigen and the protein flagellar H antigen[1].

Salmonella produce acid on glucose fermentation, reduce nitrates and do not produce cytochrome oxidase. They are non-spore forming and facultative anaerobe. They are motile by peritrichous flagella and produce H_2S on sugar fermentation. The salmonella are divided into serogroups (A, B, C1, C2,D,E) based on reactivity to somatic O-antigen antisera.

The complete genome of a multidrug resistant strain of *S. enterica* serovar typhi (CT18), isolated from a child with typhoid fever from Mekong valley basin of Vietnam has been delineated which has been found to harbour two plasmids. The larger conjugative plasmid encodes resistance to chloram-phenicol, ampicillin, trimethoprim, sulphona-mides and streptomycin. The smaller plasmid is phenotypically cryptic.

Pathogenesis

Salmonella are transmitted to humans by ingestion of food or water contaminated by fecal or urinary carriers excreting *S. enterica* serotype *typhi* orally. The infectious dose of *S. enterica* serotype *typhi* in volunteers varies between 1000 and one million organisms[2]. In the small intestine the bacteria adhere to mucosal cells and then invade the mucosa. There is not the same tendency to mucosal damage as occurs with shigella infections but ulceration of lymphoid follicles may occur. Initially *S. typhi* proliferates in the second part of the Peyer's patches of the lower small intestine from where systemic dissemination occurs, to the liver, spleen, and reticuloendo-thelial system. After penetration the invading microorganisms translocate to the intestinal lymphoid follicles and the draining mesenteric lymph nodes and some pass on to the reticulo-endothelial cells of the liver and spleen. The salmonella organisms are able to survive and multiply within the mononuclear phagocytic cells of the lymphoid follicles, liver and spleen[3]. At a critical point, which is probably determined by the number of bacteria, their virulence and the host response, the organisms are released from this sequestered intracellular habitat into the blood stream[2]. The incubation period is usually 7–14 days. In the bacteremic phase the organism is widely disseminated commonly to liver, spleen, bone marrow, gall bladder and Peyer's patches of the terminal ileum. Organisms excreted in the bile either reinvade the intestinal wall or are excreted in the feces[2,3].

The surface Vi capsular antigen interferes with phagocytosis by preventing the binding of C3 to the surface of bacterium. The ability of bacteria to survive within macrophages after phagocytosis is an important virulence trait[4]. After the macrophages have been activated by sensitized lymphocytes, an inflammatory reaction takes place and results in swelling, necrosis and ulceration of Peyer's patches, which in most cases heals uneventfully[5,6]. Typhoid fever induces systemic and local humoral and cellular immune responses but these confer incomplete protection against relapse and reinfection[6].

Pathology

Pathology in the Peyer's patches can be divided into four phases. These phases correspond approximately to the weeks of disease if treatment has not been given.

Phase 1: Hyperplasia of lymphoid follicles.

Phase 2: Necrosis of lymphoid follicles during the second week involving both mucosa and submucosa.

Phase 3: Ulceration in the long axis of the bowel with the possibility of perforation and hemorrhage.

Phase 4: Healing takes place from the fourth week onward, and unlike tuberculosis of the bowel with its encircling ulcers, does not produce strictures.

Although the ileum is the classical seat of typhoid pathology, lymphoid follicles may be affected in parts of the gastrointestinal tract, such as the jejunum and ascending colon. The ileum usually contains larger and more numerous Peyer's patches than the jejunum, but this is not an invariable finding. It is not generally appreciated that such lymphoid follicles are also found in the large intestine. The number of solitary follicles in large intestine decreases with age. Ulceration during paratyphoid B infection may involve stomach and large intestine as well.

The reticuloendothelial system, enlargement and congestion of the spleen and mesenteric nodes are characteristic finding.

The hepatosplenomegaly due to recruitment of mononuclear cells and the development of a cell-mediated immune response to *S. typhi* colonization and erosion of blood vessels thereafter may cause intestinal hemorrhage and extension of necrosis through the bowel wall may result in perforation.

Typhoid nodules, which are foci of macrophages and lymphocytes, can be detected in a large number of organs. Cloudy swelling of the liver and kidney occurs and renal failure may occur in some cases due to immune complex disease.

Various neuropsychiatric complications are common in typhoid fever, the exact pathogenesis of which is not known. However, these mechanisms have been postulated:

i. Non-specific allergic demyelinating form of encephalomyelitis which may occur as reaction to a number of bacterial and viral illnesses.

ii. An 'endarteritis obliterans' may produce thrombosis and ultimately paraplegia.

Typhoid induces systemic and local humoral and cellular responses, but these confer incomplete protection against relapse and reinfection.

References

1. ParkhillJ DG, James JD, *et al*.Complete genome sequence of a multiple drug resistant *Salmonella enterica* serovar typhi CT18. *Nature* 2001;413:848-52.

2. Afroza S. Typhoid fever in children–an update; *J Bangladesh Coll Phys Surg* 2003; 21:141-8.

3. Singh S. Pathogenesis and laboratory diagnosis: *J Indian Acad Clin Med* 2001;2:17-20.

4. Eggleton FC, Santoshi B, Singh CM. Typhoid perforationof bowel. *Ann Surg* 1979;190:31-6.

5. Shetty PB, Broome DR, Shetty PB, Broome DR.Sonographic analysis of gall bladder findings in salmonella enteric fever: *J Ultrasound Med* 1998;17:231-7.

6. Everest P, Wain J, Roberts M, Rook G, Dougan G, Everest P, *et al*. The molecular mechanisms of severe typhoid fever: *Trends in microbiology* 2001; 9:316-20.

3

Clinical Features and Differential Diagnosis of Typhoid Fever

Parang N Mehta

Typhoid fever is a systemic bacterial disease caused by *Salmonella typhi*, and is a common cause of fever in our country. Though it can be eliminated by good environmental sanitation and a safe drinking water supply, it continues to have a high incidence. Familiarity with its clinical features and differential diagnosis is therefore important for all who deal with children's health. This disease, which has been known for centuries, is now posing fresh problems because of the phenomenon of multidrug resistance. While it is almost non existent in developed countries, typhoid is a major cause of sickness among children in our country.

Typhoid fever usually manifests itself one to two weeks after the infection[1,2], but the incubation period may vary from 3 to 40 days[3]. This depends on the native immunity of the child, the virulence of the organisms, and the size of the infecting dose. The clinical features of typhoid fever vary with the age group, and from patient to patient and between geographical locations. The disease often has no definite distinguishing features, and diagnosis is sometimes made after several days, by a process of exclusion.

Salmonella paratyphi also cause disease similar to typhoid fever. Disease caused by other salmonella species is less severe than that caused by *Salmonella typhi*, and the case fatality rate is lower. Untreated typhoid fever has been reported to have a mortality of 10%.

Clinical Features

Fever

Fever is the most common manifestation of enteric fever, being present in nearly all patients[4-6]. The onset of fever is gradual, and parents often find it difficult to say when exactly the fever started. The fever increases from day to day, and by the end of one week, the child usually has high grade continuous fever. This fever may be as high as 40°C (104°F), and some children have chills and shivering[4]. The fever is often accompanied by bodyache, headache, and anorexia, though young children do not complain of these. Some children become very lethargic.

During the second week, high fever persists, and the child appears acutely ill, with marked anorexia, fatigue, and prostration. The high fever may be associated with delirium and stupor. Sometimes, the fever changes to the intermittent pattern, with high spikes mainly at night[7]. The fever and other symptoms will persist for the next 3–4 weeks, if undiagnosed and untreated.

Gastrointestinal system

Abdominal manifestations are common in typhoid fever. Among these, the most common are abdominal pain, splenohepatomegaly, anorexia, vomiting, and diarrhea[6,8]. A soft spleen becomes palpable under the costal margin, and enlarges in the second week. About 60% of children with typhoid fever will have splenomegaly. Hepatomegaly is also common, and occurs in about 40% of children[9]. In children below two years, however, hepatomegaly may be more common than splenomegaly[10].

Diarrhea is a common part of typhoid fever. This diarrhea is watery and does not usually cause dehydration[11]. Sometimes, the diarrhea may be foul smelling and thicker (Pea soup stools"). Diarrhea usually starts 3 days after the fever, and lasts for a few days. Later in the course of the disease, constipation is more likely[1], especially in older children and adults. Constipation can also be a sign of intestinal perforation or other abdominal complications.

Most children with typhoid have loss of appetite, and this can be severe in some children. Though nausea and vomiting are common in typhoid fever, they should not be ignored. If occurring in the second week (or third), they may signify an abdominal complication.

There may be some abdominal distension, with diffuse tenderness in most children with typhoid. Marked abdominal distension, constipation, and poor bowel sounds are usually associated with an intestinal complication.

Respiratory system

Many children with typhoid have cough. The onset of typhoid fever can be very much like bronchitis, with cough, fever, and scattered rhonchi and crepitations. Breathlessness occurs in a few children[4].

Skin

The "rose spots" of typhoid fever are much described, but not easy to see in Indian complexions. Even in Caucasians, they are seen in only half of patients[1]. They are sometimes seen on fair skinned children in our population.

Rose spots are macular or maculopapular rash which appears on the 7th to 10th day of fever. These spots are 1 to 5 mm in diameter, discrete, painless and mostly seen on the lower chest and abdomen. Blanching on pressure occurs, thereby differentiating them from petechiae. This rash lasts 2–4 days, and gradually fades, leaving a brownish discoloration of the skin.

Other manifestations

Relative bradycardia is considered a classical sign of typhoid fever. The heart rate is slow, in comparison to the expected rate for the degree of fever. However this sign is seen in less than half of cases, even in adults[5,12]. However relative bradycardia is not a usual feature of pediatric typhoid[13].

Loss of appetite can be severe and prolonged, and children often have significant weight loss after an attack of typhoid.

Among all clinical features of this disease, a few are diagnostically important. A history of a gradual rise of temperature, loose motions, coated tongue, and relative bradycardia are reliable markers of typhoid. Headache, hepatomegaly and splenomegaly are also markers of this disease[14].

Typhoid Fever at Different Ages

The newborn period

The disease is uncommon in newborns, but can occur as a result of vertical transmission from the mother. The baby usually develops fever 2–3 days after birth, and this may go up to 40.5°C (105°F). Other clinical manifestations at this age are jaundice, refusal to feed, hepatomegaly, vomiting, diarrhea, seizures, weight loss, and abdominal distension. It must be emphasized, however, that typhoid fever is very rare in newborn babies.

Typhoid fever below 5 years

The disease is said to be rare in this group, but in our country, at least, it makes up a significant proportion of pediatric typhoid fever. About a quarter of cases are seen in children below five years, and about 10% are below the age of 2 years[9,10,15]. One study has even found 44% of cases of typhoid fever in the community to be in children under 5 years of age[16]. Thus, it is unwise to rule out this diagnosis on the basis of the child's young age. In these young children, typhoid often presents as a non specific fever, and goes undiagnosed[17].

In younger children, diarrhea is often a presenting feature, in addition to fever. More than half of these children have cough. Young children are known to have seizures with typhoid fever[10,17].

Multidrug Resistant Typhoid

It is difficult to give a clear answer whether multidrug resistant typhoid differs clinically, from classified typhoid. Some authors from India found no clinical features that differentiated the two groups[18-22]. One study has even reported that children with chloramphenicol resistance were usually "less toxic", and encephalopathy was seen in this small study only in chloramphenicol sensitive typhoid fever[7].

On the other hand, a few authors have reported a higher incidence of gastrointestinal, CNS, and cardiovascular complications[4,15,23]. Most of these studies have been small, and no definite conclusion is as yet available.

Differential Diagnosis

Malaria

The disease often mimics malaria, with its high fever, chills and rigors, and hepatomegaly. Malaria though, has an abrupt onset in contrast to the insidious onset of typhoid fever. However, it can sometimes be very difficult to definitely diagnose the two conditions, and laboratory studies, may be needed to rule out malaria.

Viral hepatitis

Typhoid fever manifests with reduced appetite, fever, and hepatomegaly. Although jaundice is not common, it does occur in some children, and even liver function tests may be deranged[4]. A blood culture study for salmonella will help in making the correct diagnosis.

Bronchopneumonia

The onset of typhoid fever is sometimes with fever and cough, and examination shows crepitations and rhonchi all over the chest. These children are difficult to diagnose, but attention to the other clinical features, particularly abdominal, and the pattern of the fever, guide the clinician to the correct diagnosis.

Typhoid has to be differentiated from all other acute and subacute febrile illnesses. Deep abscesses, tuberculosis, amebic liver abscess, leptospirosis, infectious mononucleosis, endocarditis, visceral leishmaniasis, and connective tissue diseases all need to be considered in the differential diagnosis. Most of these diseases present with fever and no localising symptoms at first and so are very like typhoid fever. As the disease evolves, its particular clinical features will become evident.

References

1. Cleary TG. Enteric fever. In: Behrman RE Kliegman RM, Jenson HB, eds. Nelson Textbook of Pediatrics, 17th edition. Philadelphia, Saunders, 2004;916-19.

2. Olsen SJ, Bleasdale SC, Magnano AR, Landrigan C, Holland BH, Tauxe RV, *et al*. Outbreaks of typhoid fever in the United States, 1960-99. *Epidemiol Infect* 2003;130:13-21.

3. Egoz N, Shihab S, Leitner L, Lucian M. An outbreak of typhoid fever due to contamination of the municipal water supply in northern Israel. Israel *J Med Sci*. 1988;24:640-3.

4. Mishra S, Patwari AK, Anand VK, Pillai PK, Aneja S, Chandra J, *et al*. A clinical profile of multidrug resistant typhoid fever. *Indian Pediatr* 1991;28:1171-4.

5. Su CP, Chen YC, Chang SC. Changing charac-teristics of typhoid fever in Taiwan. *J Microbiol Immunol Infect* 2004 ;37:109-14.

6. Kabra M, Kabra SK, Talati A, Soni N, Patel S, Modi RR. Multidrug-resistant typhoid fever. *Trop Doct* 2000;30:195-7.

7. Sen S, Goyal RS, Dev R. Ciprofloxacin in the management of multiple drug resistant typhoid fever. *Indian Pediatr* 1991;28:417-9.

8. Wongsawat J, Pancharoen C, Thisyakorn U. Typhoid fever in children: Experience in King Chulalongkorn Memorial Hospital. *J Med Assoc Thailand*. 2002;85:1247-50.

9. Buch NA, Hassan MU, Kakroo DK. Enteric fever – a changing sensitivity pattern, clinical profile, and outcome. *Indian Pediatr* 1994;31:981-85.

10. Garg RA, Krashak R. Typhoid fever before two years of age. *Indian Pediatr* 1993;30:805-8.

11. Dutta P, Mitra U, Rasaily R, Saha MR, Manna B, Chatterjee MK, *et al*. Multidrug resistant typhoid

fever with diarrhea. *Indian Pediatr* 1997;34:891-9.

12. Hoshino Y, Masuda G, Negishi M, Ajisawa A, Imamura A, Hachimori K, *et al*. Clinical and bacteriological profiles of patients with typhoid fever treated during 1975-1998 in the Tokyo Metropolitan Komagome Hospital. *Microbiol Immunol* 2000;44:577-83.

13. Davis TM, Makepeace AE, Dallimore EA, Choo KE. Relative bradycardia is not a feature of enteric fever in children. *Clin Infect Dis* 1999;28:582-86.

14. Haq SA, Alam MN, Hossain SM, Ahmed T, Tahir M. Value of clinical features in the diagnosis of enteric fever. *Bangladesh Med Res Council Bull*. 1997;23:42-6.

15. Sharma A, Gathwala G. Clinical profile and outcome in enteric fever. *Indian Pediatr* 1993;30: 47-50.

16. Sinha A, Sazawal S, Kumar R, Sood S, Reddaiah VP, Singh B, *et al*. Typhoid fever in children aged less than 5 years. *Lancet* 1999;354:734-37.

17. Parry CM, Hien TT, Dougan G, White NJ, Farrar JJ. Typhoid Fever. *New Engl J Med* 2002; 347:1770-82.

18. Deshmukh C T, Nadkarni U B, Karande S C. An analysis of children with typhoid fever admitted in 1991. *J Postgrad Med* 1994;40:204-07.

19. Arora RK, Gupta A, Joshi NM, Kataria VK, Lall P, Anand AC. Multidrug resistant typhoid fever: Study of an out break in Calcutta. *Indian Pediatr* 1993;29:61-6.

20. Dutta TK, Beeresha, Ghotekar LH. Atypical manifestations of typhoid fever. *J Postgrad Med* 2001;47:248-51.

21. Singh M. The challenge of multidrug resistant typhoid fever. *Indian Pediatr* 1991;28:329-32.

22. Agarwal KS, Singh SK, Kumar N, Srivastav R, Rajkumar A. A study of current trends in enteric fever. *J Commun Dis*. 1998;30:171-4.

23. Koul PB, Murali MV, Sharma PP, Ghai OP, Ramchandran VG, Talvar V. Multi-drug resistant *Salmonella typhi* infection: Clinical profile and therapy. *Indian Pediatr* 1991;28:352-6.

4

Diagnosis of Typhoid Fever

Tapan Kumar Ghosh

The correct and rapid diagnosis of enteric fever is of paramount importance for instituting appropriate therapy and also for avoiding unnecessary therapy.

Complete Blood Count (CBC)

For practical purposes the CBC in enteric fever is unremarkable. The hemoglobin is normal in the initial stages but drops with progressing illness. Severe anemia is unusual and should make one suspect intestinal hemorrhage or hemolysis or an alternative diagnosis like malaria. The WBC count is normal in most cases and leukocytosis makes the diagnosis less probable. Leukopenia perceived to be an important feature of typhoid fever and has been reported in only 20–25% cases[1]. The differential count is usually unremarkable except for eosinopenia. Eosinopenia often absolute may be present in 70–80% cases[2,3]. Presence of absolute eosinopenia offers a clue to diagnosis but does not differentiate enteric fever from other acute bacterial or viral infections. Conversely a normal eosinophil count does make typhoid fever a less likely possibility. Platelet counts are normal to begin with and fall in some cases by the second week of illness. Overall prevalence of thrombocytopenia is around 10–15%[4].

Cultures

Blood culture

Blood cultures are the gold standard diagnostic method for diagnosis of enteric fever[5]. The sensitivity of blood culture is highest in the first week of the illness and reduces with advancing illness[6]. Overall sensitivity is around 50% but drops considerably with prior antibiotic therapy[5]. Failure to isolate the organism may be caused by several factors which includes inadequate laboratory media, the volume of blood taken for culture, the presence of antibiotics and the time of collection. For blood culture it is essential to inoculate media at the time of drawing blood.

Salmonella can be easily cultured in most microbiologic laboratories with use of routine culture media (Hartley's media, blood agar and MacConkey agar). Automated blood culture systems such as BACTEC certainly enhance the recovery rate. Sufficient amount of blood should be collected for culture as the median bacterial count in the peripheral blood is only 0.3 CFU/ml (interquartile range 0.1 to 10; range, 0.1 to 399)[7]. At least 10 ml of blood in adults and 5 ml in children should be collected. Dilution should be appropriate in order to adequately neutralize the bactericidal effect of serum and a ratio of 1:5 to 1:10 of blood to broth is recommended. Clot cultures, wherein the inhibitory effect of serum is obviated have not been found to be of superior sensitivity as compared to blood cultures in several clinical studies[8-10]. In the laboratory, blood culture bottles should be incubated at 39°C and checked for turbidity, gas formation and other evidence of growth after 1, 2, 3 and 7 days. For days 1, 2 and 3 only bottles showing signs of positive growth are cultured on agar plates. On day 7 all bottles should be subcultured before being discarded as negative.

There are considerable advantages of routine blood cultures in investigation of suspected enteric fever. Not only are they 100% specific, but they also provide information on the antimicrobial sensitivity of the isolate. This is vital in today's scenario of multidrug resistance. Moreover alternative methods for diagnosis particularly serology are rather unsatisfactory as will be discussed later. Blood cultures may actually turn out to be cheaper and very cost effective in the long run, as positive cultures unequivocally establish the diagnosis of enteric fever and all other investigations for PUO can be safely deferred.

Bone marrow culture

Salmonella typhi is an intracellular pathogen in the reticuloendothelial cells of the body including the bone marrow[5]. Studies have revealed that the median bacteremia in the bone marrow is 9 CFU/ml (IQR, 1 to 85; range, 0.1 to 1,5805) compared to 0.3 CFU/ml (IQR, 0.1 to 10; range, 0.1 to 399) in blood. This bone marrow: peripheral blood ratio which is around 4.8 (IQR, 1 to 27.5) in the first week of the illness increases to 158 (IQR, 60 to 397) during the third week owing to disappearance of bacteria from the peripheral blood[7]. The overall sensitivity of bone marrow cultures ranges from 80–95% and is good even in late disease and despite prior antibiotic therapy[5,11-13].

The invasive nature of bone marrow aspiration deters from its use as a first line investigation for diagnosis of typhoid fever. It is however a very useful and valid investigation in evaluation of PUO wherein the marrow should be inoculated in the culture bottle at the bedside.

Stool, urine and other cultures

Stool specimen should be collected in a sterile wide mouthed container. Specimens should preferably be processed within 2 hours after collection. If there is a delay the specimen should be stored in a refrigerator at 4°C or in a cool box with freezer packs. The sensitivity of stool culture depends on the amount of feces cultured, and the positivity rate increases with the duration of the illness. Rectal swabs should be avoided as these are less successful. Stool cultures are positive in 30% of patients with acute enteric fever[5]. For the detection of carriers, several samples should be examined because of irregular shedding of salmonella. Urine cultures are not recommended for diagnosis in view of poor sensitivity[5,14]. Other methods such as duodenal string and skin strip culture of rose spots have been reported to be more efficacious than blood cultures but are mainly of academic importance[14-16].

Antimicrobial Sensitivity Testing

The crucial issue here pertains to fluoroquinolone susceptibility testing. Fluoroquinolones were introduced in 1989 and during the past decade there has been a progressive increase in the MIC's of ciprofloxacin in *Salmonella typhi* and *paratyphi*[5]. Since the current MIC's are still below the National Committee for Clinical Laboratory Standards (NCCLS) susceptibility breakpoint, laboratory reports will continue to report *Salmonella typhi/paratyphi* as ciprofloxacin/ofloxacin sensitive[17]. However use of fluoroquinolones in this scenario is associated with a high incidence of clinical failure[5,17]. It has also been demonstrated that resistance to nalidixic acid is a surrogate marker for high ciprofloxacin MIC's, predicts fluoroquinolone failure and can hence be used to guide antibiotic therapy (i.e. if culture results show resistance to nalidixic acid irrespective of the results of ciprofloxacin/ofloxacin sensitivity, quinolones should not be used or if used high doses should be given)[18]. Since MIC testing is not within the scope of most laboratories, nalidixic acid susceptibility testing is mandatory to help guide choice of antibiotics.

Serologic Tests

Widal test

This test first described by F Widal in 1896, detects agglutinating antibodies against the O and H antigens of *Salmonella typhi* and H antigens of *S paratyphi* A and B[19]. The "O" antigen is the somatic antigen of *Salmonella typhi* and is shared by *Salmonella paratyphi* A, *paratyphi* B, other Salmonella species and other members of the Enterobacteriaceae family[20]. Antibodies against the O antigen are predominantly IgM, rise early in the illness and disappear early[20]. The H antigens are flagellar antigens of *Salmonella typhi, paratyphi* A and *paratyphi* B. Antibodies to H antigens are both IgM and IgG, rise late in the illness and persist for a longer time[19,20]. Usually, O antibodies appear on day 6–8 and H antibodies on days

10–12 after the onset of disease. The test is usually performed on an acute serum (at first contact with the patient). A convalescent serum should preferably also be collected so that paired titration's can be performed.

Conventionally, a positive Widal test result implies demonstration of rising titers in paired blood samples 10–14 days apart[19]. Unfortunately this criterion is purely of academic interest. Decisions about antibiotic therapy cannot wait for results from 2 samples. Moreover antibiotics may dampen the immune response and prevent a rise in titers even in truly infected individuals. Therapeutic decisions have to be generally based on results of a single acute sample. In endemic areas, baseline anti O and anti H antibodies are present in the population owing to repeated subclinical infections with *Salmonella typhi/paratyphi*, infections with other enterobacteriaceae and other tropical diseases such as dengue and malaria[19-21]. These antibody titers vary with age, socioeconomic strata, urban or rural areas and prior immunization with the TAB vaccine. Establishing appropriate cut offs for distinguishing acute from past infections is thus important for the population where the test is applied. In one study from Central India, anti O and anti H titer of more than 1:80 was seen in 14% and 8% respectively of a study sample of 1200 healthy blood donors[22].

While interpreting the results of the Widal test, both H and O antibodies have to be taken into account. There is controversy about the predictive value of O and H antibodies for diagnosis of enteric fever. Certain authorities claim that O antibodies have superior specificity and positive predictive value (PPV) because these antibodies decline early after an acute infection[23]. Other studies report a poorer positive predictive value of O antibodies probably due to rise of these antibodies in other salmonella species, gram-negative infections, in unrelated infection and following TAB vaccination[21]. For practical purpose and for optimal result this test should be done after 5–7 days of fever by tube method and level of both H and O antibodies of 1 in 160 dilution (four fold rise) should be taken as cut off value for diagnosis. H antibodies once positive can remain positive for a long time.

The Widal test as a diagnostic modality has suboptimal sensitivity and specificity[19-21]. It can be negative in up to 30% of culture proven cases of typhoid fever. Suboptimal sensitivity results from negativity in early infection, prior antibiotic therapy and failure to mount an immune response by certain individuals[19]. Poor specificity, an even greater problem and is a consequence of preexisting baseline antibodies in endemic areas, cross reactivity with other gram-negative infections and non-typhoidal salmonella, anamnestic reactions in unrelated infections and prior TAB or oral typhoid vaccination. The purity and standardization of antigens used for the Widal test is a major problem and often results in poor specificity and poor reproducibility of test results[19]. The slide Widal test should also be discouraged owing to high rate of false positives[20].

Notwithstanding these problems, the Widal test may be the only test available in certain resource poor set ups for diagnosis of enteric fever. In Vietnam, using a cutoff of >1/200 for the O agglutinin or >1/100 for H agglutinin test performed on acute-phase serum the Widal test could correctly diagnose 74% of blood culture positive typhoid fever, however 14% results would be false positive and 10% false negative[21]. Hence, it is important to realize the limitations of the Widal test and interpret the results carefully in light of endemic titers so that both over diagnosis and under diagnosis of typhoid fever and the resulting consequences are avoided[24].

Other serologic tests

In view of the limitations of the Widal test and need for a cheap and rapid diagnostic method, several attempts to develop alternative serologic tests have been made. These include rapid dipstick assays, dot enzyme immuno-assays and agglutination inhibition tests[25-27].

Enzyme immunoassay (EIA) test or typhidot test—A dot enzyme immunoassay that detects IgG and IgM antibodies against a 50 KD Outer Membrane Protein distinct from the somatc (O), flagellar (H) or capsular (Vi) antigen of *Salmonella typhi* is commercially available as typhidot[27]. The sensitivity and specificity of this test has been reported to vary from 70–100% and 43–90% respectively[28-33]. This dot EIA test offers simplicity, speed, early diagnosis and high negative and positive predictive values. The detection of IgM reveals acute typhoid in the early phase of infection, while the detection of both IgG and IgM suggests acute typhoid in the middle phase of infection. In areas of high endemicity where the rate of typhoid transmission is high the detection of specific IgG increase. Since IgG can persist for more that 2 years after typhoid infection[34] the detection of specific IgG cannot differentiate between acute and convalescent cases. Further more, false positive results attributable to previous infection may occur. On the other hand IgG positivity may also occur in the event of current reinfection. In cases of reinfection there is a secondary immune response with a significant boosting of IgG over IgM, such that the later cannot be detected and its effect masked. A possible strategy for solving this problem is to enable the detection of IgM by ensuring that it is unmasked[35]. The original typhidot test was modified by inactivating the total IgG in the serum samples. Studies with modified test, typhidot M, have shown that inactivation of IgG removes competitive binding and allows the access of the antigen to the specific IgM when it is present.

The typhidot M that detects only IgM antibodies of *Salmonella typhi* has been reported to be slightly more specific in a couple of studies[26,33].

IDL tubex test—The tubex test is easy to perform and takes approximately 2 minutes time[36]. The test is based on detecting antibodies to a single antigen in *S. typhi* only. The 09 antigen used in this test is very specific found in only sero group D salmonellae. A positive result always suggest a salmonellae infection but not which group D salmonella is responsible. Infection by other serotypes like *S. paratyphi* A give negative result. This test detects IgM antibodies but not IgG which is further helpful in the diagnosis of current infections.

IgM dipstick test[26]—The test is based on the binding of *S. typhi* specific IgM antibodies to *S. typhi* lipopolysaccharide (LPS) antigen and the staining of the bound antibodies by an antihuman IgM antibody conjugated to colloidal dye particles. This test will be useful in places where culture facilities are not available as it can be performed without formal training and in the absence of specialized equipments. One should keep in mind that specific antibodies appear a week after the onset of symptoms so the sensitivity of this test increases with time.

Antigen detection tests—Enzyme immunoassay's, counterimmune electrophoresis and co-agglutination tests to detect serum or urinary somatic/flagellar/Vi antigens of *Salmonella typhi* have been evaluated[37-40]. Sensitivity of Vi antigen has been found to be superior to somatic and flagellar antigen and has been reported as ranging from 50 to 100% in different studies[37-40]. Similarly specificity estimates have been reported to vary from 25 to 90%[37-40]. The suboptimal and variable sensitivity and specificity estimates, inability to detect *Salmonella paratyphi* infection and Vi antigen negative strains of *S typhi* are serious limitations of the Vi antigen detection tests.

Molecular Methods

The limitations of cultures and serologic tests advocate for development of alternative diagnostic strategies. PCR as a diagnostic modality for typhoid fever was first evaluated in 1993 when Song *et al* successfully amplified the flagellin gene of *S typhi* in all cases of culture proven typhoid fever and from none of the healthy controls[41]. Moreover some patients with culture negative typhoid fever were PCR positive suggesting that PCR diagnosis of typhoid may have superior sensitivity than cultures. Over the next 10 years a handful of studies have reported PCR methods targeting the flagellin gene, somatic gene, Vi antigen gene, 5S-23S spacer region of the ribosomal RNA gene, invA gene and hilA gene of *Salmonella typhi* for diagnosis of typhoid fever[42-50]. These studies have reported excellent sensitivity and specificity when compared to positive (blood culture proven) and healthy controls. The turnaround time for diagnosis has been less than 24 hours.

These reports should be viewed within the context of certain limitations. Clinical utility of PCR tests has been inadequately evaluated. Performance of the test in individuals with febrile illnesses other than typhoid, in those with past history of typhoid, carriers of *S typhi*, and those vaccinated with typhoid vaccine is not known. Patients with a clinical diagnosis of typhoid fever who are culture negative but PCR positive may in fact be false positives. Comparison of PCR to bone marrow cultures as a gold standard may be a superior way of evaluating the sensitivity and specificity of these tests, but has not been done. The tests claim to detect as few as 10 organisms, but it should be remembered that in typhoid the median bacteremia is 0.3 CFU/ml of blood[7].

Using small volumes of blood for DNA extraction may significantly lower the sensitivity of these tests. The cost and requirement for sophisticated instruments is also a potential drawback of molecular methods.

Conclusions

The complete blood count is the logical first investigation. Presence of a normal or low leukocyte count with eosinopenia points to possible enteric. It also helps in evaluation of alternative diagnoses such as malaria, dengue and other bacteremias. Blood cultures remain the most effective investigations for diagnosis of enteric fever till date. They should be sent early in the course of the illness and prior to starting antibiotic therapy. Susceptibility testing for nalidixic acid should be routinely done for all isolates to aid choice of antibiotics. Bone marrow culture is a highly sensitive diagnostic test even in late stages of the illness and with prior antibiotic therapy. It should be performed in all patients with prolonged pyrexia if routine investigations have failed to establish a diagnosis. The Widal test has several limitations and should be requested for in the second week of the illness and its results interpreted with caution. Data on baseline titers in the local population should be generated by appropriate studies to help in determining appropriate cut offs for the Widal test. The modified Widal test, typhidot, tubex and Vi antigen tests need to be evaluated further before their routine use can be recommended. Molecular methods are still experimental.

References

1. Abdool Gaffar MS, Seedat YK, Coovadia YM, Khan Q. The white cell count in typhoid fever. *Trop Geogr Med* 1992;44:23-7.

2. Deshmukh CT, Nadkarni UB, Karande SC. An analysis of children with typhoid fever admitted in 1991. *J Postgrad Med* 1994;40:204-7.

3. Pandey KK, Srinivasan S, Mahadevan S, Nalini P, Rao RS. Typhoid fever below five years. *Indian Pediatr* 1990;27:153-6.

4. Chiu CH, Tsai JR, Ou JT, Lin TY. Typhoid fever in children: A fourteen-year experience. *Acta Pediatr Taiwan* 2000;41:28-32.

5. Parry CM, Hien TT, Dougan G, White NJ, Farrar JJ. Typhoid Fever. *N Engl J Med* 2002;347:1770-82.

6. Ananthanarayan R, Panikar CKJ. Textbook of Microbiology. Chennai: Orient Longman 1999; 244–9.

7. Wain J, Pham VB, Ha V, *et al.* Quantitation of bacteria in bone marrow from patients with typhoid fever: Relationship between counts and clinical features. *J Clin Microbiol* 2001;39:1571-6.

8. Hoffman SL, Edman DC, Punjabi NH, Lesmana M, Cholid A, Sundah S. Bone marrow aspirate culture superior to streptokinase clot culture and 8 ml 1:10 blood-to-broth ratio blood culture for diagnosis of typhoid fever. *Am J Trop Med Hyg* 1986;35:836-9.

9. Simanjuntak CH, Hoffman SL, Darmowigoto R, Lesmana M, Soeprawoto, Edman DC. Streptokinase clot culture compared with whole blood culture for isolation of *Salmonella typhi* and *S. paratyphi* A from patients with enteric fever. *Trans R Soc Trop Med Hyg* 1988;82:340-1.

10. Escamilla J, Florez-Ugarte H, Kilpatrick ME. Evaluation of blood clot cultures for isolation of *Salmonella typhi, Salmonella paratyphi-A* and *Brucella melitensis. J Clin Microbiol* 1986;24:388-90.

11. Farooqui BJ, Khurshid M, Ashfaq MK, Khan MA. Comparative yield of *Salmonella typhi* from blood and bone marrow cultures in patients with fever of unknown origin. *J Clin Pathol* 1991;44:258-9.

12. Duthie R, French GL. Comparison of methods for the diagnosis of typhoid fever. *J Clin Pathol* 1990;43:863-5.

13. Akoh JA. Relative sensitivity of blood and bone marrow cultures in typhoid fever. *Trop Doct* 1991;21:174-6.

14. Gilman RH, Terminel M, Levine MM, Hernandez-Mendoza P, Hornick RB. Relative efficacy of blood, urine, rectal swab, bone-marrow, and rose-spot cultures for recovery of *Salmonella typhi* in typhoid fever. *Lancet* 1975; 31;1:1211-3.

15. Vallenas C, Hernandez H, Kay B, Black R, Gotuzzo E. Efficacy of bone marrow, blood, stool

and duodenal contents cultures for bacteriologic confirmation of typhoid fever in children. *Pediatr Infect Dis* 1985;4:496-8.

16. Benavente L, Gotuzzo E, Guerra J, Grados O, Guerra H, Bravo N. Diagnosis of typhoid fever using a string capsule device. *Trans R Soc Trop Med Hyg* 1984;78:404-6.

17. Crump JA, Barrett TJ, Nelson JT, Angulo FJ. Reevaluating fluoroquinolone breakpoints for *Salmonella enterica* serotype *typhi* and for non-typhi salmonellae. *Clin Infect Dis* 2003;37:75-81.

18. Kapil A, Renuka, Das B. Nalidixic acid susceptibility test to screen ciprofloxacin resistance in *Salmonella typhi*. *Indian J Med Res* 2002;115:49-54.

19. Olopoenia LA, King AL. Widal agglutination test-100 years later: still plagued by controversy. *Postgrad Med J* 2000;76:80-4.

20. Rodrigues C. The Widal test more than 100 years old: abused but still used. *J Assoc Physicians India* 2003;51:7-8.

21. Parry CM, Hoa NT, Diep TS, Wain J, Chinh NT, Vinh H, *et al*. Value of a single-tube Widal test in diagnosis of typhoid fever in Vietnam. *J Clin Microbiol* 1999;37:2882-6.

22. Shukla S, Patel B, Chitnis DS. 100 years of Widal test and its reappraisal in an endemic area. *Indian J Med Res* 1997;105:53-57.

23. Schoeder SA. Interpretation of serologic tests for typhoid fever. *J Am Med Assoc* 1968;206:839-40.

24. Nsutebu EF, Ndumbe PM, Koulla S. The increase in occurrence of typhoid fever in Cameroon: overdiagnosis due to misuse of the Widal test? *Trans R Soc Trop Med Hyg* 2002;96:64-7.

25. Jesudason M, Esther E, Mathai E. Typhidot test to detect IgG and IgM antibodies in typhoid fever. *Indian J Med Res* 2002;116:70-2.

26. Hatta M, Goris MG, Heerkens E, Gooskens J, Smits HL Simple dipstick assay for the detection of Salmonella typhi-specific IgM antibodies and the evolution of the immune response in patients with typhoid fever. *Am J Trop Med Hyg* 2002;66:416-21.

27. Gasem MH, Smits HL, Goris MG, Dolmans WM. Evaluation of a simple and rapid dipstick assay for the diagnosis of typhoid fever in Indonesia. *J Med Microbiol* 2002;51:173-7.

28. Khan E, Azam I, Ahmed S, Hassan R. Diagnosis of typhoid fever by Dot enzyme immunoassay in an endemic region. *J Pakistan Med Assoc* 2002;52:415-7.

29. Cardona-Castro N, Agudelo-Florez P. Immuno-enzymatic dot-blot test for the diagnosis of enteric fever caused by *Salmonella typhi* in an endemic area. *Clin Microbiol Infect* 1998;4:64-9.

30. Handojo I, Dewi R. The diagnostic value of the ELISA-Ty test for the detection of typhoid fever in children. *Southeast Asian J Trop Med Pub Hlth* 2000;31:702-7.

31. Bhutta ZA, Mansurali N. Rapid serologic diagnosis of pediatric typhoid fever in an endemic area: a prospective comparative evaluation of two dot-enzyme immunoassays and the Widal test. *Am J Trop Med Hyg* 1999;61(4): 654-7.

32. Jackson AA, Ismail A, Ibrahim TA, Kader ZS, Nawi NM. Retrospective review of dot enzyme immunoassay test for typhoid fever in an endemic area. *Southeast Asian J Trop Med Pub Hlth* 1995;26:625-30.

33. Choo KE, Davis TM, Ismail A, Tuan Ibrahim TA, Ghazali WN. Rapid and reliable serological diagnosis of enteric fever: comparative sensitivity and specificity of Typhidot and Typhidot-M tests in febrile Malaysian children. *Acta Tropica* 1999;72:175-83.

34. Saha SK, Talukdar SY, Islam M, Saha S. A highly ceftriaxone resistant *Salmonella typhi* in Bangladesh. *The Ped Infect Dis J* 1999;18:297-303.

35. Bhutta ZA. Impact of age and drug resistance on mortality in typhoid fever. *Arch Dis Child* 1996;75: 214-7.

36. Lim PL, Tam FC, Cheong YM, Jegathesan M. One-step 2-minute test to detect typhoid-specific antibodies based on particle separation in tubes. *J Clin Microbiol* 1998;36:2271-8.

37. Rao PS, Prasad SV, Arunkumar G, Shivananda PG. *Salmonella typhi* Vi antigen co-agglutination test for the rapid diagnosis of typhoid fever. *Indian J Med Sci* 1999;53:7-9.

38. Sharma M, Datta U, Roy P, Verma S, Sehgal S. Low sensitivity of counter-current immuno-electrophoresis for serodiagnosis of typhoid fever. *J Med Microbiol* 1997;46:1039-42.

39. Pandya M, Pillai P, Deb M. Rapid diagnosis of typhoid fever by detection of Barber protein and Vi antigen of Salmonella serotype typhi. *J Med Microbiol* 1995;43:185-8.

40. Chaicumpa W, Ruangkunaporn Y, Burr D, Chongsa-Nguan M, Echeverria P. Diagnosis of typhoid fever by detection of *Salmonella typhi* antigen in urine. *J Clin Microbiol*. 1992;30: 2513-5.

41. Song JH, Cho H, Park MY, Na DS, Moon HB, Pai CH. Detection of *Salmonella typhi* in the blood of patients with typhoid fever by polymerase chain reaction. *J Clin Microbiol* 1993;31:1439-43.

42. Sanchez-Jimenez MM, Cardona-Castro N. Validation of a PCR for diagnosis of typhoid fever and salmonellosis by amplification of the hilA gene in clinical samples from Colombian patients. *J Med Microbiol* 2004;53:875-8.

43. Cocolin L, Manzano M, Astori G, Botta GA, Cantoni C, Comi G. A highly sensitive and fast non-radioactive method for the detection of polymerase chain reaction products from Salmonella serovars, such as *Salmonella typhi*, in blood specimens. *FEMS Immunol Med Microbiol* 1998;22:233-9.

44. Chaudhry R, Laxmi BV, Nisar N, Ray K, Kumar D. Standardisation of polymerase chain reaction for the detection of *Salmonella typhi* in typhoid fever. *J Clin Pathol* 1997;50:437-9.

45. Zhu Q, Lim CK, Chan YN. Detection of *Salmonella typhi* by polymerase chain reaction. *J Appl Bacteriol* 1996;80:244-51.

46. Hashimoto Y, Itho Y, Fujinaga Y, Khan AQ, Sultana F, Miyake M, *et al.* Development of nested PCR based on the ViaB sequence to detect *Salmonella typhi*. *J Clin Microbiol* 1995;33:775-7.

47. Hirose K, Itoh K, Nakajima H, Kurazono T, Yamaguchi M, Moriya K, *et al.* Selective amplification of tyv (rfbE), prt (rfbS), viaB, and fliC genes by multiplex PCR for identification of Salmonella enterica serovars typhi and paratyphi A. *J Clin Microbiol* 2002;40:633-6.

48. Haque A, Ahmed N, Peerzada A, Raza A, Bashir S, Abbas G. Utility of PCR in diagnosis of problematic cases of typhoid. *Jpn J Infect Dis* 2001;54:237-9.

49. Massi MN, Shirakawa T, Gotoh A, Bishnu A, Hatta M, Kawabata M. Quantitative detection of Salmonella enterica serovar typhi from blood of suspected typhoid fever patients by real-time PCR. *Int J Med Microbiol* 2005;295:117-20.

50. Prakash P, Mishra OP, Singh AK, Gulati AK, Nath G. Evaluation of nested PCR in diagnosis of typhoid fever. *J Clin Microbiol* 2005;43:431-2.

5

Management of Typhoid Fever including MDRTF

Vijay N Yewale

Introduction

The emergence of drug-resistance in strains of *Salmonella typhi* causing infections has become a major problem in recent years. Given the considerable morbidity associated with MDR typhoid fever (MDRTF) in children and increased mortality with delay in treatment, it is imperative that appropriate antibiotic therapy be instituted promptly.

Multidrug-resistant Typhoid Fever

Multidrug resistance (MDRTF) is defined as typhoid fever caused by the strains of *S.enterica* serovar *typhi* that are resistant to the drugs used as the first line treatment, namely chloramphenicol, ampicillin and co-trimoxazole (trimethoprim-sulphamethoxazole).

However for variety of reasons the use of first line agents to treat typhoid fever has become uncommon. This withdrawal of antibiotic pressure has led to return of susceptibility in *S.typhi* to these drugs. Thus MDRTF, as defined above, is no longer a true problem. The major problem today is the failure of response to fluoroquinolones and increasing MIC of 3rd generation cephalosporins (Ceftriaxone/cefixime).

Resistance in *S.typhi* to fluoroquinolones and 3rd generation cephalosporins.

In 2008 there were reports of high level ciprofloxacin resistant *Salmonella enterica* from many centers in India. A high level ciprofloxacin resistant *S. typhi*, 64 µg/ml, has been reported from South India[1]. Multidrug resistance (resistance to chloramphenicol, ampicillin and co-trimoxazole) sequentially increased from 34% in 1999 to 66% in 2005 in one of the studies from North India. There has been a gradual development of resistance to fluoroquinolones over the 7 years from no resistance to fluoroquinolones in 1999, to in 2005 4.4% resistance to sparfloxacin, 8.8% resistance to ofloxacin and a high resistance, 13%, to ciprofloxacin[2].

The emergence of *S. typhi* highly resistant to ciprofloxacin is a cause of concern for both clinicians and microbiologists as well as for patients. Though fluoroquinolone resistance is chromosomally mediated, selective pressures exerted by the overuse of these drugs may see such isolates becoming more common in the future.

Increasing resistance has also been noticed to the other antibiotics, especially to the cephalosporins. Moreover 8% of the *S. typhi* isolates in the study from North India were found to be presumptive extended spectrum β-lactamase producers in this prospective study. This is an alarming development and it is of paramount importance to limit unnecessary use of fluoroquinolones and third generation cephalosporins so that their efficacy against salmonella is not jeopardized further[2].

Antimicrobial resistance in salmonella species thus is of grave concern, more so in quinolone-resistant and extended-spectrum beta-lactamase (ESBL)-producing isolates that cause complicated infections. Tigecycline and the carbapenems are likely to have roles in the final stage of treatment of quinolone-resistant and ESBL-producing multidrug-resistant salmonellae[3].

Of interest, though, is the possibility of turning to an older drug such as co-trimoxazole for treatment, in case of susceptible isolates.

Drug Resistance in *Salmonella typhi*

Time line

Resistance pattern of *S. enterica* serovar *typhi* strain vary chronologically and geographically.

Chloramphenicol was recommneded for the treatment of typhoid as early as 1940. Though resistance to chloramphenicol was reported within two years, outbreak of chloramphenicol resistance were reported from early 1970s[4]. Ampicillin continued to remain effective alternative for treatment of *S.typhi* infections.

Co-trimoxazole was first described for treatment of typhoid fever in 1981.

Driven by a change in antibiotic usage, the MDR phenotype emerged gradually in *S.enterica* serovar *typhi*, as each resistant type was acquired independently.

Until 1980s, no single isolate harbored resistance to all three drugs even though resistance was reported to each drug independently. The real problem began with the emergence of multidrug-resistant (MDR) strains of *Salmonella typhi* in the mid eighties from the subcontinent. It rapidly spread assuming epidemic proportions, accounting for almost 60–90% of all cases of typhoid in some reports.

In India, by the mid 1990s, reports began to appear of treatment failures with ciprofloxacin[1] followed by reports from 2001 onwards of rising MICs (reduced susceptibility) of ciprofloxacin for *S. typhi* isolates .

With the emergence of resistance to the first line drugs, the fluoroquinolones became the treatment of choice for typhoid fever. Oral quinolones have provided an effective oral form of therapy for MDR typhoid fever in adults but are still not licensed for widespread pediatric use. Oral quinolones, because of their availability as oral agents and low cost led to their indiscriminate use and emergence of resistance to quinolones. Since 1993 there has been a global epidemic of nalidixic acid resistant *S. enterica* serovar *typhi*. The strains exhibit decreased susceptibility to ciprofloxacin and infected patients have a poorer clinical response to fluoroquinolone treatment compared to those infected with nalidixic acid susceptible strains. There has been a progressive increase in the MIC of ciprofloxacin in *S.typhi* and paratyphi[3]. These levels are not achieved with standard doses and sometimes even with highest tolerated doses of ciprofloxacin. Nalidixic acid resistance is a surrogate marker of high ciprofloxacin MICs, predict fluroquinolon treatment failure and hence can be used to guide antibiotic therapy of typhoid fever. In Mumbai 82% of 240 blood culture isolates of *S. enteric* serovar *typhi* in 2000 were nalidixic acid resistant[4].

Broad-spectrum cephalosporins have thus remained an important therapeutic alternative for the therapy of MDR typhoid in children, with excellent primary cure rates[5].

Return of susceptibility in Salmonella enterica serovar typhi to the first line agents

In recent years several regions have seen a decline in MDR *S. enterica* serovar *typhi*, attributed to a change in the use of antibiotics. In many areas the removal of the selective antibiotic pressure due to antibiotic treatment, results in loss of the resistant phenotype. Following changes in the use of antibiotics in Mumbai, plasmid-mediated resistance initially decreased from 74% in 1990 to 40% in 1994 and then stabilized at 46% until 2000 and finally fell again to 17% in 2002[4]. However concerns of toxicity have precluded the use of these first line agents for therapy of enteric fever.

Concerns with MDR Typhoid/Fever (MDRTF)

The morbidity and toxicity associated with the MDR strains is higher in children. The morbidity is perhaps due to delay in presentation and institution of appropriate therapy. The toxicity is due to greater virulence of infecting strains of MDR *Salmonella typhi*[5].

Successful therapy of MDR typhoid is critically dependent upon prompt institution of appropriate antibiotic therapy. A number of therapeutic strategies have been employed in the management of MDR typhoid infections in childhood ranging from administration of quinolones, third generation cephalosporins, and monobactams[5].

Therapeutic Options for MDRTF (Table 5.1)

1. Cephalosporins

Ceftriaxone

S.typhi is at present almost always susceptible to this agent. The average time to defervescence of fever is one week. Clinical failure rate is reported to be 5–10%. Clinical failure is defined as persistent symptoms or development of complications necessitating further antimicrobial treatment. There have been reports of occasional case of microbiologic failure, i.e. positive cultures at the end of therapy. Relapse rate is around 5–10%. Relapse rate is higher with shorter duration of treatment than with 14 days duration[8]. Cost, parenteral route and

Table 5.1: Therapeutic options for enteric fever

Drug	Dose(mg/kg/day) & duration	Time to defervescence in days (95%CI)	Clinical failure % (95% CI)	Relapse rate % (95% CI)
Ceftriaxone	75 – 100 × 14 days	6.1 (5.9–6.3)	8.7 (6.1–12)	5.3 (3.7–8.2)
Cefixime	20 × 14 days	6.9 (6.7–7.2)	9.4 (5.5–15.3)	3.1 (1.2–7.5)
Aztreonam	50 – 100 × 14 days	5.8 (5.7–5.9)	6.9 (3.1–14.2)	1 (0.06–6.2)
Ampicillin	200 × 14 days	6.4 (6.3–6.6)	7.9 (5.1–11.9)	2.2 (0.9–5.0)
Amoxicillin	100 × 14 days			
Chloramphenicol	50 – 75 × 14 days	5.4 (5.3–5.5)	4.8 (3.7–6/3)	5.6 (4.3–7.2)
Cotrimoxazole	10 (TMP) × 14 days	6 (5.8–6.2)	9.3 (6.3–13.4)	17 (0.5–4.6)
Azithromycin	10 – 20 × 7 days	4.4 (4.2–4.5)	3.2 (1.2–7.7)	0 (0–3)
Ciprofloxacin/Ofloxacin	20 × 7 days	3.9 (3.8–3.9)	2.1 (1.4–3.2)	1.2 (0.7–2.2)

hospitalization, prolonged time to defervescence and high relapse rate are the main limitations of ceftriaxone.

Cefotaxime 200 mg/kg/day in 3 divided doses or cefoperazone in a dose of 100 mg/kg/day in 2 or 3 divided doses are other options in place of ceftriaxone.

Cefixime

Used for outpatient treatment and oral switch over drug to ceftriaxone. The dose is 20 mg/kg/day. The mean fever clearance time is 1 week. The rates of clinical failure and microbiological failure range from 5–15% and 0.5–5% respectively. Relapse rate is 1–10%.

Cefpodoxime

Another 3rd generation oral cephalosporine with similar gram negative coverage as cefixime. Limited experience and higher cost compared to cefixime are the limitation for its use.

2. Aztreonam

A monobactam effective in the treatment of MDRTF in the dose of 50–100 mg/kg/day in 3 divided doses. Defervescence time is 6 days but the relapse rate is low. Clinical failure rates can be 5–15%. Experience is limited. It is useful in the treatment of severe/complicated MDRTF with serious allergy to the cephalosporins.

3. Quinolones

They produce the most dramatic response in MDRTF where in the *S.typhi* is susceptible to nalidixic acid with a shorter time to defervescence and almost zero relapse. The MIC to ciprofloxacin has risen from 0.0004–0.004g/ml to 02–1g/ml leading to increase in clinical failure rates. Therefore quinolones should not be used as empirical therapy for enteric fever in areas with high MICs for ciprofloxacin. Use of fluoroquinolones is not permitted in India by the Drug Controller General of India (DCGI) due to fear of theoretical cartilage toxicity.

4. Azithromycin

This is a macrolide with very high intracellular penetration and is a good alteranate for the therapy of MDRTF. Clinical trials have shown efficacy equivalent to ceftrixone. The dose used varies from 10 to 20 mg/kg/day for 5–7 days. Average time to defervescence is 4.4 days. Possible limitations of azithromycin include limited clinical experience, marked variability in the dose and no information on efficacy in severe typhoid or in inpatient therapy.

Empirical antimicrobial therapy of MDR typhoid fever[3,10] (Table 5.2)

This applies to those cases where enteric fever is clinically suspected but where cultures have not been sent, or results are as yet not available or when cultures are negative. Choice for empirical therapy is guided by local sensitivity patterns of *S. typhi/paratyphi* chiefly sensitivity to quinolones and first line drugs including ampicillin/ co-trimoxazole/ chloramphenicol. Other factors including the severity of the illness, inpatient/outpatient therapy, presence of complications also need to be considered.

Outpatient Treatment

If the patient is stable enough to be treated on outpatient basis empirical therapy may be started.

Here therapeutic options in light of high nalidixic acid resistance and > 80% sensitivity to first line drugs are the following oral drugs.
1. Cefixime 20 mg/kg/day or azithromycin 10–20 mg/kg/day (ceiling dose 1 g).
2. Chloramphenicol 50 mg/kg/day.
3. Amoxicillin 100 mg/kg/day.

Table 5.2: Choice of empirical therapy for enteric fever

Situation	Local susceptibility patterns	1st line	Alternative drug
Severe illness/ inpatient/ complications	High prevalence of nalidixic acid resistance and low prevalence of resistance to ampicillin/ chloramphenicol and co-trimoxazole	Ceftriaxone	Cefotaxime Aztreonam (penicillin allergy) Ampicillin Chloramphenicol
Outpatient therapy		Cefixime Azithromycin	Chloramphenicol Amoxycillin Co-trimoxazole

4. Co-trimoxazole 10 mg/kg of TMP per day.

Clinical efficacy is more or less the same with all these drugs with each drug having its own advantages and limitations. Choice would hence depend on individual preference, experience, level of comfort (especially with chloramphenicol) and cost considerations. A recent Cochrane meta analysis has reported the efficacy of azithromycin as superior to quinolones and relapse rate lower than ceftriaxone. Clinical experience with cefpodoxime is fairly limited and is unlikely to offer any advantage over the cheaper and narrower spectrum cefixime.

In areas where nalidixic acid resistance is infrequent (rare at the moment in India), scientifically thinking quinolones may be considered the drugs of first choice. However the DCGI does not permit the use of quinolones in pediatric age group.

In areas where both nalidixic acid resistance and resistance to first line drugs (amoxycillin, chloramphenicol, cotrimoxazole) is widespread, only options are oral cefixime or azithromycin.

If the local resistance pattern is unknown, in such situation chances of failure are likely to be least if either cefixime or azithromycin are used. Once culture results are available therapy can be suitably modified on basis of principles discussed earlier. The total duration of therapy with all drugs is 14 days except for azithromycin where 7 days therapy is re-commended. There is no data at present to support use of combination therapy in enteric fever.

Inpatient Treatment

For empirical therapy in severe illness with or without complications for inpatient treatment the drug of first choice is ceftriaxone 100 mg/kg/day in two divided doses. There is no benefit of using ceftriaxone- tazobactam/ cefotaxime-sulbactam or other beta lactam - beta lactamase inhibitor (BL-BLI) combinations as *Salmonella typhi/paratyphi* has rarely been shown to produce beta lactamases. The routine use of BL-BLI combinations should be avoided as they are more expensive, are likely to have more adverse effects and may cause accidental underdosing of the cephalosporine component. In patients with history of severe penicillin or cephalosporin allergy aztreonam may be used. Parenteral treatment should be continued till defervescence has occurred, oral intake has improved and complications resolved. The mean time to devervescence with ceftriaxone is usually 5-6 days but can be as long as 10 days. If defervescence has not occurred as expected, then the first step is to review the diagnosis in those patients where the diagnosis has not been confirmed by culture. There is little logic in replacing or adding to ceftriaxone as in the current day scenario more than 99% of all strains are sensitive to ceftriaxone. The use of low dose steroids to hasten defervescence should be avoided as steroids may increase the risk of relapse or mask an alternative diagnosis. If the diagnosis of enteric fever is incontrovertible (based on blood culture and the isolate is susceptible to ceftriaxone) then a patient should wait for defervescence and a search for complications such as liver abscesses made. Following defervescence, once continous therapy with ceftrioxazone to complete 14 days course. However, therapy can be switched to oral cefixime 20 mg/kg/day to complete a total duration of 14 days but there are insufficient data to support this. Therapy of shorter duration is associated with a higher risk of relapse. Other oral drugs may theoretically be also used for switch over therapy but limited experience (cefpodoxime) and a different class (azithromycin, co-trimoxazole, amoxycillin) are potential disadvantages.

If cultures are positive and show nalidixic acid sensitivity then therapy may be changed to ciprofloxacin 20 mg/kg/day as quinolones are associated with faster defervescence and lower relapse rates as compared to ceftriaxone for quinolone sensitive strains. It must be noted that quinolones are not recommended by Drug Controller General of India (DCGI) for use in children below the age of 18 years. If cultures are positive and show nalidixic acid resistance as well as sensitivity to the first line drugs (ampicillin, chloramphenicol, cotrimoxazole) it is probably prudent to continue with ceftriaxone alone rather than change as the older drugs do not offer any advantage over ceftriaxone and are more toxic.

Patients with severe enteric fever (with presence of CNS complications or shock) have been shown in two decades old studies to benefit significantly in terms of reduction of mortality from administration of high dose steroids (dexamethasone loading dose 3 mg/kg and then 1 mg/kg 6 hourly for 48 hours).

However there is no new or current data on use of steroids in patients with severe enteric fever.

Therapy of Relapses

The relapse rate varies with the type of drug and is most common with beta lactams (ceftriaxone, cefixime) especially if shorter duration of therapy is used. Relapses are however generally milder and respond well and quickly to the same drug as used for primary therapy. Hence broadly speaking relapses may be satisfactorily treated with the same drug as used for primary therapy but in right doses and for the right duration. However if the isolate is nalidixic acid sensitive and quinolones were not used for primary therapy, they should be used for treatment of the relapse. Azithromycin may also be a good therapeutic option for relapse treatment as it achieves good intracellular levels and a recent Cochrane review has reported it to be superior to ceftriaxone in prevention of relapses.

Therapy of Carriers[9]

The carrier state is uncommon in children and testing for chronic carriage 3 months after an episode of enteric in children is not routinely recommended. However if chronic carriage is demonstrated then treatment with amoxycillin 100 mg/kg/day with probenacid 30 mg/kg/day or cotrimoxazole 10 mg/kg/day of TMP for 6–12 weeks is recommended. If the strain is nalidixic acid sensitive then quinolones for 28 days is a better option.

Conclusion

Multidrug resistance (resistance to chloramphenicol, ampicillin and co-trimoxazole) sequentially increased from 1990s . There has been a gradual development of resistance to fluoroquinolones over the 7 years. Pattern of

S. typhi resistance is changing rapidly. MDRST and strains resistant to ciprofloxacin and ceftriaxone are a major threat in developing world. Proper steps must be taken to avoid emergence of *Salmonella typhi* strains resistant to most of the pertinent antibiotics. Of interest, though, is the possibility of turning to an older drug such as co-trimoxazole for treatment, in case of susceptible isolates. ESBL in *S.typhi* is an alarming development and it is of paramount importance to limit unnecessary use of fluoroquinolones and third generation cephalosporins so that their efficacy against salmonella is not jeopardized further. Local epidemiology and antibiotic sensitivity pattern must be taken into consideration when treating enteric fever empirically.

References

1. Narasimha B, Menezes GA, Sarangapani K, Parija SC. A case report and review of the literature: Ciprofloxacin resistant *Salmonella enterica* serovar *Typhi* in India. *J Infect Developing Countries* 2008;2:324-27.

2. Kumar S, Rizvi M; Berry N. Rising prevalence of enteric fever due to multidrug-resistant *Salmonella*: an epidemiological study. *J Med Microbiology*, 2008:57:1247-50.

3. Capoor MR, Nair D, Singhal S, Deb M, Aggarwal P, Pillai P. Minimum inhibitory concentration of carbapenems and tigecycline against Salmonella spp. J. *Medical Microbiol* 2009:58;337-41.

4. Rodrigues C, Shenai S, Mehta A. Enteric fever in Mumbai, India: the good news and the bad news. *Clin Infect Dis* 2003;36:535.

5. Bhutta ZA. Editorial: The Challenge of Multidrug Resistant Typhoid in Childhood: Current Status and Prospects for the Future. *Indian Pediatr* 1999;36:129-31.

6. Bhutta ZA. Failure of short course chemotherapy for multidrug resistant typhoid fever in children: a randomized controlled trial in Pakistan.

7. Singhal T. Antimicrobial therapy of enteric fever. In: Shah N, Singhal T, eds. Rational Antimicrobial Therapy in Pediatrics. Mumbai:Indian Academy of Pediatrics, 2006.

8. Kundu R, Ganguly N, Ghosh TK, Yewale VN, Shah RC, Shah NK, IAP Task Force Report: Diagnosis of Enteric Fever in Children. *Indian Pediatr* 2006;43:875-83.

9. Jog S, Soman R, Singhal T, Rodrigues C, Mehta A, Dastur FD. Enteric fever in Mumbai—clinical profile, sensitivity patterns and response to antimicrobials. *J Assoc Physicians India.* 2008; 56:237-40.

10. Singhal T. Enteric fever. Pediatric Infectious Disease 2009;1:7-13.

6

Complications of Typhoid Fever

Shivananda

Enteric fever represents a spectrum of acute systemic febrile illness of prolonged duration, characterized by hectic rise of temperature, bacteremia and various systemic manifestations[1]. There is an extensive, but not exhaustive, list of complications of enteric fever. Most of these are rare and most likely to be encountered in children who present with untreated disease of 2 or more week's duration.

With declining incidence of enteric fever in developed counties, along with easy accessibility to health care facilities has decreased the incidence of complications in these countries. But in developing countries like India, enteric fever and its complications are still a major health problem. Factors which increase the incidence of the complications in enteric fever are inadequate and inappropriate treatment, late initiation of the antimicrobial agents, lack of early diagnostic facilities, poor accessibility to health care facility, other associated illness like sickle cell disease and HIV, innate immune deficiency in children and in community where incidence of multi drug resistance *Salmonella typhi* is high.

Untreated Enteric Fever

After ingestion of the organisms 10 to 20% children develop transient diarrhea. These patients as well as others remain asymptomatic during incubation period, which lasts for 7 to 14 days. As the stage of bacteremia develops at the end of incubation period, fever appears which classically increases daily in a stepwise fashion but may be remittent or sustained. At this point of time patients will have flu like symptoms with headache, sore throat, anorexia, nausea, abdominal pain, malaise and myalgia. The symptoms noticed at the time of hospitalization are listed in Table 6.1 and signs in Table 6.2[2].

Clinical Course

The clinical course of the enteric fever is quite variable as many patients lack some of the features varying from completely afebrile course occurring in debilitated patients, to high spiking fever from day one in children, to a focal presentation like pneumonia or nephritis, to a severe course during relapses. Infants are at high risk of developing massive

29

Table 6.1: Symptoms at the time of hospitalization

Symptoms	%
Fever	99
Weakness	99
Anorexia	85
Headache	85
Dizziness	80
Abdominal pain	50
Nausea	50
Chills	50
Diarrhea	45
Constipation	40
Cough or chest discomfort	35
Vomiting	35
Myalgia/arthralgia	35
Confusion	25
Sore throat	20
Decreased hearing	15
Malena	12
Epistaxis	10
Dysuria	2
Seizures	2

Table 6.2: Physical signs at the time of hospitalization

Common sign	%	Less common sign	%
Fever	98	Disorientation	25
Coated tongue	95	Relative bradycardia	15
Apathy	70	Rales or rhonchi	15
Hepatomegaly	50	Delirium	15
Abdominal pain	45	Severe toxicity	10
Rose spots	0–50	Decreased hearing	10
Moderate illness	45	Stiff neck	10
Toxicity	45	Stupor	2
Splenomegaly	35	Focal neurological findings	1

hepatomegaly, thrombocytopenia and other complications[3]. The mortality is high in neonatal period[4]. Infants and toddlers have a nondescript febrile illness misinterpreted as viral fever. In young children of less than 2 years of age, fever may last for as little as 1 to 5 days despite blood culture for salmonella is positive. Low grade fever and cough may be the only findings in such children[5]. Prolonged hypothermia can occur in such children during convalescence.

In pregnant women salmonella infection increases the risk of spontaneous abortion and/or premature labor[6-8]. Typically, premature labor occurs during second to fourth week of untreated maternal enteric fever[9]. This can be prevented by early diagnosis and prompt initiation of treatment as early as possible. Transmission of salmonella *in utero* is extremely rare[10]. If infection occurs late in gestation and is treated appropriately, the infant may survive intact.

Severe enteric fever

These patients represent an important subgroup of enteric fever who have high mortality rate (50%) and can be identified on the basis of mental state or cardiovascular status. The criteria for severe typhoid were marked mental confusion, delirious, obtunded, stuporous and comatose or shock defined by systolic BP of less than 80 mm of Hg with evidence of decreased skin, cerebral or renal perfusion[11-14].

Complications and unusual manifestations[15]

Most of these complications occur during second or third week of illness. Incidence of complications in developing countries may be as high as 30%. Table 6.3 gives the list of complications of enteric fever.

Gastrointestinal complications

Intestinal perforation—This is most feared complications of enteric fever occurring in 1–5% of patients[16]. Intestinal perforation is more common in children of more than 10 years (older children). The usual site is terminal ileum 75% of the cases are single perforation.

Table 6.3: Complications of typhoid fever

A. *Abdominal:*
1. Intestinal perforation
2. Intestinal hemorrhage
3. Hepatitis
4. Cholecystitis
5. Spontaneous splenic rupture
6. Rupture and hemorrhage from the mesenteric nodes
7. Pancreatitis

B. *Genitourinary:*
1. Retention of urine
2. Glomerulonephritis
3. Pyelonephritis
4. Cystitis
5. Orchitis

C. *Cardiovascular:*
1. Myocarditis
2. Pericarditis
3. Endocarditis
4. Asymptomatic ECG changes
5. Phlebitis and arteritis
6. Deep vein thrombosis
7. Gangrene
8. Shock
9. Sudden death

D. *Respiratory:*
1. Bronchitis
2. Laryngeal ulceration
3. Glottial edema
4. Pneumonia

E. *Neurophyschiatric:*
1. Delirium
2. Psychotic states
3. Depression
4. Deafness
5. Meningitis
6. Encephalomyelitis
7. Transverse myelitis
8. Signs of upper motor neuron lesions
9. Signs of lower motor neuron lesion
10. Impairment of coordination
11. Optic neuritis
12. Peripheral and cranial nerves involvement
13. Guillian Barré syndrome
14. Pseudotumor cerebri

F. *Hematological:*
1. Disseminated intravascular coagulation (usually subclinical)
2. Anemia
3. Hemolysis
4. Hemolytic uremic syndrome

G. *Focal infections:*
1. Abscess of brain, spleen, breast, thyroid, muscles, lymph nodes
2. Parotitis
3. Pharyngitis
4. Osteitis, especially tibia, ribs, spine
5. Arthritis

H. *Others:*
1. Myopathy
2. Hypercalcemia
3. Decubitus ulceration
4. Abortion
5. Relapse
6. SIADH

It usually occurs in the third week of illness, but can happen in first week as well as 2nd week also[17,18]. The clinical presentation may be acute or subacute. The patient with perforation presents with symptoms of typhoid and complains of severe abdominal pain localized to the right lower quadrant. Bowel sounds are absent in 50% of patients and 75% will have rebound tenderness and rigidity. Vomiting is almost always present. The perforation causes sudden rise in the pulse, fall in the blood pressure and severe pain. Some patients will have absence of hepatic dullness. Evidence of peritonitis occurs within 6–8 hours. However in about 25% of patients, the classical signs of peritonitis and perforation are absent and in these patients the diagnosis is difficult. Some times it may be difficult to differentiate between perforation, impending perforation and abdominal pain due to enteric fever. In appropriate clinical setting a rising WBC count with shift to the left is suggestive of perforation which is seen in less than 50% of patients[19].

X-ray abdomen may show pneumo peritoneum which may take several hours to appear. A chest radiograph may show gas under diaphragm. Ultrasonography of abdomen may be useful for demonstrating and aspirating pockets of feculent fluid in the peritoneum[20].

Intestinal hemorrhage—Intestinal hemorrhage can occur in up to 15% of cases. Hemorrhage may be slight or massive[21]. It may be frank bleeding or altered blood in stools. Severe hemorrhage occurs in 3% of cases. It occurs usually in the third week of the illness due to sloughs separating from the Peyer's patches. If blood loss is replaced, the hemorrhage is a self limiting process and does not require surgery. Clinically it presents with rise in pulse rate and fall in blood pressure. The lack of pain and rigidity and persistence of liver dullness are the main feature which differentiate hemorrhage from perforation[22].

Other gastrointestinal complications

Paralytic ileus is not uncommon in toxic cases. The onset is insidious which helps in differentiating it from perforation[23].

Mild asymptomatic elevations of transaminases (anicteric hepatitis) are common in enteric fever[24, 25]. Jaundice with or without major elevations of hepatic enzymes occurs in 1–2% of cases. Hepatic abscess can present as one of the rare complications of enteric fever[26].

Acute or chronic cholecystitis may occur months to years after an episode of enteric fever[2].

Rarely spontaneous spleen rupture can occur as a complication of enteric fever[27].

Genitourinary complications

About 25% of the patients excrete *Salmonella typhi* in urine at some point of time during their illness[21,24]. Transient proteinuria is most common urinary abnormality and may be due to immune complex mediated glomerulonephritis. Rarely glomerulonephritis may present as renal failure or nephritic syndrome and in these cases the prognosis is poor. Glomerulonephritis occurs in less than 2% of cases[2].

In severely ill patients acute tubular necrosis may develop. Pyelonephritis as well as cystitis also occurs in enteric fever patients[2]. Retention of urine can rarely occur in seriously ill patients[16].

Cardiovascular complications

Nonspecific ECG changes are the most common cardiac complications occurring in 10–15% of patients. ECG changes includes, low voltage tracings with flat or depressed ST segments and inverted T waves[24,25].

In 1–5% of patients myocarditis is seen. These patients may be asymptomatic or may have chest pain, congestive heart failure, arrhythmias or cardiogenic shock. When myocarditis occurs in young children, it is frequently a serious complication.

Pericarditis is rarely seen in enteric fever patients. Peripheral vascular collapse without cardiac finding has been increasingly seen. Patients surviving from such acute circulatory collapse will recover completely in due course. Femoral vein thrombosis is a frequent complication in the fourth week of illness. An increase in the pulse rate along with the slight rise in temperature in the fourth week of illness should lead to examination of the calf for the tenderness or swelling. Much less common but more serious complication is arterial thrombosis due to arteritis leading to pain, numbness and gangrene of the extremities[16].

Respiratory complications[16]

Bronchitis is usual and bronchopneumonia or less often lobar pneumonia may appear at any stage of the illness. Pulmonary emboli secondary to deep vein thrombosis may complicate during convalescent period.

Pharyngeal ulceration due to involvement of post arytenoids region results in hoarse voice, stridor and pain on swallowing is rarely seen now a days.

Neuropsychiatric complications

A wide spectrum of neuropsychiatric complication can occur in enteric fever and these complications are seen in more than 50% of patients[28].

The most common complication is disturbance in the level of consciousness that range from the disorientation to delirium, obtundation, stupor, and coma. Apathy is a rule in enteric fever[16]. Delirium is the earliest neurological symptom observed. Delirium, stupor and coma are grave prognostic signs associated with case fatality rate of more than 40% especially delirium persisting after temperature and metabolic abnormality has returned to normal.

Convulsions are unusual in enteric fever. Meningitis or encephalitis with or without paralysis has been seen in few cases. Post typhoid confusion state may persist for weeks or months but recovery is a rule. Peripheral neuritis with tender, painful nerves, mild muscle weakness and depressed reflex is seen during convalescent period[16].

Other less common complications are GBS, transverse myelitis with spastic paraplegia, extrapyramidal symptoms and cranial neuritis. However in India, cerebellar ataxia is one of the commonest neurological manifestations seen during enteric fever.

Brain abscess multiple or single are rarely seen as complication of enteric fever[29].

Psychiatric syndromes seen during enteric fever include schizophrenia like illness, mania, depression and catatonia. These complications are more common in developing countries like Africa[2].

The mechanisms responsible for the neurological manifestations of typhoid fever are hyperpyrexia, fluid and electrolytic disturbances, typhoid neurotoxin, vasculitis with perivascular cuffing, autoimmune mechanism, pressure effect on blood vessels resulting in cerebral infarction and acute disseminated encephalomyelitis[30].

CSF analysis in most of these conditions has no abnormality except for increased opening pressure[30].

Hematological complications

Anemia is seen in most of the patients especially in children less than 2 yrs of age[31]. The cause for anemia may be due to hemolysis, bone marrow suppression, intestinal hemorrhage or disseminated intravascular coagulation[16].

Hemolysis may be intravascular or extravascular. Intravascular hemolysis may be microangiopathic or due to toxins. Extra vascular hemolysis may be due to extensive reticuloendothelial involvement which is very common but never very severe. Hemolysis usually ceases during convalescent period[16].

Disseminated intravascular coagulation is rarely of clinical importance, but thrombocytopenia, hypofibrinogenemia, elevated prothrombin and partial thromboplastin times and elevated levels of fibrin degradation products are found in most of the patients[2].

Leukopenia with neutropenia (25%) and a relative lymphocytosis is common findings in enteric fever. WBC count has got no predictive value for complications of enteric fever. Absolute lymphocytosis is rarely seen, in fact lymphopenia is more commonly seen (75%)[32].

Focal abscess

Because of sustained bacteremia, focal infections can develop at any sites of the body. The incidence of these abscesses is low. The most common sites are bones (extremities, spine, and ribs) but also seen in brain, liver, spleen, muscles, thyroid, salivary glands, and cervical lymph nodes. In the past thrombophlebitis, parotitis and decubitus ulcers were common complications but now rarely seen[2].

Relapse

Relapse occured in 5–10% of patients in the preantibiotic era. But still relapse is a major problem in developing countries like India. Fever generally returns about 2 weeks after the cessation of the antibiotic therapy or in untreated patients about 2 weeks after defervescence. It has also been reported several months after the initial illness. Relapse is usually, but not always, milder than the initial attack. It should be differentiated from the multiple recurrences of septicemic salmonella with metastatic foci described in association with sickle cell disease and HIV infection[32].

Enteric fever in children less than 5 years of age

S. typhi infection has been documented in neonates who have been acquired congenitally. The clinical presentation in children less than 5 years especially less than 1 year is less predictable than in older children[33]. It can range from extremely mild illness like viral fever to severe enteric fever with high mortality reaching 30%. Children with enteric fever frequently have diarrhea and vomiting, and up to 20% may have convulsions. Enteric meningitis is exclusive disease of children of less than 5 years though reported in adults. The incubation period in children is shorter and onset tends to be more acute than in older children. Most often onset may mimic gastroenteritis. Complications tend to be less common, but when they do occur they progress rapidly. Dehydration and mineral loss may be particularly severe and need urgent treatment.

Chronic carriers

A person who excretes the organism in the stool 1year after the initial illness is considered to be a carrier. 20% of the patients will excrete the organism for 2 months after the onset of the initial illness and 10% for 3 months, only 3% go on to become carriers[34]. The prevalence is more common in females and in the elderly and is probably correlated with the prevalence of cholelithiasis and is also more common in children younger than 5 years and in patients with biliary tract disease. Most carriers are asymptomatic and up to 25% will not have preceding history of acute enteric fever. Up to 10⁶ organisms per gram of feces may be excreted[35]. Persons with genitourinary tract abnormality like tuberculosis, hydronephrosis, strictures, pyelonephritis or stones have much incidence of urinary carriage than those with a normal urinary tract. The significance of such chronic carrier is that they serve as a source of infection to their contacts[36,37].

Management of Complications (Table 6.4)

Both outpatients and inpatients with typhoid fever should be closely monitored for the development of complications. Timely intervention can prevent or reduce morbidity and mortality. The parenteral fluoroquinolones are probably the antibiotics of choice for severe infections but there have been no randomized antibiotic trials[38]. In severe typhoid the fluoroquinolones are given for a minimum of 10 days. Typhoid fever patients with changes in mental status, characterized by delirium, obtundation and stupor, should be immediately evaluated for meningitis by examination of the cerebrospinal fluid. If the findings are normal and typhoid meningitis is suspected, children should immediately be treated with high-dose intravenous dexamethasone in addition to antimicrobials[39]. Dexamethasone is given in an initial dose of 3 mg/kg by slow IV infusion over 30 minutes and after six hours, 1 mg/kg is administered and subsequently repeated at six-hourly intervals for 48 hours, mortality can be reduced by some 80–90% in these high-risk patients. Hydrocortisone in a lower dose is not effective[40]. High-dose steroid treatment can be given before the results of typhoid blood cultures are available if other causes of severe disease are unlikely.

Management of intestinal perforation

Generalized peritonitis and large amount of pus is seen in patients with perforation of intestine. If a well trained surgeon, anesthesiologist and operating room staff and necessary equipment are available, operative management is indicated[21,22]. In the absence of these, the choice between operative and non operative management should be individualized. There are no randomized control trials comparing operative and medical management.

In all cases, appropriate antibiotics, nasogastric suction, resuscitation with IV fluids, blood, oxygen and if severely toxic corticosteroids should be administered. Antibiotic should cover gram negative rods and anerobes of intestinal flora apart from Salmonella. If perforation is confirmed, surgical repair should not be delayed longer than six hours. Metronidazole and gentamicin or ceftriaxone should be administered before and after surgery if a fluoroquinolone is not being used to treat leakage of intestinal bacteria into the abdominal cavity.

It is preferable to stabilize the patients before surgery but surgery should not be delayed for more than several hours after diagnosis.

At surgery ileum, cecum and proximal large bowel should be examined for the perforation. One of the several procedures should be done for example, intestinal resection and primary anastamosis or wedge excision or debridement of the ulcer with primary closure of the perforation. Most surgeons will suture future site of perforation with serosa to serosa approximation. The peritoneal cavity is then lavaged and abdominal cavity is closed with or without drainage.

As the interval between perforation and surgery increases and preoperative status worsens and the case fatality rate increases. Mortality rate of 10–32% have been reported[41].

Management of intestinal hemorrhage

Patients with intestinal hemorrhage need intensive care, monitoring and blood transfusion. Intervention is not needed unless there

Table 6.4: Drug therapy of complicated cases

Susceptibility	Optimal parenteral drug			Alternative effective parenteral drug		
	Antibiotic	Daily doses mg/kg	Days	Antibiotic	Daily doses mg/kg	Days
Fully sensitive	Fluoroquinolone e.g., oflaxacin	15	10–14	Chloramphenicol Amoxycilin TMP-SMX	100 100 8–40	14–21 14 14
Multidrug resistant	Fluroroquinolone	15	10–14	Ceftriaxone Cefotaxime	60 80	10–14
Quinolone resistant	Ceftriaxone or Cefotaxime	60 80	10–14	Fluroquinolone	20	7–14

is significant blood loss. Surgical consultation for suspected intestinal perforation is indicated. If the patient does not have abnormal level of mental status or shock then case fatality rate is less than 1%[2].

Management of other complications

Renal failure, pneumonia, respiratory failure, myocarditis, arrhythmias, cardiac failure, shock, meningitis, localized abscess, arthritis, osteomyelitis, hemolytic anemia and cholecystitis are all occasionally encountered and should be managed with antimicrobials and standard medical or surgical practices[24].

DIC may sometimes be clinically significant, in which case platelet, blood and clotting factor transfusion may be necessary. There is no evidence that heparin therapy is of any help in enteric fever[2].

Management of relapse

Relapses involving acute illness occur in 5–10% of typhoid fever cases that have apparently been treated successfully. Cultures should be obtained and standard treatment should be administered.

Management of carriers

If cholelithiasis is present the patient probably requires cholecystectomy in addition to antibiotics in order to achieve bacteriological cure. In order to eradicate *S. typhi* carriage, amoxycillin or ampicillin (100 mg per kg per day) plus probenecid (1 g orally or 23 mg per kg for children) or TMP-SMZ (160 to 800 mg twice daily) is administered for six weeks; about 60% of persons treated with either regimen can be expected to have negative cultures on follow-up. A cure rate of 80–90% can be obtained with combination of surgical and antimicrobial treatment. Clearance of up to 80% of chronic carriers can be achieved with the administration of 750 mg of ciprofloxacin twice daily for 28 days or 400 mg of norflo-xacin in adults. Other quinolone drugs may yield similar results[42,43]. Carriers should be excluded from any activities involving food preparation and serving, as should convalescent patients and any persons with possible symptoms of typhoid fever. Although it would be difficult for typhoid carriers in developing countries to follow this recommendation, food handlers should not resume their duties until they have had three negative stool cultures at least one month apart. Vi antibody determination has been used as a screening technique to identify carriers among food handlers and in outbreak investigations. Vi antibodies are very high in chronic *S. typhi* carriers[44].

Prognosis

The prognosis depends on the patient population and geographic area. In an epidemic in developed countries patients will be generally seen and treated promptly, have case fatality rate of less than 1%. The majority of patients in the endemic area will be treated as outpatients and have case fatality and complication rates comparable to those expected in epidemic in developed countries.

Factors associated with poor prognosis are late diagnosis and late initiation of treatment, extremes of age (children of less than 2 years and elderly) MDR organism, associated conditions like HIV infection, sickle cell disease, complications (seizures, perforation, pneumonia, delirium or coma and shock) and its late identification and management.

Four baseline variables such as abdominal pain, low systolic blood pressure, hypoalbuminemia and laboratory evidence of disseminated intravascular coagulation are independently associated with complication and can be used as prognostic indicators[45].

In developing countries like India, severe typhoid is common among hospitalized patients. These patients have mortality rate as high as 50% if not treated with high doses of dexamethasone[11,13,14,18].

A delay in appearance of agglutinins may indicate severe illness. Toxemic circulatory failure is the commonest cause of death which can be relieved by the steroids. Second most common and serious cause of death is intestinal perforation[16].

The prognosis for the neurological deficit is usually good. In most of the cases the recovery is slow and complete, but in some cases deficit may persists for long[30].

Periosteitis may cause symptoms for months but recovery usually ensues. Post enteric mania has good ultimate prognosis. Immunity following enteric fever is partial. But second attacks are rare[16].

References

1. Lakohotia M, Gehlot RS, Jain P, Sharma S, Bhargava A. Neurological manifestation of enteric fever. *J Indian Acad Clin Med* 2003;4:196-9.

2. Thong P Le, Hoffman SL. Typhoid fever. In: Guerrant RL, Walker DH, Weller PF, eds. Tropical Infectious Diseases. Philadelphia : Churchill livingstone, 1999:277-95.

3. Rajajee S, Anandi, Shubha TB, *et al.* Nasocomial *S typhimurium* epidemic in infants. *J Trop Pediatr* 1994;41:52-54.

4. Reed RP, Klugman KP. Neonatal typhoid fever. *Pediatr Infect Dis* 1994;13:774-7.

5. Ferrico C, Levine MM, Manterola A, *et al.* Benign bacteremia caused by *S. typhi* and *S.paratyphi* in children younger than 2 years. *J Pediatr Infect Dis* 1984;104:899-901.

6. Michel J, Malpuach G, Godeneche P, *et al.* Clinical and bacteriological study of salmonellosis epidemic in a hospital. *Pediatr* 1970;25:13-9.

7. Stuart BM, Pullen RL. Typhoid. Clinical analysis of 360 cases, *Arch Intern Med* 1946;78: 629.

8. Seoud M, Saade G, Uwaydah M, *et al.* Typhoid fever in pregnancy. *Obstet Gynecol* 1988;71:711-4.

9. Griffith JPC, Ostheimer M. Typhoid fever in children. *Am J Med Sci* 1902;124:868-88.

10. Chin KC, Simmons EJ Tarlow MJ. Neonatal typhoid fever. *Arch Dis Child* 1986;61:1228-30.

11. Kholsa SN. Changing patterns of typhoid fever. *Asian Med J* 1982;25:185-98.

12. Gulati PD, Saxena SN, Guptha PS, *et al.* Changing profile of typhoid fever. *Am J Med* 1968;45:544-8.

13. Hoffman SL, Punjabi NH, Kumala S. Reduction in cholramphenicol treated severe typhoid by high dose of dexamethasone. *N Engl J Med* 1984;310:82-8.

14. Punjabi NH, Hoffman SL, Edmand DC, *et al.* Treatment of severe typhoid fever in children with high dose of dexametha-sone. *Pediatr Infect Dis J* 1988;7:598-600.

15. Richens J. Typhoid Fever. In: Weatherall DJ, Ledingham JGG, Warrell DA, eds. Oxford Textbook of Medicine. 3rd ed. New York: Oxford University Press, 1996:560-8.

16. McKendrick GDW. Salmonella Infections. In: Scott RB, ed. Price's Textbook of the Practice of Medicine, 12th ed. Norfolk: The English Language Book Society, 1978:39-44.

17. Bitar R, Tarpley J. Intestinal perforation in typhoid fever: A historical and state of the art review. *Rev Infect Dis* 1985;7:257-71.

18. Eustache JM, Hreis DJ. Typhoid perforation of the intestine. *Arch Surg* 1983;118:1269-71.

19. Butler T, Islam A, Kabir I, *et al.* Patterns of morbidity and mortality in typhoid fever dependent on age and gender : Review of 552 hospitalized patients with diarrhea. *Rev Infect Dis* 1991;13:85-90.

20. Kapoor VK, Mishra MC, Ardhanari R, Chattopadhyay TK, Sharma LK. Typhoid enteric perforations. *Infection* 1987;15:359-62.

21. Meier DE, Imediegw OO, Tarpley JL. Perforated typhoid enteritis: operative experience with 108 cases. *Am J Surg* 1989;157:423-7.

22. Kim JP, Oh SK, Jarrett F. Management of ileal perforation due to typhoid fever. *Ann Surg* 1975; 181:88-91.

23. Edelman R, Levine MM. Summary of an international workshop on typhoid fever. *Rev Infect Dis* 1986;8:329-49.

24. Woodward TE, Smadel JE. Management of typhoid fever and its complications. *Ann Intern Med* 1964;60:144-57.

25. Rowland HAK. The complications of typhoid fever. *J Trop Med Hyg* 1961;64:143-8.

26. Soni PN, Hoosen AA, Pillay DG. Hepatic abscess caused by *Salmonella typhi*. A case report and review of the literature. *Dig Dis Sci* 1994;39:1694-6.

27. Julia J, Canet JJ, Lacasa XM, Gonzalez G, Garau J. Spontaneous spleen rupture during typhoid fever. *Int J Infect Dis*. 2000;4:108-9.

28. Osuntokum BO, Bademosi O, Ogunremi K, *et al*. Neuropsychiatric manifestations of typhoid fever in 959 patients. *Arch Neurol* 1972;27:7-13.

29. Hanel RA, Araujo JC, Antoniuk A, da Silva Ditzel LF, Flenik Martins LT, Linhares MN. Multiple brain abscesses caused by *Salmonella typhi*: case report. *Surg Neurol* 2000;53:86-90.

30. Vidyasagar S, Nalloor S, Shashikiran U, Prabhu MM. Unusual neurological complication of typhoid fever. *Calicut Med J* 2004;2:e3.

31. Palacios Malmaceda PG, Vela Acosta JJ, Gutierez Arrasco W. Typhoid fever in children under 2 years of age. *Bol Med Hosp Infant Mex* 1981;38:473-83.

32. Abdool Gaffar MS, Seedat YK, Coovadia YM, Khan Q. The white cell count in typhoid fever. *Trop Geogr Med* 1992;44:23-7.

33. Rubin RH, Weinstein L. Salmonellosis: Micro-biologic, Pathologic and Clinical Features. New York, Stratton Intercontinental, 1997.

34. Hoffman TA, Ruiz CJ, Counts GW, *et al*. Water-borne typhoid fever in Dade county, Florida: Clinical and therapeutic evaluations of 105 bacteremic patients. *Am J Med* 1975;59;481-87

35. Merselies JG, Kaye D, Connolly CS, *et al*. Quantitative bacteriology of typhoid carrier state. *Am J Trop Med Hyg* 1964;13:425.

36. Farid Z, Bassily S, Kent DC, *et al*. Chronic urinary *Salmonella* carriers with intermittent bacterimia. *J Trop Med Hyg* 1970;73:153-7.

37. Rocha H, Kirk JW, Hearey CD. Prolonged Salmonella bacteremia in patients with *Schistosoma mansoni* infection. *Arch Intern Med* 1971;128:254-7.

38. Dutta P, Rasaily R, Saha MR, *et al*. Ciprofloxacin for treatment of severe typhoid fever in children. *Antimicrobial Agents Chemother* 1993;37: 1197-9.

39. Punjabi NH, Hoffman SL, Edman DC, *et al*. Treatment of severe typhoid fever in children with high dose dexamethasone. *Pediatric Infect Dis J* 1988;7: 598-600.

40. Rogerson SJ, Spooner VJ, Smith TA, Richens J. Hydrocortisone in chloramphenicol-treated severe typhoid fever in Papua New Guinea. *Trans Roy Soc Trop Med Hyg* 1991;85:113-6.

41. Van Basten JP, Stockenbrugger R. Typhoid perforation. A review of the literature since 1960. *Trop Geogr Med* 1994;46:336-9.

42. Ferreccio C, *et al*. Efficacy of ciprofloxacin in the treatment of chronic typhoid carriers. *J Infect Dis* 1988;157:1235-9.

43. Gotuzzo E, *et al*. Use of norfloxacin to treat chronic typhoid carriers. *J Infect Dis* 1988;157: 1221-5.

44. Lanata CF, Levine MM, Ristori C, *et al*. Vi serology in the detection of chronic *Salmonella typhi* carriers in an endemic area. *Lancet*, 1983;ii: 441-3.

45. Khan M, Coovadia Y, Connolly C, Sturm AW. Risk factors predicting complications in blood culture-proven typhoid fever in adults. *Scand J Infect Dis* 2000;32:201-5.

7

Typhoid Vaccines

Nitin K Shah

Introduction

Enteric fever is common in developing countries like India, affecting mainly school going children and young adults due to poor measures of hygiene and sanitation. It leads to significant morbidity and even mortality. Evolution of multidrug resistance *Salmonella typhi* strains has led to more morbidity, mortality and has made the treatment more expensive. In this scene, mass immunization against typhoid fever is an interim solution. Though the whole cell inactivated typhoid vaccines were efficacious and cheap, they used to lead to severe toxicities, which led to these vaccines falling in disrepute. Unfortunately the existing so called newer typhoid vaccines though safe are not efficacious enough to arouse interest in the public health authorities. Recent reports of excellent immunogenicity, safety and efficacy of Vi conjugate vaccines have been very encouraging and they hold promise to be included in the routine vaccination schedule if proved to be as efficacious in some more studies, especially in infants.

Typhoid Fever – The Need for Routine Vaccination

Disease burden

It is estimated that per year 16 million cases of enteric fever occur with 600,000 deaths world over. This seems to be an underestimate and the number of cases is likely to at least double, i.e. 33 million cases[1]. Before the antibiotics were available, enteric fever was a dreaded disease with 10–30% mortality and even with the effective antibiotic treatment available now the case fatality may be as high as 1–2%[2,3]. Enteric fever peaks in school going children and in young adults. However from studies done in India and Vietnam it is now realized that it often occurs in younger children too including infants. In one study in India nearly 20% of enteric fever occurred in children < 2 year of age[4]. The incidence is estimated to be 1–2 million cases per year in India.

Drug resistance

Of late there has been the problem of multidrug resistant typhoid fever, including significant resistance to fluroquinolones like

39

ciprofloxacin. The recent epidemic of enteric fever in Tajikistan reported 24,000 cases of enteric fever where 92% of the strains were multidrug resistance including 82% resistance to ciprofloxacin[5]. This leaves us with ceftriaxone as the drug of choice now which means more cost of therapy. Isolated cases of late response to ceftriaxone are disturbing as it means development of resistance to even 3rd generation cephalosporins in near future!

Prevention

In the developing countries enteric fever is still rampant due to heavy contamination of the drinking water with the sewage and by the carriers of *S. typhi*. Till such time that sanitation can improve in the entire country, the only hope is simultaneous effective typhoid vaccination programs for children. Whatever may be the efficacy of the current typhoid vaccines, there is very strong case to consider routine typhoid vaccination of all the school going children in India. This has been the stand even of the Indian Academy of Pediatrics Committee on Immunization.

Typhoid Vaccines

The first typhoid vaccine was whole cell inactivated typhoid vaccine invented in 1896 by Wright[3]. The WHO sponsored large scale field trials of these vaccines in 1950s to 1960s. Though found to have high efficacy in the trials, these vaccines fell in disrepute due to high incidence of severe side effects and occasional but significant report of deaths following the vaccines. The need of having effective and safe vaccine was always felt. A breakthrough occurred when Germanier and Fuer invented the Ty21a mutant typhoid strain in 1970s which led to the availability of the live oral typhoid vaccine[3] and subsequently invention of Vi vaccine by Dr. Robbins group. These two so called newer vaccines showed limited efficacy but better safety

profile. None of these vaccines were shown to be effective in children younger than 5 years. Of late there are attempts made to develop Vi conjugate vaccine. This was successfully done with conjugation of the Vi antigen with the recombinant exotoxin. A protein of the *Pseudomonas aerugenosa* organism leading the conjugate–Vi vaccine Vi rEPA. This vaccine has been highly successful in the 2 trials published so far and probably will be the vaccine of the future[6,7]. Recently Vi conjugate vaccine using tetanus toxoid as carrier protein has been marketed in India with very limited data though.

Characteristics

A recent meta-analysis has compared 3 commonly used typhoid vaccines, i.e. injectable whole cell inactivated vaccine, oral Ty21a vaccine and injectable Vi vaccine[8].

Parenteral whole cell inactivated vaccines

Two whole cell inactivated typhoid vaccines have been found to be the best in efficacy trials, i.e. acetone inactivated vaccine and heat inactivated phenol preserved vaccine. In past this vaccine was combined with paratyphi A/B. It is a ready to use liquid vaccine and contains 10^9 inactivated *S. typhi* organisms per 1.0 ml. It is suspended in 0.5% phenol solution[3]. It used to be manufactured by Haffkine institute in India, however it is no more available.

Oral Ty21a vaccine

This makes this strain immunogenic but not pathogenic[9]. This vaccine was available in 3 forms, gelatin-$NaHCO_3$ capsule, enteric coated capsule and liquid vaccine, of these the enteric coated capsules are commercially available. The enteric coated capsule contains $2 – 6 \times 10^9$ CFU of Ty21a organisms per capsule and $5 – 50 \times 10^9$ nonviable Ty21a organisms[9].

However, of late this vaccine is not available and probably withdrawn from the Indian market.

Vi vaccine

The current Vi vaccines are very pure and contain less than 5% impurity with LPS making them as very safe vaccines. It is a ready to use liquid formulation containing 25 μg of Vi antigen in 0.5 ml volume[8]. It is widely available in India from various pharma companies.

Immunogenicity

The immunity against typhoid fever is always relative to the quantum of organisms ingested which means no amount of immunity can protect against development of disease after ingestion of large infective dose of organisms. There are no clear serological correlates of protection and one has to conduct field efficacy trials to understand efficacy of these vaccines.

Parenteral whole cell inactivated vaccines

The major antibodies that protect against disease are the serum anti-flagellar, i.e. anti-H antibodies. There is hardly any secretory antibody response or cellular immune response

following these vaccines. Study done in Guyana[9] showed that acetone inactivated vaccine had better and higher antibody response and hence also better efficacy than heat inactivated vaccine as shown in Table 7.1.

Vi vaccine

Vi vaccine leads to development of anti-Vi antibodies. There is hardly any secretary or cellular immune response as expected. Pure Vi vaccines also fail to elicit significant anti-O antibody response. Table 7.1 shows the immune response following Vi vaccine (Aventis Pasteur) as studied in various studies[9].

Oral Ty21a vaccine

Oral Ty21a vaccine is Vi negative and yet it shows good efficacy in field trials. This is because it leads to good serum and secretary antibody response and even cellular immune response. The serum anti-O antibody responses are shown in Table 7.2 which clearly shows that the seroconversion occurs in 60–70% of the vaccinees[9]. However it is the secretary anti-O IgA antibody response which protects against the disease and it is shown to develop in almost all the vaccinees by the recently developed test ELISPOT.

Table 7.1: Immunogenicity of Vi typhoid vaccines in children[9]

Study	Vaccine	Age (year)	N	Anti-Vi antibody (μg/ml) GMT		
				Pre	Post	SC%
Nepal	Vi 1 dose	45–55	8	0.5	4.4	63
		15–44	43	0.4	3.7	79
		5–14	65	0.2	1.9	77
Indonesia	Vi 1 dose	>22	22	0.8	11.3	68
		5–12	80	0.3	5.0	88
		2–4	54	0.2	5.8	96
Kenya	Vi 1 dose	5–15	97	0.3	2.0	76
Vietnam	Vi rEPA Conjugate	2–5	76	0.11(EU/ml)	72.9(EU/ml)	100%

Safety of Typhoid Vaccines

A meta-analysis compared the side effects seen with the commonly used typhoid vaccines as shown in Table 7.3.

Parenteral whole cell inactivated vaccines

Common side effects seen following these vaccines include fever, pain, swelling, redness, malaise, etc. The reactions were more common with acetone inactivated vaccine than heat inactivated vaccine. Often this led to work absenteeism in many of these vaccinees. There were also reports of severe adverse drug reactions including the reports of septic shock like picture and sudden deaths following these vaccines. All these led to the withdrawal of these vaccines from the market in most of the countries including India in spite of showing excellent clinical efficacy in the field trials.

Vi polysaccharide vaccine

Withdrawal of the parenteral vaccines led to the invention of the so called newer vaccines which include the oral Ty21a vaccine and the injectable Vi vaccine. Both these vaccines were shown to be quite safe in various studies. High fever almost never develops after Vi vaccine and mild fever is seen only in 2–3% of cases. Even other local side effects are seen in less number of cases and are very mild. There are no serious side effects reported with this vaccine in its rich experience of using more than 22 million doses over last 15 years. This along with the need of single dose to vaccinate an individual makes it more acceptable vaccine.

Oral Ty21a vaccine

Oral Ty21a vaccine too is a very safe vaccine. Common side effects seen include diarrhea, vomiting, abdominal discomfort, fever, etc. These side effects are seen in less than 5% of the vaccinees and in fact are comparable to the placebo in most cases.

Efficacy of the Typhoid Vaccines in the Field Trials

Parenteral whole cell inactivated vaccines

In 1960s WHO initiated field efficacy trials of parenteral whole cell inactivated vaccines in the countries where typhoid disease was

Table 7.2: Immunogenicity of oral Ty21a typhoid vaccines: anti-O antibodies[9]

Vaccine formulation	No of doses	Seroconversion(N)	Seroconversion%	Efficacy in field trials
Enteric capsule	3	61/96	64	67
	2	22/50	44	47
	2	9/50	18	18
Gelatin capsule	3	99/195	50	21

Table 7.3: Side effects following typhoid vaccines – pooled analysis of studies[8]

Pooled estimate(95% CI)	Fever %	Swelling %	Vomiting %	Diarrhea %	Missed school/work %
Ty21a Vaccine(5 studies)	2.0(0.7–5.3)	NA	2.1(0.6–7.8)	5.1(1.7–14.5)	ND
Vi vaccine(5 studies)	1.1(0.1–12.3)	3.7(1.3–9.6)			0
Whole cell inactivated vaccines(10 studies)	15.7(11.5–21.2)	20.0(12.9–29.7)			10.0(6.0–16.2)

endemic like USSR, Yugoslavia, Guyana, Indonesia, Poland, etc.[10-14]. Acetone inactivated vaccine was better than heat inactivated vaccine (79–88% vs. 51–66% efficacy). The efficacy differed in different countries. Two doses were better than single dose. The vaccine was effective in all age group including smaller children of 2–6 years of age.

Vi polysaccharide vaccine

Only 2 randomized controlled trials are available for this vaccine. Table 7.4 summarizes the results of these studies[7-9]. Efficacy of Vi vaccine was 72% over 17 months follow up in Nepal study[15]. In South Africa the follow up was longer and the efficacy was 55% at the end of 3 years[16]. There is one study using the 30 µg of Chinese Vi vaccine made by the Shanghai Institute which shows 69% efficacy at the end of 19 months. Unfortunately all these studies were done on children above 5 years of age and no study is available in 2–5 year age group. There have been some doubts that wide spread use of Vi vaccine will lead to replacement with Vi negative strains which are obviously not protected by the Vi vaccine and are capable of leading to clinical typhoid cases. However, fortunately no study has actually found this to be a clinical problem.

Oral Ty21a vaccine: This vaccine has been tried in Egypt, Chile and Indonesia[17-20]. It was concluded that the enteric coated capsule formulation was better than the gelatin capsule and showed efficacy of 67% at the end

of 21/2 years and it was maintained at 62% at 7 years follow up. Giving the capsules at 2 days interval, as is recommended now, was better than giving them at 7 days interval. In another study it was shown that three doses were better than 2 doses or a single dose. In fact 2 doses did show efficacy for only the first 2 years. One more study in Chile compared 2 vs. 3 vs. 4 doses of enteric coated capsule formulations[21]. The results showed that the efficacy of 4 doses was 40% more than that of 3 doses given at 2 days interval. Unfortunately there was no control arm to compile the efficacy of the individual arms. Lastly a new liquid formulation was tested against the enteric coated capsule formulation in Chile and Indonesia[19,20]. This vaccine was similar to the original liquid formulation tested in Egypt study. It involved two packets one containing the lyophilized vaccine and the other the buffer. The contents of both the packets are diluted in 100 ml of water on the spot and ingested by the vaccinee. The study showed that the efficacy of the liquid formulation was statistically superior to that of the enteric coated capsule.

Meta-analysis of the Pooled Randomized Controlled Trials

Engels EA *et al.* did a meta-analysis of the pooled randomized controlled trials of typhoid vaccines where the follow up was for at least 3 years[8]. The results of the analysis showed that the 3 year pooled efficacy of 2

Table 7.4: Clinical efficacy in the field trials with Vi typhoid vaccines[7,8]

Study	Age (year)	FU (year)	Incidence control per 10^5	Vaccine	No. of doses	No. of subjects	Efficacy (95% CI)
Nepal	5–44	1.4	655	Vi (25 µg)	1	3457	72 (41–87)
SA	5–16	3.0	387	Vi (25 µg)	1	5692	55 (30–710
China	5–19	1.7		Vi (30 µg)	1	65948	69 (28–87)
Vietnam	2–5	2.3	930	Vi rEPA (conjugate)	2	5525	91.5 (77.1–96.6)

doses of the parenteral vaccine was 73% (65–80% CI), one dose of Vi vaccine was 55% (30–71% CI) and 3 doses of oral Ty21a vaccine was 51% (35–63% CI). This means that the whole cell inactivated vaccine were the best but for their side effects. However there were some flaws in this study as results were combined for different formulations which are not recommended today. The efficacy for the liquid formulation of oral Ty21a vaccine was 74% (41–89% CI), of the enteric capsule of the oral Ty21a vaccine was 47% (32–59% CI), the acetone inactivated whole cell vaccine was 80% (61–90% CI) and that of the heat inactivated whole cell vaccine was 58% (34–73% CI).

Duration of immunity

Seven years long follow up is available with two studies using the parenteral vaccines, i.e. Guyana and Tonga studies[11,12]. In Guyana studies the acetone inactivated vaccine showed 88% efficacy at 7 years where as the heat inactivated vaccine showed 77% efficacy at 3 years which fell to 47% for the last 4 years of follow up. Tonga study had used a derivative of the acetone inactivated vaccine and it showed moderate protection for 5 years. The longest follow up available for Vi vaccine is 3 years from the South Africa study where the efficacy was 55% at 3 years[16]. The longest follow up for the oral Ty21a vaccine available is 7 years in the Chile study where the enteric coated capsule formulation showed efficacy of 67% at 3 years and 62% at 7 years[18]. Similarly the original liquid formulation in the Egypt study showed efficacy of 93% at 3 years[17]. A similar liquid formulation in Chile showed efficacy of 77% at 3 years of follow up and 78% efficacy at 5 years follow up[19].

Herd immunity

Two studies have shown presence of herd immunity with mass typhoid vaccination program. In Thailand heat inactivated vaccine was used in 1980s in school based vaccination program. The incidence of typhoid in non-vaccinated children fell by 10 fold after few years suggesting development of herd immunity[22]. Similarly in Chile trial more than 200,000 children were given the oral enteric coated capsule vaccine. The incidence of enteric fever fell in the control placebo group by 70% after 3 years of the initiation of the vaccine drive[18].

Comparison with the natural infection

Development of immunity following the natural infection is weak and incomplete. This leads to relapses in patients who have suffered from enteric fever in past. In fact the protection is seen in only 33% of those who develop natural infection[9]. This is in contrast to 60–70% protection with the vaccines. In that sense the vaccines are far better than the natural infection in inducing immunity.

Dose, Schedule and Cost of Vaccination

Parenteral whole cell killed vaccines

The whole cell killed vaccines are given as IM injection. The dose is 0.25 ml for a child less than 6 years and 0.5 ml for older children and adults. It is given as 2 doses at 2–4 weeks interval. It can be given from 6 months of age onwards. It is to be stored in refrigerator at 2–8°C and it should not be frozen. If frozen by mistake, it should be discarded. The shelf life is usually 2 years. It is not available now in India. It was very cheap and used to cost Rs. 2 per dose. It does not lead to T cell memory and hence revaccination has to be carried out every 3–5 years.

Vi vaccine

The Vi vaccine is given as IM or deep SC injection. The dose is 25 μg in 0.5 ml. It is given as a single dose. It can be given from 2 years of age. It is to be stored in refrigerator at 2–8°C and it should not be frozen. If frozen by mistake, it should be discarded. The shelf life is usually 2 years. It is widely available in India from various companies. It costs from Rs. 50–125 per dose. It does not lead to T cell memory and hence revaccination has to be carried out every 3 years.

Oral Ty21a vaccine

It is given as enteric coated capsule orally. The capsule should not be opened and should be swallowed intact. It is given one capsule on alternate day for a total of 3 capsules in endemic countries and 4 capsules in US. Care should be taken not to take too much of hot or cold items half an hour before and after the dose. Antibiotics that act against enteric fever should be avoided for 5 days before the immunization, 5 days during the immunization and 5 days after the immunization[8]. As it has to be swallowed as intact capsule, it is recommended only in those who can swallow capsules, i.e. usually after the age of 6 years. It has to be stored in the refrigerator at 2–8°C like any other vaccine and this should be stressed to the parents who tend to keep 'capsules' in the cupboard! (this was a frequent mishap in the ill famous so called school based campaigns in the past). It should not be frozen and if frozen by mistake, it should be discarded. It is not available in India anymore. It used to cost Rs. 175 per course of 3 capsules. If the child chews any of the doses, a new pack has to be purchased as it is not available loose.

Comparison of the 3 vaccines

The ideal typhoid vaccine should be oral, cheap, effective with minimum number of doses, safe, immunogenic, protective in a large number of vaccinees for a long period of time.

However none of the current vaccines satisfies all these criteria. These vaccines are compared in the Table 7.5.

Indications

As typhoid disease is severe illness with high morbidity and potentially high mortality, the best way would be to prevent the disease. Improved sanitation is the only long term measure to prevent enteric fever; however it is a dream come true for many developing countries. The only way out then is its prevention through vaccination. Ideally mass vaccination of all the children should be the target to control the disease; however it does not seem to be possible as the ideal vaccine is still evading us. As the governments in many endemic countries do not appear to be interested in spending on Vi or oral vaccine for mass vaccination, there are very few reports of its use for mass vaccination like in Thailand or Chile.

Children and young adults in endemic areas

Most of the time the typhoid vaccine is used in the private market where the parents have to spend the money on vaccination. The stress has been on the local manufacturing of the Vi vaccine to make the vaccine highly cost effective. The vaccine is especially indicated routinely in school going children and adolescents as they are the most affected age group and for whom the efficacy is best shown in the field trials.

Travelers

International travelers from west tend to develop enteric fever when they travel to endemic countries where the risk is low ($20/10^5$) but definite. This risk is more when they travel to countries like India or Bangladesh. This is more important as many of these countries have high drug resistant strains making treatment more difficult.

Table 7.5: Comparison of typhoid vaccines

Characteristic	WCK vaccines	Ty21a Capsule vaccine	Ty21a Liquid vaccine	Vi vaccines	Vi conjugate
Type	Killed	Live	Live	Subunit	Subunit
Route	IM	Oral		IM	IM
Doses	2	3	3	1	2
Revaccination	3–5 yr	3–5 yr	3–5 yr	3 yr	?
Immunogenicity	+	+		+	+++
Efficacy	51–79%	35–67%	55–96%	55–72%	91%
Duration of efficacy (in years)	65 % at 7 yr	62 % at 7 yr	75% at 5 yr	55% at 3 yr	91% at 2.3 yr
Herd immunity	?	Yes	Yes	?	?
Side effects	++++	+		+	+
Age	> 6 mo	> 6 yr		> 2 yr	> 6 wk
Boosting	–	–		–	++
Cost/per course	Rs 10	Rs. 175	?	Rs. 50	?
Mass vaccination	Unsuitable	Suitable	Suitable	Suitable	?
Availability	No	No	No	Yes	No

Military personnel

Military personnel posted in endemic areas form a special group of "travelers" and are at high risk especially if posted for a long period of time. They should be vaccinated routinely from time to time.

Food handlers

Food handlers can spread the disease if they are short or long term carriers and need to be vaccinated routinely.

Patient recovered from enteric fever

Natural infection does not lead to good immunity and hence these patients should be vaccinated 4 weeks after they recover from the disease.

Laboratory personnel

In west accidental infections in laboratory personnel forms 33% of the total cases of enteric fever and they are advised vaccination routinely.

Contraindications

The whole cell killed parenteral vaccines and Vi vaccines are contraindicated only in those who have shown severe adverse reaction with the previous doses of the same vaccine. Oral Ty21a vaccine is contraindicated in immune-compromised host as it is a live vaccine. It is also contraindicated during pregnancy. Antibiotics acting against *S. typhi* should be avoided during the vaccination with oral Ty21a vaccine. Similarly one should avoid proguanil as it interferes with the immunogenicity.

Future vaccines

Many newer vaccines are being investigated in search of the ideal typhoid vaccine. Besides the various studies on oral live vaccines using different attenuated strains, the foremost in the race is the conjugated Vi vaccine.

Vi conjugate vaccine

A major breakthrough in the field of vaccino-logy has been the method of conjugation of polysaccharide carbohydrate antigens. The advantages of conjugate polysaccharide vaccines are many. They make the polysaccharide antigen T cell dependant. This leads to strong and long lasting IgG response and T cell memory which leads to boosting with subsequent doses. It also means that the vaccine can be used before the age of 2 years, i.e. from 6 weeks of age onwards. It also improves the overall immunogenicity and efficacy of the vaccine. It may also lead to local IgA response which helps bring down carrier rate like in Hib disease. The first and the most successful conjugate vaccine has been the conjugate Hib vaccine. Since then the technique of conjugation has been mastered which has led to the development of the conjugate pneumococcal vaccine, conjugate meningococcal vaccine and now conjugate Vi typhoid vaccine.

Vi rEPA vaccine

Earlier Vi conjugate vaccines used tetanus toxoid, as the carrier which had technical difficulties due to large molecular mass of the Vi antigen. Subsequently Szu *et al* successfully conjugated Vi antigen with the non toxic recombinant exotoxin A of the *Pseudomonas aeruginosa* leading to the development of the vaccine Vi rEPA[5,6]. In the earlier study done by Kossaczka *et al.* in Vietnam, this vaccine had enhanced immunogenicity and T cell dependant properties as it led to booster response in children 2–4 years old whose antibody levels were 3 times as high as those elicited by Vi in children of 5–14 years old[5]. The vaccine was also found to be highly safe. The vaccine using SPDP as the linker was found to be inferior to the one where adipic acid dihydrazide was used as a linker.

Subsequently this vaccine was studied in a field trial in Vietnam in children of 2–4 years of age by Feng *et al*[6]. The vaccine had 22.5 µg of Vi antigen and 22 µg of rEPA in 0.5 ml of phosphate buffer saline per dose. 13,766 children were enrolled from the Dong Thap province of Vietnam. Two doses of the vaccine were given at 6 weeks interval to the subjects. Vaccinees were followed for 27 months for development of enteric fever as diagnosed on the basis of blood culture. The results of this study are shown in Tables 7.1 and 7.4. Immunogenicity studies was done in 76 of the subjects which showed that the vaccine was highly immunogenic in these young children with 100% of them showing at least 10 fold increase in the anti-Vi antibody level. Mean increase in the titers was 575 fold in the vaccinees. On follow up the titers persisted at high level even at 2 years. There were 4 cases of typhoid in the vaccinees as compared to 47 in placebo group which means the vaccine had efficacy of 93% at 27 months follow up. Even if the vaccinee had received only one dose it showed 91% efficacy. None of those who developed typhoid in the vaccinees needed hospitalization as compared to 35% of those who developed enteric fever in the placebo group which means that the enteric fever was mild in the vaccinees. These figures are amazing and unprecedented and far better than unconjugated Vi vaccine as can be seen in the Table 7.4. If these results are duplicated in other studies and may be even in infants, this vaccine has the potential to replace all the existing typhoid vaccines and could enter the immunization schedule of infants in the endemic countries. What is needed is the commercial interest in mass production of this vaccine and further confirmation studies. Severe fever was almost not seen and less than 2% had mild fever. Similarly less than 1% of the vaccinees had local side effects like pain and swelling. This proves that this is the most safe and effective typhoid vaccine.

Vi-TT (Pedatyph[R])data and product monogram

Recently a Vi conjugate vaccine using tetanus toxoid as the carrier protein has been marketed in India under the brand name of *Pedatyph*[R]. However, this vaccine has no field efficacy data and has only one immunogenecity trial done in only one population, i.e. in India. The only study done on *Pedatyph*[R] vaccine is on 169 Indian subjects > 12 weeks old for safety and 145 for immunogenicity study compared to a control group of 37 children > 2 years old given Vi vaccine studied for safety and 29 for immunogenicity; totally unmatched for number of subjects (and obviously for the age group)[23]. The vaccine showed near 100% seroconversion for all the Vi-T subjects with GMCs of 70.32 Elisa units (exact units not mentioned in the results). This immunogenecity data is extrapolated to efficacy data of the Vi-rEPA vaccine which is not correct as they are two different vaccines, used in different age groups and different countries. Besides this, the vaccine was tried as 1 dose schedule in the study in children > 12 weeks and yet recommended as two doses from 12 weeks of age onwards with a booster at 2.5 years for 3 month–2 year old children (followed by a booster every 10 years for all age groups)! These recommendations seem arbitrary and not based on sound scientific data. To best of belief, the study data is neither published in peer reviewed journal nor available for critical review. The only source of data is the product monogram and even there the data available is piecemeal and not complete as the safety and immunogenecity data are not available for the subjects receiving unconjugated Vi vaccine (control) arm for comparison with those receiving *Pedatyph*[R]) vaccine. Again one is misled to believe that *Pedatyph*[R] vaccine is same as the Vi-rEPA vaccine by repeated highlights of work done by Szu *et al* and Kossaczka *et al* (which is for Vi-rEPA vaccine), stating field efficacy data of Vi-rEPA vaccine (which is different from *Pedatyph*[R] and then linking it to *Pedatyph*[R] which in fact is totally different vaccine than the Vi-rEPA)[23].

References

1. Richards LG, Margaret K. Polysaccharide conjugate typhoid vaccine. *N Engl J Med* 2001;344: 1322-3.

2. Hessel L, Fletcher L, Dumas R. Experience with Salmonella typhi Vi capsular polysaccharide vaccine. *Eur J Clin Microbiol Infect Dis* 1999;18:609-20.

3. Gupta A, Jalla S, Sazawal S, Bhan MK. Advances in vaccines for typhoid fever. *Indian J Pediatr* 1994;61:321-39.

4. Patnai KC, Kapoor PN. A note on the incidence of typhoid fever. *Indian J Med Res* 1967;55:288-40.

5. Tarr PE, Kuppens L, Jones TC, *et al*. Considerations regarding mass vaccination against typhoid fever as an adjunct to sanitation and public health measures: potential use in an epidemic in Tajikistan. *Am J Trop Med Hyg* 1999;61:163-70.

6. Kossaczka Z, Lin FY, Ho AV, *et al*. Safety and immunogenicity of Vi conjugate vaccines for typhoid fever in adults, teenagers, and 2-4-year-old children in Vietnam. *Infect Immun* 1999;67: 5806-10.

7. Lin FY, Vo AH, Kheim HB, *et al*. The efficacy of a *Salmonella typhi* Vi conjugate vaccine in two-to-five-year-old children. *N Engl J Med* 2001;344: 1263-9.

8. Engels EA, Matthew EF, Joseph L, *et al*. Typhoid fever vaccines: a meta-analysis of studies on efficacy and toxicity. *British Med J* 1998;316:110-16.

9. Levine MM. Typhoid fever vaccines. *In* Poltkin SA, Orenstein WA (eds): Vaccines. USA, Saunders, 2004:1057-95.

10. Yugoslav Typhoid Commission. A controlled field trial of the effectiveness of the acetone-dried and inactivated and heat-phenol-inactivated typhoid vaccines in Yugoslavia. *Bull WHO* 1964;30:623-30.

11. Ashcroft MT, Singh B, Nocholson CC *et al*. A seven-year field trial of two typhoid vaccines in Guyana. *Lancet* 1967;ii:1056-59.

12. Tapa S, Cvjetanovic B. Controlled field trial on the effectiveness of one and two doses of acetone-inactivated and dried vaccine. *Bull Who* 1975;52: 75-80.

13. Polish Typhoid Committee. Controlled field trials and laboratory studies on the effectiveness of the typhoid vaccines in Poland, 1961-64. Final Report. *Bull WHO* 1966;34:211-22.

14. Hejfec LB, Salmin LV, Letzman MZ, *et al.* A controlled field trial and laboratory study of five typhoid vaccines in the USSR. *Bull WHO* 1966;34: 321-39.

15. Acharya IL, Lowe CU, Thapa R, *et al.* Prevention of typhoid fever in the Nepal with the Vi capsular polysaccharide of *Salmonella typhi*: A preliminary report. *N Engl J Med* 1987;317:1101-4.

16. Klugman KP, Koornhof HJ, Robbins JB, *et al.* Immunogenicity, efficacy and serological correlate of protection of *Salmonella typhi* Vi capsular polysaccharide vaccine three years after immunization. *Vaccine* 1996;14:435-38.

17. Wadhan MH, Serie C, Cerisier Y, *et al.* A controlled field trial of live salmonella typhi strain Ty21a oral vaccine against typhoid: three years results *J Infect Dis* 1982;145:292-95.

18. Levine MM, Ferrecio C, Black RE, *et al.* Large scale field trial of Ty21a live oral typhoid vaccine in enteric coated capsule formulation. *Lancet* 1987;i:1049-52.

19. Levine MM, Ferreccio C, Cryz S, *et al.* Comparison of enteric–coated capsules and liquid formulation of Ty21a typhoid vaccine in randomized controlled field trial. *Lancet* 1990;336:891-4.

20. Simanjuntak CH, Paleologo FP, Punjabi NH, *et al.* Oral immunization against typhoid fever in Indonesia with Ty21a vaccine. *Lancet* 1991;338: 1055-59.

21. Ferreccio C, Levine MM, Rodrigues H, *et al.* Comparative efficacy of two, three or four doses of Ty21a live oral typhoid vaccine in enteric coated capsules: a field trial in endemic area. *J Infect Dis* 1989;159:766-69.

22. Bodhidatta L, Taylor DN, Thisyakorn U, *et al.* Control of typhoid fever in Bangkok, Thailand, by annual immunization of school children with parenteral typhoid vaccine. *Rev Infect Dis* 1987;9:841-45.

23. Protection to infants against typhoid. Peda Typh Vi conjugate vaccine. Product Monogram, Bio Med Pvt. Ltd.

Section 2
Tuberculosis

8

Epidemiology of Tuberculosis in Children: Current Perspective

Monjori Mitra, Soumya Swaminathan

Tuberculosis (TB) remains the number one killer infectious disease affecting adults in developing countries. In the World Health Organization (WHO) report of 1990 on the global burden of disease TB was ranked as the 7th most morbidity-causing disease in the world, and expected it to continue in the same position up to 2020[1]. This is deplorable when one considers that various cost-effective tools that can cure tuberculosis have existed since the 1960s.

An increasing morbidity and mortality from tuberculosis (TB) in the near future is forecast for the world at large, with the number of newly occurring cases predicted to increase from 7.5 million a year in 1990 to 8.8, 10.2 and 11.9 million in the years 1995, 2002 and 2005 respectively; an increase amounting to 58.6% over a 15-year period[2]. The proportion of tuberculosis cases co-infected with human immunodeficiency virus (HIV) was also found to be rising, being 2–10 times greater for the 1997 estimates than for 1990[3]. The association with HIV and increasing multi drug resistant tuberculosis (MDRTB) appears to be a serious issue, especially for the developing nations. The following factors, e.g. chronicity, ability of bacilli to stay alive in body for years, increase in life expectancy, high level of endemicity in ethnic groups even in the midst of affluence in the western world, increases the emergence of MDRTB.

Global Incidence of TB

The global incidence rate of TB (per capita) was growing at approximately 1.1% per year, and the number of cases at 2.4% per year. The growth in case notifications has been much faster in African countries with high human immunodeficiency virus (HIV) prevalence and in eastern Europe. Directly observed therapy, short course (DOTS) programmes have notified 3 million new TB cases in the year 2002, of which 1.4 million were smear-positive, 28% of the additional smear-positive cases reported under DOTS in 2002 were found in India[4].

There were smaller but apparently significant improvements in case detection in South Africa (contributing 12% of the total increase), Indonesia (10%), Pakistan (4%), Bangladesh (3%), and the Philippines (3%). These 6 countries together accounted for over 60% of the additional cases detected in 2002. The ranking of countries by the number of TB cases has drawn attention to the 22 countries that account for roughly 80% of the world's burden of TB, of which India tops the list. Among the 15 countries with the highest estimated TB incidence rate per capita, 13 were in Africa and, in most, the prevalence of HIV infection among TB patients is high[4].

Nearly 40 million children are likely to be exposed to the risk of TB and nearly 3–4 million children below 5 years are estimated to be infected and may progress to disease[3]. Among infants (<1 year), 43% of those infected will develop the disease compared to 24% of children 1–5 years, 15% of adolescents, and 5–10% of adults over a lifetime[5]. In addition, children <5 years of age are at increased risk of developing disseminated forms of TB, including miliary TB and TB meningitis (TBM), which are frequently associated with high morbidity and mortality.

Host immunity was considered to be one of the risk factor for disease development following infection. Infants with immature immune system were at increased risk with 30–40% developing pulmonary disease and 10–20% TBM or miliary disease. The risk decreases as the age increases reaching the lowest level at 5–10 years of age. Bronchial disease was the predominant manifestation in < 5 years of age and pleural effusion at 5–10 years of age. Adolescents are more prone to develop adult type of pulmonary disease (10–20%). The risk and the type of disease that followed primary infection are summarized for specific age groups (Table 8.1)[6].

In 1989, WHO estimated that there were 1.3 million annual cases and 450,000 deaths due to TB among children less than 15 years of age[6]. In 1994, it was estimated there were 7.5 million total TB cases, of which 650,000 (9%) occurred in children[7]. As per the Global TB

Table 8.1: Average age specific risk for disease development following primary infection

Age at primary infection	Immune competent children	Risk of disease following primary infection (%)
< 1 year	No disease	50
	Pulmonary disease	30–40
	(Ghon focus, lymph node, or bronchial)	
	TBM or miliary disease	10–20
1–2 years	No disease	70–80
	Pulmonary disease (Ghon focus, lymph node or bronchial)	10–10
	TBM or miliary disease	2–5
2–5 years	No disease	95
	Pulmonary disease (lymph node, or bronchial)	5
	TBM or miliary disease	0.5
5–10 years	No disease	98
	Pulmonary disease (lymph node, bronchial, effusion or adult-type)	2
	TBM or miliary disease	< 0.5
> 10 years	No disease	80–90
	Pulmonary disease (effusion or adult type)	10–20
	TBM or miliary disease	< 0.5

Control Report 2002, children aged 0–14 years constituted about 0.8–10.5% of the total reported smear positive cases as against 0.6–6.9% observed in the year, 2000 (Table 8.2)[2]. Table 8.3 shows the sex wise distribution of children <14 years of age who were sputum smear positives as reported by WHO in 2004. It was observed that there was no difference between the sexes. This is unlike adults where the number of reported TB cases among males was 3–4 times that among females.

TB Epidemic in India

About 40% of the Indian population is infected with TB bacillus. Every year 1.8 million people in India develop TB, of which 0.8 million are infectious. 778 million people (almost 70% of the total population) had access to DOTS services and about 358,496 new smear positives are put on DOTS by the year 2003. The notification rate of all TB cases in India has been falling at an average of 2% per year for the past decade, which may reflect a real decline in incidence. TB claims > 400,000 lives every year in India[8].

One of the main factors contributing to the importance of childhood tuberculosis in developing communities is the shape of the population pyramid, where about 40–50% of the population may be under the age of 15 years. In India, almost 3.4 million children have TB disease (40% of them contract TB by the age of 6 and 80% by the age of 16)[9].

In 2002, of the 245,051 new smear positive pulmonary TB cases initiated on treatment under revised national tuberculosis control programme (RNTCP), 4,159 (1.7%) were aged 0–14 years. From a survey of RNTCP implementing districts, pediatric cases were seen to make up 3% of the total load of new cases registered under RNTCP. Lymph node TB cases predominated (>75%) among the pediatric extrapulmonary cases registered under RNTCP. Of those pediatric cases treated under RNTCP, cure and completion rates were both above 90% as versus 80% and 70% for those cases treated not under RNTCP (central TB division, Unpublished data)[10].

TB is more common among the disadvantaged and vulnerable groups in each society and the impact of overcrowding, undernutri-

Table 8.2: Proportion of patients <14 years with sputum smear positive TB reported by (WHO 2002)

WHO region	DOTS			Non DOTS		
	Total cases	No.	%	Total cases	No.	%
Africa	381,488	17,397	4.6	9,621	1,006	10.5
America	57,221	1,822	3.2	48,077	1,190	2.5
Eastern Mediterranean	64,962	2,959	4.6	389	22	5.7
Europe	41,261	357	0.9	37,525	194	0.5
SEAR	404,845	7,281	1.8	112,812	2,727	2.4
Western Pacific	305,695	2,280	0.7	31,453	244	0.8

Table 8.3: Sexwise distribution of <14 years old population with sputum smear positive TB (WHO 2002)

WHO region	DOTS			Non DOTS		
	Total No.	Male	Female	Total No.	Male	Female
Africa	17,397	7,926	9,471	1,006	467	539
America	1,822	834	988	1,190	594	596
Eastern Mediterranean	2,959	1,415	1,544	22	16	6
Europe	357	156	201	194	110	84
SEAR	7,281	2,741	4,540	2,727	1,284	1,443
Western Pacific	2,280	1,000	1,280	244	132	112

tion and poverty is particularly severe on children. The actual global disease burden of childhood TB is not known, but it has been assumed that about 10% of the total TB case load is found among children. Tuberculosis in children is of great importance as it is a major cause of infectious disease morbidity and mortality among children and indicates recent TB transmission and impact of TB control measures. Further children with untreated latent TB infection are reservoir of future cases and serve as the fountainhead of adult TB.

In adults, the predominant manifestation is the pulmonary form of the disease. In children, however, manifestations involving more than one system are common. The major differences between adult and childhood TB are detailed in Table 8.4[11].

Difficulties in Estimating the Burden of TB in Children

Since most children acquire the organism from adults in their surroundings, the epidemiology of childhood tuberculosis follows that in adults. Because of the difficulty of confirming the diagnosis, the global burden of childhood tuberculosis in the world is unclear. Another important reason is that children do not make a significant contribution to the spread of tuberculosis. Several estimates make use of an arbitrary calculation assigning 10% of the tuberculosis burden to children. Available data linking the incidence of tuberculosis to the proportion of the tuberculosis case load represented by children suggest an exponential rise in the proportion of the tuberculosis case load caused by children. Following are the limitations in estimation of TB burden in children.

1. *Difficulty in diagnosis*—Vague signs and symptoms, doubtful value of tuberculin skin test in high endemic areas, over emphasis on chest radiography, difficulty in collecting specimen, paucibacillary

Table 8.4: Tuberculosis in children compared to adults

Feature	Adults	Childhood
Symptoms	Cough, fever, chest pain, hemoptysis, loss of weight	Negligible symptoms at the time of primary infection
Lesion	Apical, upper lobes most commonly involved	Peripheral, often middle and lower lobe
Cavitation	Common	Uncommon seen in infancy and adolescence
Glands (Hilar or mediastinal)	Uncommon	Very common
Dissemination	Uncommon	Common
Healing	Fibrosis, less than one third heal spontaneously	Calcification, most often heals spontaneously
Infectivity	Patients with smear-positive pulmonary tuberculosis are infectious to others	Paucibacillary disease, usually not infectious

condition leading to either under or over diagnosis of TB. This picture is further complicated by the co-existing HIV infection.

2. The increased presence of extrapulmonary disease in young children.

3. Lower public health priority given to childhood TB compared to adult TB.

Risk Factors of TB in Children

The risk of developing infection are attributed to the following factors namely, type and duration of exposure to the source case, bacterial load in the sputum of the source case, poverty and overcrowding and being an immigrant or from an immigrant family. The concentration of tubercular bacilli around 5,000 per ml in the sputum gives a reasonable chance for a sputum smear examination being identified as positive. With 10,000 bacilli per ml, there is a 95% probability of a correct identification of a positive result [12]. This is the reason why smear microscopy is a sensitive test for identifying infectious cases and is used as the mainstay diagnostic tool in tuberculosis control in India.

During the period 1985-94, in the two urban communities of Cape Town, South Africa, the case notification rate of TB in children aged 0–5 years was 3,588/100,000, that is 3.5 times the case notification in adults. Children of 0–14 years accounted for 39% of the total caseload. In that study, childhood TB case notification rates correlated with low parental education, annual household income and crowding.[13] A study from the Bronx also showed that the overall TB case rate among children increased as crowding increased.[14] The risk for progression from TB infection to disease in children may be related to age, race and ethnicity, host factors, host immunity, and HIV infection status. Hence efforts to improve TB control must not only target adults but also screen children, particularly the vulnerable group in the lower socioeconomic classes in each country.

Childhood TB and HIV

Nearly, 5 million people (4.2 million adults and 700 000 children) are newly infected with HIV each year, more than 95% of them belong to developing countries. It is estimated that there are 40 million people living with HIV/AIDS worldwide and of these 2.5 million are children less than 15 years of age[14]. In India, there are an estimated 5.1 million HIV infected persons of whom 160,000 are children (NACO 2003 Report). It is estimated that 50–60% of HIV-infected persons in India will develop TB[15].

A prospective cohort study of children with TB diagnosed in Addis Ababa from December 1995 to January 1997 in which HIV-positive children were compared with HIVnegative children, reported that HIV-positive children were younger, more underweight and had a 6-fold higher mortality than HIV-negative children[16]. The tuberculin skin test was less sensitive and chest radiography was less specific in HIV-infected patients. Adherence to treatment was high (96%), and the cure rate was 58% for HIV-positive and 89% for HIV-negative pediatric TB patients. The study concluded that HIV-positive children are at risk of diagnostic error as well as delayed diagnosis of TB. Clinical manifestations were more severe and progression to death was more rapid in HIV-positive children than in HIV-negative children. Weight for age may be used to identify children at high risk of a fatal outcome[16]. In a retrospective study of 118 culture proven tuberculosis patients in Durban, South Africa; 57 (48%) children were detected to be HIV-1 infected, 44 (37%) non-HIV-1-infected, and in 17 (14%) HIV-1 status was not determined[17]. In contrast to previous studies, this study has shown that TB-HIV coinfection in children is common (48% of all culture proven cases), the presentation of tuberculosis may be acute (43%), and supportive tests are individually useful in confirming the diagnosis in a-third of cases. All culture for *M. tuberculosis* were positive by 8 week. Hospital-related mortality was higher (17.5%) in HIV-1-infected children compared to that in noninfected group (11.4%). The changing pattern of presentation of childhood tuberculosis and the high prevalence of TB in HIV endemic areas have made it imperative to maintain a high index of suspicion, with culture evaluation being an important part of clinical practice[12]. There are not many studies from India on proportion of children co-infected with HIV and TB. In a small study from Mumbai[13], 18% of children with disseminated tuberculosis (N = 50) were HIV seropositive. Reported co-infection of HIV and TB in various Indian studies was 16–68%[18-20]. Since follow up data of HIV infected children are not available, it is very difficult to estimate annual infection rate of tuberculosis in HIV positive patients.

The lifetime risk of developing TB disease in TB-infected, HIV-non-infected people is 10% as against 50% in TB and HIV co-infected people [15]. HIV is the most powerful risk factor for progression of TB infection to disease.

Tuberculosis causes depletion of CD4 T cell even in the absence of HIV infection and increased expression of HIV co-receptors on CD4 cells causing progression of HIV infection. CD4 T-cells that are vital for immunity against TB infection are diminished in HIV infected patients creating an increased susceptibility to TB as HIV progresses[21].

Children with HIV often have other lung disease related to their HIV infection, including PCP, lymphocytic interstitial pneumonitis (LIP), and other viral or bacterial pneumonias making the diagnosis difficult.

TB Mortality in Children

Globally about 500 children die every day from TB. Mortality in children has been shown to correlate with the socioeconomic status of the population. The annual TB mortality rate among children in an urban slum in Chennai was 239/100,000 compared to 52 and 55/100,000 for the same age group in the rural areas of Tamil Nadu and Bengaluru.

Mortality from disseminated forms of TB disease such as TB meningitis (TBM) causes the highest case-fatality in early childhood. Chakraborthy has estimated that against an ARI of 1% (incidence of infection), the TBM mortality rate in the ages of 0–4 years could be 1.5/100,000. The outcome of TB also depends on age. The case fatality ratio for all

forms of TB in children in South Africa from 1970-1980 was 7% in <1 year, 3% in 1–4 years and 1% in 5–9 years of age. Hence, mortality due to TB in children is linked both to the age and as well as the socioeconomic status of the family[22].

Conclusion

TB remains a public health problem in many countries of the developing world and is exacerbated by the HIV epidemic. Treatment of adults with infectious TB is the most effective way of preventing TB in children. A high index of suspicion is required to diagnose TB in young children as progression from infection to disease is much more rapid. Mortality from TB is high in children as they develop more disseminated forms of TB. Table 8.1 shows age specific risk factors for development of primary infection of tuberculosis. Table 8.2 depicts proportion of patients <14 years of smear positive TB in various WHO region in DOTs and nonDOTs group. Sexwise distribution of patients <14 years with smear positive TB in various WHO region is shown in Table 8.3.

References

1. Murray, CJL, Lopez AD: The global burden of disease: a comprehensive assessment of mortality and disability from diseases, injuries and risk factors in 1990 and Geneva: WHO projected to 2020: Summary Geneva: WHO, 1996; W 74 96GL-1/1996.

2. Dolin PJ, Raviglione MC, Kochi A. A review of current epidemiological data and estimation of future tuberculosis incidence and mortality. WHO/TB/93.173. Geneva: World Health Organization; 1993.

3. Dye C, Scheele S, Dolin, P, Pathania V, Raviglione MC. Global burden of tuberculosis: estimated incidence, prevalence and mortality by country. WHO Global Surveillance and Monitoring Project. *JAMA* 1999;282:677-86.

4. WHO. Global Tuberculosis Control, Surveillance, Planning, Financing. WHO Report 2004.

5. Ministry of Health and Family Welfare. TB India 2002: RNTCP status report. New Delhi: Central TB Division, Directorate General of Health Services, Ministry of Health & Family Welfare; 2000.

6. World Health Organisation. Expanded Program on Immunization. Update August, 1989. Geneva, Switzerland:WHO, 1989.

7. Dolin PJ, Raviglione MC, Kochi A. Global tuberculosis incidence and mortality during 1990-2000. *Bull WHO* 1994;72:213-20.

8. RNTCP Status Report Central TB Division. Delhi: TB India 2004.

9. Singh V. Tuberculosis in children: Some issues. *Health Millions* 1995;21:27-8.

10. Management of Pediatric TB under the Revised National Tuberculosis Control Programme (RNTCP). A Joint Statement of the Central TB Division, Directorate General of Health Services, Ministry of Health and Family Welfare, and Experts from Indian Academy of Pediatrics. New Delhi, August 2003.

11. Rie A, Beyers N, Gie RP, Kunneke M, Zietsman L, Donald PR. Childhood tuberculosis in an urban population in South Africa: burden and risk factor. *Arch Dis Child* 1999;80:433-7.

12. Frieden T (ed) Toman's Tuberculosis: case detection, treatment and monitoring – question and answers, 2nd ed). World Health Organization, Geneva, Switzerland, 2004.

13. Drucker E, Alcabes P, Bosworth W, Sckell B. Childhood tuberculosis in the Bronx, New York. *Lancet* 1994;343:1482-5.

14. World Health Organisation. Fight Stigma and Discrimination. New Delhi: WHO SEARO, 2003.

15. Cotton MF, Schaaf HS, Hesseling AC, Madhi SA. HIV and childhood tuberculosis: the way forward. *Int J Tuberc Lung Dis* 2004;8:675-82.

16. Schaaf HS, Geldenhuys A, Gie RP, Cotton MF. Culture positive tuberculosis in human immuno-deficiency virus type 1-infected children. *Pediatr Infect Dis J* 1998;17:599-604.

17. Schaaf HS, Gie RP, van Rie A, Seifart HI, van Helden PD, Cotton MF. Second episode of tuberculsos in an HIV-infected child: Relapse or reinfection? J Infect Dis 2000;41:100-3.

18. Kassa-Kelembho E, Bobossi-Serengbe G, Takeng EC, Nambea-Koisse TB, Yapou F, Talarmin A. Surveillance of drug-resistant childhood tuberculosis in Bangui, Central African Republic. *Int J Tuberc Lung Dis* 2004;8:574-8.

19. Merchant RH, Oswal JS, Bhagwat RV, Karkare J. Clinical profile of HIV infection. *Indian Pediatr* 2001;38:239-46.

20. Lodha R, Singhal T, Jain Y, Kabra SK, Seth P, Seth V. Pediatric HIV infection in a tertiary care center in north India: early impressions. *Indian Pediatr* 2000;37:982-6.

21. Dhurat R, Manglani M, Sharma M, Shah NK. Clinical spectrum of HIV infection. *Indian Pediatr* 2000;37:831-6.

22. A.K. Chakraborty Epidemiology of tuberculosis: Current status in India. *Indian J Med Res* 2004; 120:248-76.

9

Pathogenesis of Tuberculosis

Anju Aggarwal, Jaydeep Choudhury

Clinical consequences of infection with *Mycobacterium tuberculosis* depend on number of host factors, especially the immune system, environmental factors and the microorganism.

Etiologic Agent

Robert Koch discovered tubercle bacillus in 1882. Lehmann and Newman coined the term mycobacterium in 1896. *M. tuberculosis* is obligate aerobe, non-motile, non-spore-forming. Its most conspicuous feature is its waxy content, which makes it impermeable to the usual stains. It slowly takes up heated stains-carbol fuchsin in the Ziehl-Neelsen method. Once stained the bacilli cannot be decolorized even by strong acids and alcohols. Thus, it is also classified as acid-fast and alcohol-fast. Acid fastness is mainly due to the organisms' high content of mycolic acids, long-chain cross-linked fatty acids and other cell wall lipids[1].

M. tuberculosis is very resistant to drying. It can survive in dust for several months. It is very sensitive to the effect of ultraviolet radiation and is rapidly killed in sunlight. It is relatively resistant to chemical disinfectants. It is destroyed by tincture of iodine in five minutes and by 80% ethanol in 2–10 minutes. The latter is recommended as a disinfectant for skin, rubber gloves and clinical thermometers[4].

Antigenic Properties

Mycobacterial cell wall is highly immunogenic[2]. **Lipid components** as muramyl dipeptides and mycolic acids cause granuloma formation, phospholipids and metalloproteinases induce caseation necrosis and cord factor confers virulence.

Certain **protein components** are highly species specific for *Mycobacterium tuberculosis* as 14 kDa. Their classification is based on different molecular weights .These proteins will have implications in serodiagnosis as well. Previously non specific proteins as PPD were used in serodiagnosis, which have now been replaced by antigen[5,6] which are specific for *Mycobacterium tuberculosis* and have a strong immunogenicity. Antigen 5 has 38kDa protein. Protein antigens are type specific.

Group specificity is due to polysaccharide components which induce delayed hypersensitivity. Following infection by *M. tuberculosis*, delayed type hypersensitivity is developed to the protein of the bacillus known as tuberculin.

Host Factors

Age of infection, immune status of the child, specific immunodeficiency states, malnutrition, HIV infection and genetic factors.

Immune Mechanism (Fig 9.1)

Cell mediated immunity deals with intracellular organisms as *Mycobacterium tuberculosis*. T lymphocytes and macrophages play an important role by contributing to protection and for survival of pathogens and pathogenesis. Immunity to tuberculosis may be innate in some population or genetically related. Cell-mediated immunity is beneficial to the host whereas delayed hypersensitivity reaction is adverse. Activated macrophages kill mycobacteria by production of TNF, interferon, and nitric oxide. Other cytokines produced are IL-1 which causes fever, IL-6 mediate hyperglobulinemia, IL-10 inhibits cytokine production. TNF alpha induces granuloma formation, fever, weight loss and tissue necrosis.TNF beta suppresses T cell proliferation hence prevents excessive inflammation and tissue damage. Relative activation of the two pathways determines the pathogenesis of the disease[3-5].

Pathophysiology

The pathophysiology of tuberculosis in children evolves through various stages.[6]

1. *Onset*—After inhalation tubercular bacilli are ingested by alveolar macrophages and destroyed.
2. *Symbiosis*—If not destroyed by macrophages they multiply for 7–21 days till delayed hypersensitivity develops.

Droplets of aerosolized pulmonary secretion containing viable *M. tuberculosis* are released by an infected adult while coughing or sneezing

↓

A small part of the inhalant reaches the terminal bronchiole and alveoli

↓

The bacilli begin to multiply within the macrophages. Interlukin-12 is generated by the macrophages

↓

This causes sensitization of CD4+ cells and T$_H$1 cells and they re-circulate at the site of infection

↓

Antigen from the tubercle bacilli reaches draining lymph nodes and is presented to T cells

↓

Sensitized CD4+ cells release cytokines when exposed to antigens at the site of infection

↓

Monocytes are recruited and activated to kill or inhibit the growth of the organism

↓

The rapid growth of bacteria quickly kills the macrophage which lyses

↓

The bacilli also spread to the regional lymph nodes resulting in lymphatic and hematogenous dissemination

↓

The lymphocytes start appearing from second week onwards

↓

Two host responses: tissue-damaging response and macrophage-activating response. Balance between the two determines the form of tuberculosis that will develop subsequently.

Fig. 9.1: Immunopathogenesis of tuberculosis

3. *Initial caseous stage*—Host becomes tuberculin positive, caseous material, necrotic material is formed. Clotting

pathway, etc. are activated, reactive oxygen radicals are released. Depending on the dose of surviving bacilli lesions may heal or progress. Hematogenous spread may occur within 2–3 weeks.

4. Stage of interplay between tissue damage and macrophage activating immune response.

5. Liquefaction and cavity formation usually occur in immunocompetent individuals, not in infants and immunosuppressed. This leads to spread of tuberculosis in the community.

Infection, Resistance and Immunity

Following infection with *M. tuberculosis* it is seen that sometimes there is healing by fibrosis of a small caseous focus, and on other occasions, it progresses to florid disease. Even the disease may rapidly spread with fatal outcome. The factors that determine the tissue response are:

1. The dose and virulence of the organism.
2. The innate and acquired resistance of the body. The risk of developing disease after being infected depends largely on endogenous factors, such as the individual's innate susceptibility to disease and level of function of cell-mediated immunity. Disease directly following infection is primary infection. It is common among children up to 4 years of age. Though, this form is often severe and disseminated, it is usually not transmissible. Gender affects resistance. Females appear to be more susceptible during adolescence. General health of the individual is also of great importance. Certain co-morbid conditions favour the development of tuberculosis. The most potent risk factor is HIV co-infection, which actually suppresses cellular immunity. With the emergence of HIV, tuberculosis has come up as the most important re-emerging infection even in the developed countries. Other conditions known to increase the risk of active tuberculosis among persons infected with *M. tuberculosis* include silicosis, lymphoma, leukemia and other malignancies, hemophilia, chronic renal failure and hemodialysis, immunosuppressive treatment and malnutrition[7].

Portal of Entry

The tubercle bacillus is usually inhaled. The interaction of *M. tuberculosis* with human host starts as soon as the droplet nuclei containing the bacillus from infectious patients are inhaled. Majority of the inhaled bacilli are trapped in the upper airway and expelled by ciliary movement of mucosal cells. A small fraction, usually less than 10%, reach the alveoli.

Ingestion accounts for a small percentage of primary pulmonary foci and for some gastrointestinal tuberculosis. Contamination of a superficial skin or mucous membrane lesion, such as an abrasion, an insect bite, ritual circumcision or infection of the vulva, may lead to infection. Few cases of infection by inoculation with a sputum-contaminated syringe have been reported. Congenital infection may occur as a result of either lymphohematogenous spread in the mother during pregnancy or endometritis[8,9].

Variations in the Reaction to Tubercle Bacilli

The common type of reaction described above is called productive or proliferative, because its main components are cells rather than fluid exudate. Another type of lesion is exudate form of tuberculosis. It is characterized by the outpouring of an inflammatory exudates rich in fibrin. There is a considerable infiltration of lymphocytes and often polymorphs, but epitheloid and giant cells are scanty. Exudative lesions are typical of tuberculosis of serous cavities.

In a minority of cases, the macrophage activating response is weak. Mycobacterial growth can be inhibited only by intensified delayed-type hypersensitivity reaction which leads to tissue destruction. Surrounding tissues are progressively damaged as lesions tend to increase further. Bronchial walls and blood vessels are invaded and destroyed. Cavities are formed[9].

The Fate of Tuberculous Lesion

The caseous focus may either cease to progress and heal by fibrosis, or it may soften and spread.

The hallmark of healing is fibrous tissue. It is produced by the proliferating fibroblasts at the periphery of the lesion. Eventually a solid fibrous nodule may replace the area of caseation. Sometimes the central mass of caseation undergoes slow dystrophic calcification. In this calcareous nodule organisms can survive. Years later when resistance of the host breaks down, they may become active again. Sometimes the nodule ossifies.

The hallmark of activity is caseation and softening. If the lesion is spreading, bacilli are carried by macrophages into the surrounding lymphatics and tissue spaces. There they set up satellite follicles. They may fuse and produce conglomerate tubercle follicle.

Sometimes the caseous material liquefies. It is associated with spread, and the liquefied debris contains many bacilli. This whole lesion is called cold abscess.

Spread of Tuberculosis in the Body

1. *Local spread*—Mainly by macrophages.
2. *Lymphatic spread*—It is the continuation of local spread. The regional tuberculous lymphadenitis with lymphangiitis is called primary complex.
3. *Hematogenous spread*—In the initial stage of infection, bacilli are usually transported by macrophages to regional lymph nodes, from which they disseminate to various organs and other tissues. In children with poor natural immunity, hematogenous dissemination may result in fatal miliary tuberculosis or tuberculous meningitis.
4. *Spread in serous cavities*—Lung lesions may lead to pleural effusion. Other examples are localized peritonitis around tuberculous salpingitis, and tuberculous meningitis.
5. *Spread along epithelial-lined surfaces*—Intrabronchial spread of tuberculosis occurs when sputum is inhaled into adjacent lung segments. Similarly tuberculous laryngitis or when swallowed it may produce tuberculous enteritis. Tuberculosis of kidney may spread to bladder tuberculosis and tuberculous salpingitis may produce endometritis.

Pathogenesis of Tuberculosis in Various Organs

Endothoracic primary complex and its complications

Primary tuberculosis is the form of disease that develops in a previously unexposed and therefore, unsensitized person[1]. In childhood the primary focus (Ghon focus) is a small, wedge-shaped area situated at the periphery of the lung field usually in the mid-zone. This subpleural focus may heal, or the infection spreads to the hilar nodes. A primary complex is the result. It includes three elements: the primary focus, lymphangiitis and regional lymphadenitis.

The development of tuberculin hyper sensitivity within 3 to 12 weeks after initial infection enhances the cellular reaction throughout the primary complex. At this time the infection may spread along nearby lymphatic chains to involve more distant nodes. The lymphatic drainage of the lungs occurs predominantly from left to right[5]. The nodes in the right upper paratracheal area are the ones most often affected. Bronchial obstructions as a result of enlargement of the peribronchial lymph nodes are found. As the nodes enlarge they impinge on the neighbouring regional bronchus and compress. It may cause diffuse inflammation of its wall and even may obstruct the lumen.

The chief implications of primary tuberculosis are:

1. It induces hypersensitivity and increased resistance,
2. The foci of scarring may harbour viable bacilli for years and thus be a nidus for reactivation later,
3. Sometimes the disease may develop without interruption into progressive pulmonary tuberculosis or disseminated disease[10].

Pleural effusion—Tuberculous pleural effusion originates in the discharge of the bacilli into the pleural cavity from a subpleural pulmonary focus or from subpleural caseous lymph nodes.

Progressive pulmonary tuberculosis—The primary pulmonary focus instead of resolving or calcifying enlarges steadily and develops a large caseous center. This center then liquefies and empties into an adjacent bronchus to create a primary cavity. This is a serious complication of primary complex. The tubercle bacilli further disseminate to other parts of the lung. Rarely an enlarging primary focus ruptures into the pleural cavity and creates pneumothorax, bronchopleural fistula or into the pericardial sac.

Chronic pulmonary tuberculosis—Also known as reactivation tuberculosis, it is usually due to endogenous re-infection. It is the pattern of disease that arises in a previously sensitized host[1]. The primary focus in some patients is followed within a few years by small round foci in the lung apices probably due to hematogenous spread at the time of initial infection. They often get calcified, known as Assmann foci or Simon foci. These foci disappear spontaneously or remain visible as tiny calcifications or large round foci. If untreated this may progress to the typical lesions of chronic pulmonary tuberculosis.

Myocardial and pericardial tuberculosis—Tubercles are found in the heart in miliary tuberculosis. Myocardial caseation, though rare, is secondary to direct spread from mediastinal glands.

Tuberculous pericarditis arises by direct invasion or by lymphatic drainage from caseous lymph nodes in the subcranial area or from nodes close to the ductus arteriosus.

Lymphohematogenous spread of tuberculosis

Tubercle bacilli from the lymphadenitis of the primary complex are disseminated during the incubation period in all cases of tuberculosis. Tuberculosis can reach deep and distant organs via the bloodstream or lymphatic channels. The clinical picture produced by lymphohematogenous spread probably is determined by host susceptibility at the time of spread and by the quantity of tubercle bacilli released.

Miliary tuberculosis—It is analogous to sepsis with pyogenic bacteria. It arises from discharge of a caseous focus, often a lymph node into a blood vessel such as pulmonary vein. The factors that determine the tissue susceptibility are the number of fixed intravascular phagocytes, as well as the relative tortuosity of smaller blood vessels.

Central nervous system tuberculosis—During lymphohematogenous spread tubercle bacilli are distributed by the bloodstream into all parts of the central nervous system. They do not multiply well in nervous tissue as in other areas such as the lung. Central nervous system tuberculosis, though an early manifestation of tuberculosis, usually does not appear simultaneously with miliary spread, but days later. The various manifestations of tuberculosis of central nervous system are tuberculous meningitis, serous meningitis, tuberculoma, tuberculous brain abscess or spinal tuberculous leptomeningitis.

Tuberculous meningitis arises from caseous foci situated in the brain or meninges. These foci discharge tubercle bacilli directly into the subarachnoid space. The thick gelatinous exudates lie in the mesh of the pia-arachnoid in the brain. It infiltrates the walls of meningeal arteries and veins and produces inflammation, caseation and obstruction. The exudates can extend along small vessels into the cortex where it causes occlusion and produces infarcts. This exudates also interferes with normal flow of cerebrospinal fluid in and out of the ventricular system and with absorption of fluid.

Skeletal tuberculosis—The tubercle bacilli are usually disseminated to skeletal structures during lymphohematogenous spread of the initial infection. Each of the frequently involved bones and joints has a characteristic incubation period. It takes about 1 month for tuberculous dactilytis and about 30 months for tuberculosis of the hip to develop following initial infection.

In young children blood flow through growing bone is intense. They suffer from skeletal tuberculosis more often than the older ones. The lesion starts as an area of endarteritis in the metaphysis of the long bone, where the blood supply is particularly abundant. Lesions can be single or multiple. Bone infection can be initiated by two other mechanisms, particularly in the vertebrae. First is by direct extension via the lymphatics from a caseous paravertebral lymph node. The second is direct local hematogenous or lymphatic extension from a neighboring bone. As bone is destroyed progressively by pressure necrosis and cold abscess formation, a nearby joint may become involved.

The bones most commonly affected are the vertebrae. Others commonly affected are the knees, hip and elbow. The upper extremities and the non-weight-bearing bones such as skull, clavicle and mandible are rarely involved. Often a history of trauma is present and may play some part in activating an underlying lesion.

Cutaneous tuberculosis—The various pathogenic mechanisms of cutaneous tuberculosis in children are the following:

1. Inoculation from an exogenous source in a previously uninfected child, in a previously infected child or after inoculation with BCG vaccine.
2. Hematogenous dissemination.
3. Arising from an endogenous source.
4. Erythema nodosum.

Tuberculosis of the superficial lymph nodes—Enlargement of the superficial regional lymph nodes is an integral component of primary tuberculosis complex. The tonsillar and submandibular nodes are involved most often and probably represent extension from the paratracheal lymph nodes. Other regional lymph nodes may be enlarged in cases of tuberculosis in the corresponding drainage area.

Superficial tuberculous lymphadenitis sometimes occurs early in the course of lymphohematogenous spread. In such cases, it is often manifested as general glandular enlargement. In adolescents and young adults tuberculous adenitis may be reactivation tuberculosis who were infected months or years earlier.

Ocular tuberculosis—Phlyctenular tuberculosis is one of the hypersensitivity phenomena of childhood tuberculosis. Conjunctiva can serve as the initial portal of entry for tubercle bacilli, especially after trauma.

Cornea may also be affected similarly. Tubercles of the choroids have been found in patients with miliary tuberculosis.

Tuberculosis of the middle ear—It occurs as a primary focus in the area of the eustachian tube due to reflux up the tube. In neonates due to aspirated infected amniotic fluid and in infants who have ingested tuberculous material.

Gastrointestinal and abdominal tuberculosis—Abdominal tuberculosis may occur after ingestion of tubercle bacilli or as a part of generalized lymphohematogenous spread. When tubercle bacilli penetrate the gut wall, they do so via Peyer patches or the appendix. Here they give rise to local ulcers followed by mesenteric lymphadenitis and sometimes peritonitis.

The spleen is seeded during the initial lymphohematogenous spread. Mesenteric lymphadenitis can arise as part of an intra-abdominal primary complex or by extension from tuberculous lymph nodes. Tuberculous peritonitis can be a result of direct extension from a primary intestinal focus, adjacent mesenteric lymph nodes or tuberculous salpingitis.

Renal tuberculosis—Hematogenous dissemination can give rise to tubercles in the glomeruli with resultant caseating and sloughing, which then discharge tubercle bacilli into the tubules. Occasionally, an encapsulated caseous mass develops, it may calcify and form a cavity. Infection can spread downward to involve the bladder.

Genital tuberculosis— It is uncommon before puberty and usually arises as a metastatic lesion during lymphohematogenous spread and occasionally by direct extension from an adjacent lesion of bone, gut or the urinary tract.

Tuberculosis of external genitalia has been seen as a manifestation of child abuse. Genital tuberculosis can occur in males as primary tuberculosis of the penis after circumcision.

Timetable of Tuberculosis

The timetable concept of tuberculosis is by Wallgren[6]. It permits a realistic prognosis, the early course and timing of initial infection and complications.

Symptomatic massive lymphohematogenous spread (miliary or acute meningeal tuberculosis) has usual onset within 2 to 6 months after initial infection. Which means even before the tuberculin test becomes positive and the child develops any symptom. Endo bronchial tuberculosis develops slightly later. Lesions of bones and joints usually appear after about 1 year. Renal lesions come still later, 5 to 25 years after initial infection. The first 5 years after initial tuberculosis infection in children, especially the first year, is the time when complications usually occur. Later in life, during times of stress, a previously silent or arrested lesion may reactivate and become dangerous to the patient and highly infectious to others.

Pathogenesis of Perinatal Tuberculosis

Though only about 300 cases of perinatal tuberculosis have been reported so far, this clinical entity deserves mention due to its unique mode of transmission and pathogenesis. Perinatal tuberculosis can be acquired by the infant via one of the following routes:

1. *Transplacental spread*—From mother with primary hematogenous tuberculosis during pregnancy, spread via umbilical vein. This is true congenital tuberculosis.
2. *In uteroaspiration of amniotic fluid*—From endometritis in mother or from placental tuberculosis. This is also true congenital tuberculosis.
3. *Ingestion of infected material during delivery*—Usually amniotic fluid or secretions.

4. *Inhalation*—Soon after birth from mother or others coming in close contact. This route is probably the most common mode of transmission to newborns.
5. *Ingestion of infected breast milk or cow milk.*

References

1. Comstock GW. Epidemiology of tuberculosis. *Am Rev Respir Dis* 1982;125:8-16.
2. Seth V, Kabra SK. Immunopathogenesis: Basic aspects and their relevance to diagnosis in children. In Seth V, Kabra SK eds: Essentials of Tuberculosis in Children. 3rd ed. 2006 Jaypee Brothers, Delhi, 76-94.
3. Walter JB, Israel MS. General Pathology, 6th ed. Edinburgh: Churchill Livingstone, 1987; 261-9.
4. Bareness PF, Modlin RL, Ellner JE. T cell responses and cytokines. In: Berry Bloom, ed. Tuberculosis: Pathogenesis, Protection and control. Washington DC, 1994;417-35.
5. Starke JR, Smith KC. Tuberculosis. In: Feigin RD, Cherry JD, Demmier GJ, Kaplan SL, eds. Textbook of Pediatric Infectious Diseases, 5th ed. Philadelphia: WB Saunders, 2004;1337-9.
6. Lurie MB. Resistance to Tuberculosis: Experimental Studies in Native and Acquired Defensive Mechanisms. Cambridge, Massachus-sets Harvard University Press 1964.
7. Starke JR, Correa AG: Management of myco-bacterial infection and disease in children. *Pediatr Infect Dis* 1995;14:455-70.
8. Iseman MD. In: A Clinician's Guide to Tuberculosis, 1st ed. Philadelphia: Lippincott Williams and Wilkins, 2000;63-96.
9. Dannenberg AMJR, Rook GAW. Pathogenesis of pulmonary tuberculosis. In: Blood B, ed. Tuberculosis: Pathogenesis, Protection and Control. Washington DC: ASM Press, 1994;459-83.
10. Marais BJ, Gic RP, Schaaf HS, *et al*. A proposed radiological classification of childhood intra-thoracic tuberculosis. *Pediatr Radiol* 2004;34:886-94.

10

Laboratory Diagnosis of Tuberculosis in Children

Camilla Rodrigues

Tuberculosis remains one of the deadliest diseases today despite the availability of effective preventive measures and chemotherapy[1]. Childhood tuberculosis represents a sentinel event in a community as it suggests recent transmission. Cases among children represent approximately 5–10% in the developed nations and 15–20% in developing countries of all tuberculosis cases. Globally, accurate figures for the burden of pediatric tuberculosis are not available and perhaps this reflects the inadequacy of accurate diagnosis and lack of importance given to childhood tuberculosis.

The diagnosis of tuberculosis in children is not easy, since the distinction between latent infection and actual disease is often blurred. Also childhood tuberculosis is a paucibacillary disease unlike adults where sputum smear and culture is the mainstay in diagnosis. The relatively higher frequency of extrapulmonary disease and nonspecific clinical signs and symptoms in children only serve to compound the problem. Traditionally, history of contact with an infectious case, chest radiography and TST form the basis for diagnosis of tuberculosis.

Tuberculin Skin Test (TST) — Mantoux Test

We have celebrated more than 100 years of the TST (developed in the late 1800's) and it is based on the fact that M. tuberculosis caused cutaneous reactivity to a concentrated filtrate from heat-killed cultures of M. tuberculosis. The immunologic basis of this lies in the fact that infection with M. tuberculosis produces a delayed type hypersensitivity (DTH) to certain antigenic components contained in the extract of the culture filtrates.

Since it was first introduced, the tuberculin test has undergone continual refinement in its formulation, standardization, and dosage, as well as its interpretation and indications for use. New guidelines have replaced universal screening with targeted testing and rigid definition of positivity with individualized criteria. The standard skin test dose for RT-23 (WHO – Statens Serum Institute) is 2 TU and this has been matched for bioequivalence to 5TU of Purified Protein Derivative PPD-S (USA)[2].

As in adults, a Mantoux test of 5TU of PPD-S or 2TU of RT-23 is used for tuberculin skin tests in infants and children. Universal testing of children, including screening in school-based programs, has a low yield of positive results and a large proportion of false-positive results, resulting in the inefficient use of health care resources. ATS/CDC guidelines advocate the replacement of universal screening with targeted skin testing of selected groups at increased risk. Prior BCG vaccination is not contraindication to an indicated TST. The interpretation of TST results in children is based on a Bayesian approach analogous to that in adults.

Methods—The test is administered as 0.1 ml of 2 Tuberculin Units (2TU) RT 23 intra cutaneously on the volar surface of the forearm. The reaction is read 48 to 72 hours later. The size is determined by measurement of induration (not erythema). The criterion for interpreting the reaction as positive is dependent on certain characteristics of the person being tested.

Heaf and Tine tests are multipuncture methods in which the inoculation of purified protein derivative solution is placed on the skin and subsequently inoculated in the Heaf test by spring-loaded gun which dives six needles into the skin. In the Tine test, the PPD is dried onto four spikes on a small single-using disposable unit.

For persons with latent TB infection with normal immune responsiveness the sensitivity is 100%. However, false positives occur in persons with non-tuberculous mycobacteria and on children recently immunized with BCG. Tuberculin reactivity caused by BCG generally wanes with passage of time but can be boosted by the TST.

No reliable method has been developed to distinguish tuberculin reactions caused by vaccination with BCG from those, which caused by natural mycobacterial infections. Several studies have consistently demonstrated that >90% of BCG vaccines develop induration >10mm, 8–12 weeks after vaccination. However, in those vaccinated in the neonatal period this reactivity wanes rapidly and all have indurations <10 mm within a year after vaccination and no reactivity 5 years after vaccination. Highly positive reactions of > 20 mm induration are not likely caused by BCG.

A PPD positive in a child less than 2 years of age is highly suggestive of recent infection and must be treated. Beyond 2 years of age, a positive test along with history of contact, symptoms and signs and risk factors increase the risk of natural infection. Without prophylaxis, it is believed that 40–50% of infants and 15% of older children with infection will develop disease in 1–2 years. In adults, this distinction is clearer and separated by years before reactivation[3].

A PPD positive is regarded as induration of more than 10 mm irrespective of BCG vaccine status[4] (Table 10.1). If results are inconclusive, repeat TST should be performed on the other forearm. Upto 10 % of otherwise normal children with culture positive tuberculosis may not react to PPD suggesting that the disease itself may contribute to immunosuppression. False negative TST also occurs in children with severe tuberculosis, debiliation, malnutrition and immune suppression[5].

Keeping in mind the concepts of sensitivity, specificity, positive predictive value (PPV) and negative predictive value (NPV), the TST has different recommended cutoffs in different scenarios. The PPV is dependent on the disease prevalence as well as the specificity of the test. In populations as India with high prevalence of disease the PPV will remain high even if the cutoff is low. The US recommendations cannot be extrapolated to India as we are high prevalence country. The IAP consensus group recommendations are that the cut off to define a positive TST be set at >10 mm[4]. The concept of interpreting the skin test on the basis of

Table 10.1: Summary of interpretation of positive TST results for PPD in children

Indian academy of pediatrics	British thoracic society	WHO	American academy of paediatrics
Mantoux test (5TU) Positive >10 mm Irrespective of BCG	Mantoux test (10TU) Positive: 5–14 mm (no BCG) >15 mm	Mantoux test Positive: >10 mm (no BCG)> 15 mm	Mantoux test Positive: >5 mm and one or more of the following: Children in close contact with known or suspected contagious case of tuberculosis disease, i.e. households with active or previously active cases if treatment cannot be verified as adequate before exposure, treatment was initiated after the child's contact, or reactivation of latent tuberculosis culosis infection is suspected, or Children suspected to have tuberculosis disease, i.e. chest radiograph consistent with active or previosuly active tuberculosis; or clinical evidence of tuberculosis disease, or Children receiving immuno-suppressive therapy or with immunosuppressive conditions including HIV infection Positive >10 mm, and one or more of the following: Children at increased risk of disseminated disease, i.e. younger than 4 years of age; or other medical condition, including Hodgkin's disease, lymphoma, diabetes mellitus, chronic renal failure, or malnutrition, or Children with increased exposure to tuberculosis disease, i.e. born or whose parents were born in high-prevalence regions of the world; or frequently exposed to adults who are HIV-infected, homeless, users of illicit drugs, residents of nursing homes, incarcerated or institutionalized, and migrant farm worker. Positive > 15 mm, and children 4 years of age or older without any risk factors

predictive value and risk of disease instead of just the size of induration is worth bearing in mind. A positive skin test in association with other features supports the diagnosis of tuberculosis disease but a negative skin test does not rule it out.

Etiological Diagnosis

The definitive diagnosis of TB demands that tubercle bacilli are isolated and identified. A proper sample collection is vital. Sputum, gastric lavage, urine, body fluids and tissues should be examined.

Specimen collection

- *Sputum*—Three sputum cultures in older children is likewise the gold standard and all attempts must be made to isolate the organism.
- *Gastric aspiration*—This may require in children who cannot produce sputum. At least 50 ml of gastric contents should be aspirated early in the morning after patient has fasted for at least 8–10 hours. These should be neutralized immediately on collection with sodium bicarbonate 100 mg/ 5–10 ml. In children with radiographic evidence of pulmonary disease, *M. tuberculosis* can be recovered in about 40% of cases with a single sample. Three consecutive morning aspirates yield *M. tuberculosis* on 30–50% of cases and may be as high as 70% in infants[6]. Gastric aspiration requires admission and is inconvenient and uncomfortable. The culture yield from random outpatient samples is unclear. However, every attempt to elicit a culture should be made. Nasopharyngeal aspirates can also be tried and in a single study have been compared to gastric aspirates[7].

Laryngeal swabs have been reassessed and found to be positive in 25% of children with pulmonary tuberculosis[8].

- *Sputum*—Induced sputum is convenient, non-invasive and superior to gastric aspirates[9].
- *Bronchoalveolar lavage*—Use of broncho-alveolar lavage (BAL) is not routinely recommended; it may be used for establishing a diagnosis of endobronchial tuberculosis, or in the evaluation of an immunocompromised child and whenever drug resistant tuberculosis is suspected[10,11].
- *CSF*—In tubercular meningitis bacteriologic confirmation is possible in only 10% of cases[12]. *Mycobacterium tuberculosis* is best grown using multiple large volume samples of CSF. At least 15 mL and preferably 40 to 50 ml of CSF are recommended! This volume is clearly impractical for children. Culture is positive 56% of the time on the first sample, and improved to 83% of the time if four separate samples are cultured in the volumes mentioned above[13]. Bone marrow cultures and blood cultures can be performed to diagnose disseminated mycobacterial infection, especially in cases of HIV/AIDS.
- For paucibacillary disease the culture yield from other body fluids (pleural/peritoneal fluid) or tissues, lymph nodes from children and extra pulmonary TB is usually less than 50%. Pleural biopsy culture is more rewarding with positivity ranging from 50–80%[14].
- *Urine*—Culture of urine is important in the genitourinary tract tuberculosis. Either a single, early morning, voided midstream specimen or the total first morning specimen should be collected. Multiple, single specimens may be required to obtain positive results.

Microscopy

Given the poor specificity of TST, the importance of smear and culture confirmation cannot be overemphasized.

For day-to-day work, detection of AFB in the sample is enough if the clinical and/or radiological features suggest the diagnosis. Smear examination by Ziehl-Neelson (Z/N) stain has the advantage of simplicity, availability and rapidity, but the sensitivity is affected by the skill and experience of the microscopist, the number of specimens examined and the concentration of organisms in the sputum. To detect 1–2 organisms in 300 oil immersion fields the concentration of organisms must be 5,000–10,000 per ml. Thus under operational conditions positive smears are found in 50–70% specimens. Early and timely diagnosis of tuberculosis relies heavily on microscope examination of clinical samples for acid-fast bacilli using the Ziehl Neelson (Z-N) stain. (Microscopy can detect 60–70% of culture positive samples with a lower limit of detection of 5×10^3 organisms/ml). Typical acid-fast bacilli appear as slightly curved, beaded long or short rods.

The AFB smear report is of value not only in diagnosis but also helps to grade infectivity. The scale recommended by RNTCP is as follows:

3+=   >10 AFB/ oil immersion field
2+=   1–10 AFB/ oil immersion field
1+=   10–99 AFB / 100 oil immersion fields
Exact= 1–9 bacilli / 100 oil immersion fields

Fluorochrome stains

The waxy mycolic acids in the cell walls of mycobacteria have an affinity for the fluorochromes, auramines and rhodamine. These dyes non-specifically bind to nearly all mycobacteria. The mycobacterial cells appear bright yellow or orange against a greenish background. This method can be used to enhance detection of mycobacteria directly in patients specimens. The advantage of this method is that lower magnification can be used; so wider area is covered enabling rapid

screening. However, the cost of microscope and reagents are high and a very highly trained technician only can screen the smears. Besides the quick fading of the fluorescent stains creates additional practical problems[15].

The problem is younger children with pulmonary tuberculosis rarely produce sputum and early morning gastric aspirates are often collected. In extrapulmonary tuberculosis, the yield is lower.

Culture Techniques

Conventional tests

Agar-based methods—Culture of mycobacteria is a much more sensitive test than smear examination and allows for biochemical identification of the species considering enhancing the specificity. Unfortunately the slow doubling time of *M. tuberculosis* makes culture on egg or agar-based solid media slow and time consuming. Agar-based media allow detection of colonies in 10–12 days, whereas most commonly used Lowenstein-Jensen medium (LJ) usually takes 18–24 days. Susceptibility testing can also be performed on LJ medium but the turn around time is approximately 3 months for culture and susceptibility.

Automated liquid culture methods

1. *BACTEC TB 460*—this is a sensitive, specific and rapid culture method for smear positive respiratory as well as non-respiratory specimens. Time for detection of *M. tuberculosis* complex from smear negative clinical specimens is 13–15 days. In specimens, which are difficult to obtain such as tissue biopsies and body fluids, the use of L.J. media and BACTEC TB 460 may be justified to maximize isolation of mycobacteria. Different studies of the sensitivity of TB-BACTEC in monitoring mycobacterial

growth showed that an inoculum of 200 viable *M. tuberculosis* bacilli could be detected in 12–13 days while as few as 20 viable bacilli could be detected if one waited for 14–17 days[16,17].

2. *Mycobacterial growth indicator tube (MGIT) 960 TB:* The test employs a new state of the art fluorescent technology that enables result towards positivity as rapidly as 7–10 days. It is based on oxygen quenching with fluorescent dye[18].

MGIT 960 TB is used for isolation and accurate identification of mycobacteria and also for susceptibility testing to first and second line anti-tubercular drugs by the modified proportion method.

Phage assays

The ability of mycobacteriophages to lyse and destroy mycobacteria has been explored for rapid diagnosis of TB. The assay uses specific mycobacteriophages (DNA viruses specific for *M. tuberculosis* complex) as a reporter to reflect the presence of viable TB bacilli in the clinical specimens within 48 hours[19].

Detection of Mycobacterial Antigens

Mycobacterial antigen detection has been evaluated in clinical samples from adults, but rarely from children. Two recent assays detecting *M. tuberculosis*-specific antigens yielded high sensitivity and specificity in various clinical specimens from adults with TB[3]. Measurement of tuberculo stearic acid, a mycobacterial mycolic acid, has been used to detect *M. tuberculosis* in clinical specimens. Brooks *et al.* demonstrated a sensitivity of 95% and specificity of 91% when chromatographic profile of carboxylic acids and detection of tuberculostearic acid were combined and compared with culture results and clinical findings in adults with pulmonary TB;[20] however, these techniques require technically advanced equipment and expertise, which are not available where TB in children is most common. Their sensitivity and specificity in children are unknown.

Serological Tests

The search for a rapid accurate and cheap serological test for the diagnosis of tuberculosis has become as the search for the holy grail. Of 100 immunologically normal persons infected with *M. tuberculosis* only 10% or so will develop active disease. A large number of antigens have been used in assessing the humoral response in tuberculosis, but the fact that none has emerged victorious underscores the poor sensitivity and specificity of serology in endemic areas.

The antigens used so far include antigen 5 (38 kDa antigen), A60 antigen 45/47 kDa antigen complex, BCG, 19kDa 30 kDa antigen, LipoArabinoMannan (LAM) and many more[21,22]. In majority of studies specific serologic tests for diagnosing active pulmonary tuberculosis have been addressed[17]. The diagnostic dilemmas exist not so much in pulmonary tuberculosis but in paucibacillary extrapulmonary disease where the performance of serological tests is simply not good enough.

Antigen 5 (38 kDa antigen) has been evaluated with a sensitivity ranging from 64–89 and specificity of 81%. Similarly antigen 60, a thermostable component of PPD is also present in nocardia, and corynebacteria in addition to being present in mycobacteria. The 30 kDa antigen has been used with poor sensitivity, especially for HIV positive patients demonstrating that the humoral response to TB antigen indicates a non-protective response in addition to signifying active infection. Lipoarabinomannan is a lipoglycan known to have number of immunomodulating effects showed a wide range of sensitivity varying from 21–89%.

A good serological assay should perform well in specific targeted populations, especially childhood tuberculosis, HIV positive and extrapulmonary TB. Unfortunately, the sensitivity of most serological tests falls with smear negativity—a finding attributed to the lower burden of organisms. In addition, the fact that large number of environmental bacteria have cross reactive antigens and the antigens used so far are not very species specific contrive to confuse the diagnosis.

Interferon γ assays

An alternative to the tuberculin test are the Interferon – γ assays in the immunodiagnosis of tuberculosis. These assays are based on the principle that tuberculosis antigen sensitized T cells produce γ interferon when they encounter mycobacterial antigens.

These in vitro assays employ extremely specific antigens of *M. tuberculosis* as early secretory antigenic target-6 (ESAT-6) and culture filtrate protein 10 (CFP-10) called the RD1 antigens. These antigens are not shared by BCG strains and most non tuberculous Mycobacteria. In a recent study has been shown to have little diagnostic utility in countries endemic for tuberculosis with 80% of healthy adults in Mumbai responded to this antigen compared to 0% of a similar cohort in the United Kingdom[23].

A recent meta analysis has shown the sensitivity of these assays in patients with bacteriologically confirmed active tuberculosis varied between 32–100% and in those latent tuberculosis about 80%[24]. The sensitivity was slightly lower than TST.

Two commercial assays are currently available:

• The QuantiFERON GOLD assay with both ESAT-6 and CFP-10 uses whole blood to measure γ interferon response to the above antigens.

• T SPOT–TB assay uses peripheral blood mononuclear cells (PBMCs) and detects the number of "spot forming T cells" by use of ELISPOT in response to the above RD1 antigens.

Molecular Methods

Advances in molecular medicine have provided the research and diagnostic laboratory with tools that are revolutionizing its function. Molecular methods of diagnosis are exciting new developments that are already in practice in developed countries.

1. Nucleic acid probes

Nucleic acid hybridization is a powerful and widely used technique which exploits the ability of complementary sequence in single-strand (ss) DNA or RNA to pair with each other to form a duplex. The ss nucleic acid probes used for hybridization should be complementary to the amplified sequence or the region of interest on the gene to be identified.

2. In situ hybridization

In situ hybridization is used to detect and locate specific DNA or RNA sequence(s) in tissues or chromosomes by making use of radioactive or fluorescent labelled DNA/RNA probes complementary to the required sequence. However, in paucibacillary states like tubercular meningitis and pleural effusion the number of bacilli is too low to be picked up by this technology. This technique is commercially available for the identification of *M. tuberculosis* complex, *M. avium*, *M. intracellulaire*, *M. kansasi* and *M. gordonae*. Nucleic acid probes form a useful adjunct to BACTEC cultures for confirmatory identification.

3. Nucleic acid amplification

a. *Polymerase chain reaction (PCR)*—PCR is an in vitro method for amplifying specific

DNA sequence. Starting with extremely minute amounts of a particular nucleic acid sequence from any source, PCR enzymatically generates millions or billions of exact copies thereby making genetic analysis of tiny samples a relatively simple process. Studies in children have found PCR on respiratory samples including gastric lavage to have a sensitivity of 40–60% compared to clinical diagnosis[6]. Nested PCR certainly enhances the sensitivity of PCR.

b. *Transcription mediated amplification (TMA)*—TMA uses a species specific sequence of ribosomal RNA (rRNA) as the target for reverse transcriptase. The advantage of this technology being that the dead cells have no transcription machinery hence only viable cells are picked up and amplified[25].

c. *Ligase chain reaction (LCR)*—A phenotypic change in the organism such as virulence or drug resistance, can be detected by this technique.

DNA amplification technology can amplify minute quantities of DNA to levels that can be readily seen following routine agarose gel electrophoresis. But amplification can amplify even minute quantities of contaminating DNA. False positive results are the major concern. Also the presence of an organism in a clinical specimen does not necessarily indicate disease. Various target antigens have been used IS6110, MPB64, 16S rRNA gene 65kd, etc.

Results of molecular tests demonstrate the arbitariness of TB latent infection disease and may have a useful but limited place in evaluating children for TB. A negative PCR never eliminates TB as a diagnostic possibility and a positive result does not confirm it. Its use will be in evaluating children with significant pulmonary disease, immuno-compromised children and in extrapulmonary tuberculosis. However, PCR on gastric aspirate should not be performed for children with normal chest radiographs.

In theory, nucleic acid amplification (NAA) tests are capable of amplifying a single copy of the target genomic sequence. In practice, however, these tests may have only modest sensitivity in specimens that have a low bacillary load. Data from several studies that have shown a significantly lower sensitivity in smear-negative sputum specimens, compared with smear-positive specimens, support this argument. Since specimens such as cerebrospinal fluid (CSF) and pleural fluid often have low bacillary load (i.e. they tend to be smear-negative), it is possible that NAA tests will have low yield. In a separate meta-analysis assessing the accuracy of NAA tests for tuberculous pleuritis, the summary estimate of sensitivity was only 0.62 for pleural fluid specimens tested by commercial NAA tests. Similarly in another meta-analysis the diagnostic accuracy of NAA for TBM was a low sensitivity of 0.58 and high specificity of 0.98[26].

However, a major concern with the evaluation of any test for tuberculosis meningitis is the lack of a definitive reference standard. None of the available tests can be considered "gold" or even "silver standards.

Thus, in conclusion the diagnosis of tuberculosis in children is not an easy one. Culture remains the gold standard and every attempt should be made to isolate the organism. In tubercular meningitis and pleural effusions adenosine deaminase are useful adjunctive tests[27]. Serological tests do not offer an accurate sensitivity and should not be pursued. Lastly molecular techniques certainly hold promise in diagnosis , but lack sensitivity in paucibacillary states.

Molecular methods for detection of drug resistance in TB

Genotypic methods for drug resistance in TB assess the genetic determinants of resistance rather than the resistance phenotype[28]. PCR based sequencing is used to elucidate and study mutations as it allows for detection of both previously recognized and unrecognized mutations. Unfortunately it is not readily applicable in routine practice.

Solid-phase hybridization techniques—There are currently two commercially available solid-phase hybridization techniques for the rapid detection of drug resistance in tuberculosis: The Line Probe Assay (INNO-LiPA Rif TB Assay, Innogenetics, Belgium) for the detection of resistance to rifampicin and the GenoType MTBDR assay (Hain Lifesciences, Germany) for the simultaneous detection of resistance to isoniazid and rifampicin. An inhouse Reverse Line blot Hybridization assay to simultaneously speciate mycobacteria and detect resistance to all known mutations for rifampicin, isoniazid and streptomycin has also been developed that can be performed directly on smear- positive clinical samples[29].

Real-time PCR techniques—The main advantages of real-time PCR techniques are the speed of the test and a lower risk of contamination. Real-time PCR techniques have been applied to *M. tuberculosis* strains and, more recently, directly to clinical samples. Molecular beacon assays are based on a stem and loop structure with the loop in the probe. Easier to perform, real time formats as GeneXpert are being currently evaluated directly from samples. These assays have huge potential as they are rapid , and can be performed in a real world setting out of the molecular lab.

Microarrays, also known as biochips or DNA chips, have been proposed as genotypic methods for detecting drug resistance in *M. tuberculosis*. The·· are based on the hybridization of DNA obtained from clinical samples to high density oligonucleotides immobilized on a solid support, such as miniaturized glass slides.

Despite the clear advantages that molecular methods offer for drug susceptibility testing in terms of turn around time, the cost implications have to be borne in mind for resource constrained settings as ours. Associated laboratory infrastructure including proper design, and quality control issues to avoid cross contamination and amplicon generation is paramount. Lastly, wherever the genetic basis of resistance is not fully characterized, drug resistance should be confirmed by well standardized phenotypic methods.

Lastly it is evident that along with microbiology and skin testing, maintaining a high index of suspicion, rigorous contact tracing, expert clinical skills with radiology are essential for diagnosis of childhood tuberculosis.

References

1. Starke JT, Correa AG. Management of mycobacteria infection and disease in children. *Pediatric Infect Dis* J 1995;14:455-70.

2. Lee E., Holzman RS. Evolution and current use of the Tuberculin Test. *Clin Infect Dis* 2002; 34:365-70.

3. Khan E, Starke JR. Diagnosis of tuberculosis in children: Increased need for better methods. *Emerg Infect Dis* 1995;4:115-23.

4. Amdekar YK.Consensus Statement of IAP Working Group Status Report on diagnosis of childhood tuberculosis. *Indian Paediatrics*. 2004;41:146-55.

5. Steiner P, Rao M, Victoria MS, *et al*. Persistently negative tuberculin reactions: Their presence among children culture positive for *M. tuberculosis*. *Am J Dis Child* 1980;134:745-50.

6. Shingadia D and Novelli V. Diagnosis and treatment of tuberculosis in children. *Lancet Infect Dis* 2003;3:624-32.

7. Franchi Lm Cama RI Gilman RH, Montenegro JS, Sheen P. Detection of *Mycobacterium tuberculosis* in nasopharyngeal aspirate samplesin children. *Lancet* 1998:352:1681-82.

8. Thakur A, Coulter JB, Zutshi K, *et al*. Laryngeal swabs for diagnosing tuberculosis. *Ann Trop Paediatr* 1999;19:333-46.

9. Zar HJ, Hanslo D, Apolles P, Swingler G, Hussey G.Induced sputum versus gastric lavage for microbiological confirmation of pulmonary tuberculosis in infants and young children. *Lancet* 2005;365:10-4.

10. Eamranond P, Jaramillio E. Tuberculosis in children: reassessing the need for improved diagnosis in global control strategies. *Int J Tuberc Lung Dis* 2001;5:594-603.

11. Kabra SK, Lodha R, Seth V. Some current concepts on childhood tuberculosis. *Ind J Med Res* 2004;120:387-97.

12. Garg RK. Tuberculosis of the central nervous system. *Postgrad Med J* 1999;75:133-40.

13. Seehusen D A, Reeves M M, Fomin D A. Cerebrospinal Fluid Analysis. *Am Fam Physician* 2003;68:1103-08BA.

14. Lima DM, Colares JK , da Fonseca BA.Combined use of polymerase chain reaction and detection of adenosine deaminase activity on pleural fluid improves the rate of diagnosis of pleural tuberculosis.*Chest* 2003;124:909-14.

15. Kent PT, Kubica GP. Public health mycobacteriology — a guide for the level III laboratory. Atlanta, GA: Centers for Disease Control 1985.

16. Middlebrook G Reggiardo Z, Tigertt WD. Automatable radiometric detection of growth of *Mycobacterium tuberculosis* in selective media. *Am Rev Resp Dis*. 1977;115:1066-69.

17. Anargyros P Astill DSJ, Lim ISL. Comparison of Improved BACTEC and Lovenstein Jensen Media for culture of Mycobacteria from Clinical Specimens. *J. Clin Microbiol*. 1990;28:1288-91.

18. Pfyffer GE, Welsher Hm, Kissling P, *et al*. Comparison of mycobacterial growth inducator tube (MGIT) with radiometric and solid culture for recovery of acid fast bacilli. *J. Clin. Microbiol*. 1997;35:364-68.

19. Shenai S, Rodrigues C, Mehta A. Evaluation of a new phage amplification technology for the rapid diagnosis of tuberculosis. *Ind J Med Microbiol*. 2002;20(4):194-99.

20. Brooks JB,Daneshvar MI,Harberger RL, *et al*. Rapid diagnosis of tuberculous meningitis by frequency pulsed electron captive gas-liquid chromatography detection of carboxylic acids in cerebrospinal fluid. *J.Clin Microbiol* 1999;28:989-97.

21. Daniel TM, Debanne SM. The serodiagnosis of tuberculosis and other mycobacterial diseases by enzyme linked immunosorbent assay. *Am Rev Respir Dis* 1987;135:1137–51.

22. Chan ED Heiferts L, Iseman MD. Immunologic diagnosis of tuberculosis – a review. *Tubercle Lung Disease* 2000;80:131-40.

23. Lalvani A Nagwekar P Udwadia Z *et al*. Enumeration of T Cell Specific for RD1-encoded antigens suggests a high prevalence of latent *Mycobacterium tuberculosis* Infection in healthy urban Indian *J Infect Dis* 2001;183:469-77.

24. Pai M,Riley LW, Colford JM. Interferon γ assays in the immunodiagnosis of tuberculosis; a systemic review. *Lancet Infect Dis* 2004;4:761-76.

25. Shenai S, Rodrigues C, Almeida A, Mehta AP. Rapid diagnosis of tuberculosis using Transcription Mediated Amplification. *Indian J Med Microbiol*. 2001;19:184-89.

26. Pai M, Flores LL, Pai N. Hubbard A, Riley LW, Colford JM. Diagnostic accuracy of nucleic acid amplification tests for tuberculous meningitis: a systematic review and meta analysis. *Lancet Infect Dis* 2003;3:633-43.

27. Trajman A, Kaisermann MC, Kritski AI, *et al*. Diagnosing pleural tuberculosis. *Chest* 2004;125:2366.

28. Soini H and Musser J : Molecular diagnosis of Mycobacteria. *Clin Chem* 2001;47:809–14.

29. Shenai S, Rodrigues C, Ajita Mehta: Rapid speciation of 15 clinically relevant mycobacteria with simultaneous detection of resistance to rifampicin, isoniazid,and streptomycin in *Mycobacterium tuberculosis* complex. *International Journal of Infectious Diseases Dec* 2009;13:46-58.

11

Pharmacology of Antituberculosis Drugs

Ritabrata Kundu, Nupur Ganguly, TU Sukumaran

Introduction

Tuberculosis is caused by *Mycobacterium tuberculosis*. It primarily affects lungs causing pulmonary tuberculosis; also affects other organs of the body. Tuberculosis is one of the oldest diseases known to mankind dating back to ancient Egyptian, Chinese, Hebrew literature and in the Vedas. Today tuberculosis has become a major international public health problem despite the fact that highly effective anti-TB drugs and vaccine are available.

Management of tuberculosis before the discovery of antibacterial drugs for tuberculosis was mainly aimed at increasing the patient's resistance to the disease. This consists of sanatorium regimen, which was bed rest, high calorie protein diet, good air, nursing care and collapse therapy in suitable cases. With the advent of antituberculous drugs and various chemotherapeutic drug regimens the aim of treatment has changed. For elimination of tubercle bacilli from the body by direct action of the drugs is the major therapeutic approach.

To understand the increasing burden of tuberculosis it has been estimated that between the year 2000 and 2020, nearly 1 billion will be newly infected with TB, 200 million will develop the disease and 35 million will die from it[1]. Besides population explosion, often associated with overcrowding and poverty, infection with HIV is the most important factor contributing to the resurgence of TB. HIV infected individuals are more likely to develop tuberculosis disease from latent infection than persons without HIV infection.

TB in children is an indicator of recent transmission and thus serves as a sentinel event[2]. Although TB in children is the tip of an iceberg of unrecognized transmission it is sensitive indicator to the status of TB control.

TB control programs have failed to achieve desired results chiefly due to[3]:

i. Failure to ensure accessible diagnosis and treatment services, including Direct Observation Therapy (DOT).

ii. Inadequate treatment regimen and failure to use standardized treatment regime.

iii. Lack of supervision and an information management system for the vigorous evaluation of treatment outcome of TB patient.

iv. Cuts in health budgets with reduction in financial support to peripheral health services.

To formulate the treatment of TB infection and disease it is essential to understand the basic principles of antituberculosis therapy and the rationality behind.

Bacteriological Basis of Current Chemotherapy against Tuberculosis

Mycobacterium tuberculosis is a slow growing aerobic organism with a growth doubling time of about 20 hours. In unfavorable conditions it will grow only intermittently or remain dormant for a prolonged period. Antituberculosis drugs (ATD) act only at the time of multiplication and have no action on dormant bacilli. This accounts for the need of prolonged treatment, unlike other bacterial infection, to prevent relapse. In human disease the bacilli exist in different subpopulation with each having distinct metabolic status with different vulnerability to anti TB drugs. (Table 11.1)[4,5].

Table 11.1: Different subpopulation of tuberculosis bacilli

Site	Oxygen supply	pH	Growth and multiplication
Cavitary wall	High	Neutral	Rapid
Caseous material	Poor	Neutral	Slowly with occasional spurts
Intracellular and acute inflammatory tissue	Poor	Acidic	Slow

Another subpopulation is completely dormant

In the walls of the cavitary lesion the growth condition is favorable because of high oxygen content and a neutral pH. Here the bacillary load is high and it grows rapidly.

A second subpopulation exists mainly in the caseous material where the pH is neutral but oxygenation is poor. Here the organisms grow very slowly with occasional spurts of active metabolism.

A third slow growing subpopulation exits in an acidic environment located mainly intracellularly and in areas of acute inflammation with acidic pH.

A fourth subpopulation is completely dormant.

There is probably a constant shifting between these subpopulations.

In the cavitary wall where the condition is favorable the bacilli are particularly vulnerable to INH and to a lesser degree to RIF, SM and EMB.

The second subpopulation in the caseous material, the most effective drug is RIF with INH, SM and EMB having lesser activity. PZA is particularly active in killing intracellular bacilli and in areas of acute inflammation with acidic pH whereas INH, RIF and EMB are less active. Antituberculosis drug has no action against dormant bacilli. (Table 11.2).

Table 11.2: Vulnerability to antituberculosis drugs

Drugs	Cavitary wall	Caseous material	Intracellular	Dormant
INH	+++	++	++	−
RIF	++	+++	++	−
PZA	−	−	+++	−
EMB	++	+	+	−
SM	++	+	−	−

Drug Resistance

The genes that encode for drug resistance within *M. tuberculosis* are located on a chromosome. This type of resistance is not transferred from one organism to another. The resistance to individual drug results from spontaneous mutation in the mycobacteria and the estimated frequency of this naturally drug resistant organism is about 1 out of every 10^6 bacilli but varies with individual drugs as follows:

INH	-	$1 - 10^6$
RIF	-	$1 - 10^8$
SM	-	$1 - 10^5$
EMB	-	$1 - 10^6$
INH + RIF	-	$(1 - 10^{6+8}) = 1 - 10^{14}$

If we consider a cavitary lesion containing 10^9 bacilli, 1000 bacilli ($10^9 - 10^6 = 10^3 = 1000$) will be resistant to INH, which is predictable. If we treat this population of bacilli with a single drug, say INH, at first the patient will improve as it will kill all the susceptible bacilli excepting the 1000 bacilli which are resistant to INH. With time the resistant bacilli will grow and there will be relapse of the disease now with INH resistant strain. If we would have started with 2 drugs rather than a single drug, e.g. INH and RIF, RIF would have killed those thousand organisms which are resistant to INH by spontaneous mutation and INH would have taken care of those which are spontaneously resistant to RIF. This is one of the rationalities of combining two or more drugs.

Resistance is, however, divided into two types—

a. *Primary drug resistance*—It is when the patient is infected with drug resistant organism without having received prior treatment. The infection is usually transmitted from a person suffering from drug resistant tuberculosis.

b. *Acquired or secondary drug resistance*—It is the resistance which has developed during the course of treatment. This is due to poor compliance or inadequate drugs.

On the basis of animal experiments and clinical trials way back in 1985 Mitchison categorized anti-TB drugs into three groups[4].

i. *Drugs with resistance prevention activity—* These drugs when given together can prevent emergence of resistant mutants to the companion drug. INH and RIF are the most effective combination closely followed by ETB and SM. PZA is less effective in preventing emergence of resistance.

ii. *Drugs with early bactericidal activity—* These drugs rapidly decrease the number of living bacilli at the beginning of treatment. As they quickly reduce the bacillary load and converts sputum positive patients to negative they reduce the chance of transmission.

iii. *Drugs with sterilizing activity—*These drugs have the ability to kill the tubercle bacilli, which grow very slowly with occasional spurts of active metabolism, either in the caseous material, acute inflammatory tissues or in the acidic environment of the macrophages. RIF is the most potent sterilizing drug available followed by PZA. INH is weaker whereas SM and EMP have little activity.

Case Definition[6]

Beyond the diagnosis of TB disease, the type of TB case should also be defined to allow appropriate treatment to be given and the outcome of treatment evaluated.

The four determinants of case definition are:

i. Site of TB disease.

ii. Bacteriology.

iii. Severity of TB disease.

iv. History of previous treatment of TB.

Site of TB disease

In general recommended treatment regimes are similar irrespective of site. The importance of defining site is primarily for reviewing and reporting.

Pulmonary tuberculosis (PTB)—It includes disease involving the lung parenchyma. Intrathoracic lymphadenopathy (mediastinal and/or hilar) or pleural effusion without radiographic abnormalities in the lungs should be classified as extrapulmonary TB (EPTB) [Miliary TB is classified as pulmonary TB because there are lesions in the lungs]. A patient with both PTB and EPTB should be classified as a case of PTB.

Extrapulmonary tuberculosis (EPTB)—This includes tuberculosis of organs other than lungs like pleura, lymph node, abdomen, genitourinary tract, joints and bones and meninges.

Bacteriology

The diagnosis of tuberculosis, particularly pulmonary tuberculosis, is difficult in children under the age of 6–8 years where resources are poor. This is because children present with primary rather than reactivation (cavitary) PTB and because the majority of children with PTB are too young to produce sputum for smear microscopy. The prevalence of PTB is low between the age of 5 and 12 years and increases slightly in adolescence, when PTB presents more like adult PTB. The important diagnostic features include:

1. Contact with smear positive PTB case.
2. Respiratory symptoms for more than 2–3 weeks not responding to broad spectrum antibiotics.
3. Weight loss or failure to thrive.
4. Positive test to a standard dose of tuberculin. X-ray findings are often nonspecific and certainly not diagnostic.
5. The diagnosis of EPTB is more straight forward because of the characteristic clinical features (e.g. spinal deformity, painless ascites) and infrequently, supportive microscopic findings in specimens such as CSF fluid, pleural fluid, ascitic fluid and lymph node aspiration or biopsy.

The smear examination in pulmonary cases is important because those who are positive are most infectious and usually have higher mortality. In these cases bacteriological monitoring of treatment progress is most practicable. Most of childhood pulmonary TB are smear negative and they harbour fewer bacilli.

Severity of TB disease

Bacillary load, extent of disease and anatomical sites are important considerations to determine disease severity and appropriate treatment. Involvement of a particular anatomical site if results in significant acute threat to life (e.g. pericardial TB) or risk of subsequent severe handicap (e.g. spinal TB) or both (e.g. meningeal TB) is considered severe disease. Miliary and disseminated TB is also taken as severe. The following EPTB are classified as severe— meningeal, pericardial, peritoneal, bilateral or extensive pleural effusion, spinal, intestinal, genitourinary.

Less severe tuberculosis includes lymph node, unilateral pleural effusion, bone excluding spine, peripheral joint and skin.

History of previous treatment

In order to identify those patients who are at increased risk of acquired drug resistance, history of previous TB treatment is important. Fortunately secondary resistance is rare in children because of the small size of their mycobacterial population. Therefore, most drug resistance in children is primary and patterns of drug resistance among children tend to mirror those found among adults in the same population. The main predictors of drug resistant tuberculosis among adults are history of previous antituberculous treatment, co-infection with HIV, and exposure to another adult with infectious drug resistant tuberculosis. Above mentioned factors are important in a resource poor country like ours where facility of tuberculosis culture and drug sensitivity is not available.

Tuberculosis research center studies on prevalence of primary drug resistance over last 3 decades showed that INH resistance ranges from 10–16% and for streptomycin it is from 8–13%. Rifampicin resistance started appearing from 1990s and remains at around 1% with MDR TB labels of 1% or less[7].

Outline of the Management of Childhood TB[8]

The recommended regime for the treatment of childhood TB are the same as for adults under National Tuberculosis Control programme to reduce confusion and improve compliance. The presentation of tuberculosis in children are as follows:

I. *Primary TB disease*

i. Lymphadenopathy (hilar or mediastinal) without radiographic abnormalities in the lung, i.e. without parenchymal involvement is most frequent (70–80%) and is classified as EPTB and treated as category III.

ii. Typical primary complex with lymphadenopathy and the small opacity in the lung (primary lesion). It is less frequent (20%) and is classified as PTB and treated as category III.

iii. Rarely lobar or segmental opacity combined with lymphadenopathy on the same side. A PTB case with large parenchymal involvement should be treated as category I.

II. *Acute disseminated postprimary TB*

Miliary with or without meningitis, classified as severe PTB or severe EPTB and treated as category I.

III. *Postprimary PTB*

Without cavitation smear negative or with cavitation smear positive. Treated as category I.

IV. *Post primary EPTB either category I or III depending upon severity*

Recommended regimes of different types of tuberculosis in children are shown in Table 11.3.

Table 11.3: Recommended regimes for treatment of tuberculosis in children

Clinical presentation	Category and treatment regimen
Sputum smear positive PTB,	Category I
Sputum smear negative TB with extensive parenchymal involvement (acute military, segmental/lobar opacity), Severe EPTB (disseminated acute TB, abdominal, spinal and pericardial TB)	2RHZE/4HR daily or 3 times weekly
TB meningitis	Category I 2RHZS/4HR
Sputum smear negative PTB, less severe EPTB (TB adenitis, mediastinal lymphadenopathy)	Category III 2RHZ/4RH daily or 3 times weekly

In children with TB meningitis streptomycin should be used instead of ethambutol because the latter does not cross blood brain barrier.

Thiacetazone can cause severe and fatal reactions in HIV infected children and so should not be used in HIV endemic regions. Though young children cannot report early visual deterioration following ethambutol use but it has been used safely in infants and young children in recommended doses.

Tuberculosis Infection and Disease

When the tubercle bacillus enters the host it causes infection but not all will develop tuberculosis disease. In infection the bacillary load is less and the only evidence may be a positive tuberculin test.

When the bacilli overpower the host defense and multiply it will develop disease. The bacillary load in disease is much more as compared to infection Fortunately not all infected children will develop tuberculosis disease. The likelihood of developing disease is greatest shortly after infection and declines steadily with time. Studies have shown that 40–50% of those with tuberculosis infection will develop detectable disease within 1–2 years. Infant might develop serious tuberculosis even before Mantoux becomes positive, in fact as early as 6–8 weeks. Various immunosuppressive illnesses, e.g. measles, whooping cough, PEM and HIV may facilitate progression of infection to disease. This is the basis of giving preventive therapy to children with tuberculosis infection or with contacts of infectious adults because they always have the chance to develop serious disease.

Preventive Therapy

Preventive therapy is recommended in children below 5 years in contact with smear positive adults. After a thorough screening they should be given prophylactic INH or INH+RIF combination for 6 months. The choice of 2 drugs are in places where primary INH resistance is high.

Breastfed child of a smear positive mother is the most important group for preventive therapy. Children above 5 years who are otherwise well need clinical follow up but no prophylaxis.

Basis of Intermittent Therapy

The principle of intermittent therapy is that when the tubercle bacilli are exposed to antituberculous drugs for a brief period after removal of the drug the peak concentration attained in the blood inhibits the growth of tubercle bacilli for a time period known as lag period. The lag period differs in various antituberculous drugs.

INH	-	6–9 days
RIF	-	2–3 days
PZA	-	5–25 days

It is possible to prevent further growth of bacilli if the next dose is given before the end of the lag period. This is the rationale of intermittent therapy.

WHO does not recommend twice weekly regimen. If a patient receiving twice weekly regimen misses a dose, this missed dose represents a larger fraction of total number of treatment doses than if the patient were receiving a thrice weekly or daily regimen. Thus, there is increased risk of treatment failure. With HIV positive patient twice weekly regimen is at increased risk of failure or relapse with acquired rifampicin resistant TB. Thiacetazone is the only drug, which is ineffective when given intermittently. Intermittent therapy should always take DOTS strategy.

Fixed Dose Regime

Fixed dose combinations have several advantages over individual drugs. Prescription errors are likely to be less frequent as dosage recommendations are more straight forward and adjustment according to patient's weight is easier. It encourages patient's adherence as the number of tablets is less and even if treatment is not observed patient cannot be selective in the choice of drugs. It also has some disadvantages, if prescription error is to occur, either excessive or subtherapeutic concentration of all drugs may result. Poor RIF bioavailability is seen in some fixed drug combinations. Health care workers will be tempted to evade directly observed therapy, erroneously believing that adherence is automatically guaranteed.

References

1. WHO. Global Tuberculosis Control. WHO Report 2001. Geneva : World Health Organization. 2001 WHO/CDS/TB/2001.287.

2. Bloch AB, Snider De Jr. How much tuberculosis in children must we accept. *Am J Pub Hlth*. 1986; 76:14-5.

3. WHO. Treatment of Tuberculosis: Guidelines for National Programmes, 3rd ed, World Health Organization. Geneva 2003; WHO/CDS/TB/2003;313:17.

4. Grosset J. Bacteriologic basis of short course chemotherapy for tuberculosis. *Clin Chest Med* 1980;1:231-41.

5. Mitchison DA. Mechanism of drug action in short course chemotherapy. *Bull Intern Union Against Tuberc* 1985;60:34-7.

6. WHO. Treatment of Tuberculosis : Guidelines for National Programmes 3rd ed, World Health Organization. Geneva 2003; WHO/CDS/TB/2003;313:21-5.

7. Paramasivam CN. Status drug resistant TB after the introduction of Rifampicin in India. *J Indian Med Assoc* 2003;101:155.

8. WHO. Treatment of tuberculosis: Guidelines for National Programmes 3rd ed, Geneva: World Health Organization, 2003; WHO/CDS/TB/2003;313:62-5.

12

Management of Tuberculosis including RNTPC Guidelines

M Indrasekhar Rao, AK Dutta

Tuberculosis, the biggest infectious killer, kills more than the dreaded diseases like plague and cholera. Its impact on the patient as well as the rest of the family due to risk of cross infection, stigmatization and financial drain is more real and common than with most other infectious diseases. Tuberculosis in a family has both direct and indirect implications for the children in the family or the household. Commonly the infectious sources like parents, grandparents or other adult members of the household who are sick with the disease infect the children. These infected younger ones are not only at a higher risk of developing the disease but also are more likely to develop the severe form of the disease. While most infants who get tuberculosis suffer from lung disease, yet they are more likely to develop miliary or meningeal forms with severe morbidity and sequele.

A. Currently Recommended Regimens

1. Short course chemotherapy

Most of the currently recommended regimens, lay stress on short course chemotherapy. This usually includes an intensive initial phase of 2 months with 3 or 4 drugs to be followed by a continuation phase containing 2 drugs. Rifampicin, isoniazid and pyrazinamide form the backbone of initial regimens. Fourth drug recommended is mostly ethambutol, though some still recommend using streptomycin initially. With increasing experience in usage of ethambutol in pediatric cases, confidence has now been reposed in this drug as oral formulation makes it safer, easier and cheaper than injectable streptomycin. Continuation phase usually contains rifampicin and isoniazid for a duration of 4 months except for patients with meningeal, disseminated or bone tuberculosis where some recommend 7–8 month continuation phase[1,2].

The drug dosage for various first line drugs used along with their major side effects are shown in Table 12.1.

2. Daily vs intermittent therapy

Prolonged treatment and cost of therapy has been an important factor for nonadherence to therapy resulting in treatment failure. To overcome this, intermittent therapy was

Table 12.1: Anti tuberculousis drugs and their dosages

Drug (symbol)	Daily dosages	Intermittent dosages	Major side effects
Streptomycin (S)	15–20 mg/kg/day	20–30 kg/mg/dose	Tinnitus
Rifampin (R)	10 mg/kg/day	10 mg/kg/dose	Hepatotoxicity, gastritis, flu like illness
Isoniazid (H)	5–10 mg/kg/day	10–15 mg/kg/dose	Peripheral neuropathy, hepatoxicity
Pyrazinamide (Z)	30–35 mg/kg/day	30–35 mg/kg/dose	Arthralgia, hepatoxicity, Oculotoxicity
Ethambutol (E)	20 mg/kg/day	30 mg/kg/dose	

attempted which initially faced skepticism. However, now after comparative studies, its role is established beyond doubt. Doses and schedules have been defined[3]. Directly observed therapy (DOT) under which the patient actually consumes the drug in front of treatment supervisor, as is being followed currently, becomes easier with intermittent therapy. WHO and the Government of India recommend thrice weekly regimens under revised national tuberculosis program for the country (RNTCP). However, self-administered intermittent therapy should be strongly discouraged. To formulate adequate dosage and administration of antituberculosis drugs in children medications are made available in the form of combipacks in patient-wise boxes according to the child's weight as shown in Tables 12.2 and 12.3.

Table 12.2: Formulation in RNTCP

Rifampicin	75/150 mg
Isoniazid	75/150 mg
Ethambutol	200/400 mg
Pyrazinamide	250/500 mg

Table 12.3: Weight range (in kg) for treatment of childhood tuberculosis

i. 6–10

ii. 11–17

iii. 18–25

iv. 26–30

v. 30 and above

3. Adjunctive treatment

Corticosteroids have been used as an adjunct to anti-TB therapy. It may be useful to mention that although corticosteroids are helpful in certain patients, they should not be prescribed injudiciously. Following are the specific indications for corticosteroids use:

i. Neurotuberculosis.

ii. Severely ill patients with miliary TB.

iii. Pericarditis.

iv. Massive pleural effusion.

v. Genitourinary tuberculosis.

For most situations, prednisolone 1–2 mg/kg/day for initial 4 weeks and tapering doses for next 2–4 weeks may be sufficient. The duration may be shorter in cases with pleural effusion.

B. Diagnosis of Childhood Tuberculosis

Diagnosis is difficult as children do not produce sputum and the cases are paucibacillary. Though majority of the cases are sputum negative but it is always advised to obtain sputum samples wherever possible. Any child with cough and fever for more than 3 weeks not responding to conventional antibiotics should arouse suspicion of tuberculosis. Other points favoring the diagnosis include no weight gain or weight loss and history of household contact, suspected or diagnosed case of active tuberculosis, within last 2 years. Along with history and clinical examination sputum examination whenever possible, X-ray chest and Mantoux test with 2TU of PPDRT23 or 5TU PPDS should be done. The child should be evaluated as a whole keeping in mind that positive Mantoux test neither confirms disease nor a negative test rules out the condition. Various scoring system available are not recommended for the diagnosis of childhood tuberculosis.

C. Steps in Starting Appropriate Treatment

Having decided the need for anti-TB treatment in a patient, it is extremely important to define the patient's status. Usually the patient should be evaluated for:

i. *Site of the disease*—Pulmonary, extra-pulmonary or disseminated,

ii. *Severity or extent of the disease*—As described later,

iii. *Bacillary load*—Bacillary positivity in the appropriate specimen,

iv. *Past history of treatment*—Any patient who has never had treatment for TB or who has received treatment for a period of less than a month is considered as new case while those with complete treatment and recurrence of disease are labeled as relapse and those with active disease but incomplete treatment are classified as defaulters. Patients having failed (e.g. sputum positive for TB) in spite of adequate treatment is taken as failure. Patient who have received treatment in the past are at increased risk of acquiring drug resistance. Whenever possible drug sensitivity test is recommended before treatment in failure cases.

The case definition becomes essential as it determines the regimen of chemotherapy to be used and its duration. WHO defines the various categories (Table 12.4) on the basis of site and severity of the disease, result of sputum smear examination and previous anti-TB treatment. It advocates different regimens for each category, sputum positive receiving most aggressive therapy[4].

The use of more aggressive initial treatment in some cases and / or use of more prolonged continuation phase in others is based on following factors:

i. Naturally occurring resistance to various anti-TB drugs is small but it becomes clinically significant if the resistant strains are allowed to multiply due to inadequate drug action. By using more than one drug, chances of leaving out resistant strains will be greatly minimized. Higher the bacillary load in a patient, more will be the resistant number of bacilli in the lesion hence such patients would require a combination of several drugs (3–4) to be effective rapidly.

ii. Relapse rate has been demonstrated to be lower with 3/4 drug regimen. Theoretical basis for this comes from the hypothesis that a large number of bacilli in the lesion may have initial resistance to drug(s), therefore by using several drugs at once in initial phase, more effective killing of bacilli can be achieved. A mathematical model of chances of bacilli having initial resistance has been described. This forms the basis of using aggressive therapy with four drugs for cases with serious forms of TB presumed to have higher bacillary load or in areas where initial resistance to some of the primary drugs like isoniazid is high.

According to the above hypothesis, if the number of bacilli is large, the number of organisms going in 'lag phase' (and hence protected) will be more. These cases will require a longer duration continuation phase as is recommended by some authorities. Disease of organs where the penetration of drugs may be inadequate like in bones or across meninges, may also require prolonged continuation phase.

D. Recommended Regimes

The Table 12.4 gives the modified classification and treatment protocol as agreed under

Table 12.4: IAP-RNTCP treatment categories and regimens

WHO category of treatment	Type of patients	TB treatment regimens	
		Intensive phase (thrice weekly)	Continuation phase (thrice weekly)
Category I	New sputum smear-positive PTB New seriously ill sputum smear-negative PTB New seriously ill extra-pulmonary TB	2 months of HRZE	4 months of HR
Category II	Sputum smear-positive relapse Sputum smear-positive treatment failure Sputum smear-positive treatment after default Cases who are AFB negative but considered to have active disease after complete treatment (relapse) or due to incomplete treatment (defaulter) or due to non response (failure)	2 months of SHRZE and 1 month of HRZE	5 months of HRE
Category III	New sputum smear-negatives PTB and extra-pulmonary TB not seriously ill	2 months of HRZ	4 months of HR

the IAP-RNTCP (revised national TB control program) consensus meeting. There is a practical problem in children due to their inability to bring up phlegm. Though a sincere and active effort by inducing sputum should be made in all pediatric cases for proper categorization, it may be acceptable to treat patients with extensive lesions at least as likely sputum positive as the sputum examination may not be feasible.

The following recommendations are made pertaining to treatment categories and regimens:

i. Under RNTCP these drugs are given under direct observation (DOT) on thrice weekly basis whereas for unsupervised treatment the same combination and duration of drug is used on a daily basis. The intermittent treatment is as effective as the daily treatment and should be given only under supervision.

ii. New case is a patient who is recently diagnosed and has never received anti-TB drugs or for less than 4 weeks duration.

iii. Seriously ill sputum smear-negative PTB will include all forms of pulmonary TB other than primary complex.

iv. Seriously ill extrapulmonary TB includes TB meningitis, disseminated TB, TB pericarditis, TB peritonitis and intestinal TB, bilateral or extensive pleurisy, spinal TB with or without neurological complications, genitourinary tract TB, bone and joint TB.

v. Not-seriously ill extrapulmonary TB includes isolated peripheral lymph node TB and unilateral pleural effusion.

vi. In patients with TB meningitis on category I treatment, the four drugs used during the intensive phase can either be HRZE or HRZS. WHO recommends streptomycin instead of ethambutol because ethambutol does not cross blood-brain barrier.

vii. Continuation phase of treatment in TB meningitis and spinal TB with neurological complications should be given for 6–7 months, extending the total duration of treatment to 8–9 months. Steroids should be used initially to reduce inflammation in hospitalized cases of TBM and TB pericarditis and reduced gradually over 6–8 weeks.

Table 12.5 details the recommended regimes for management of various forms of childhood tuberculosis in patients who have no history of treatment in the past or have received treatment for less than 4 weeks (New Case)[5]. Routinely no other adjunct treatment is required in most cases. Steroids are indicated in patients with CNS tuberculosis, severely ill miliary cases, pericardial and pleural tamponade and genitourinary tuberculosis.

Table 12.5: Simplified regimes for management of various types of children

Disease group	Likely WHO Category	Suggested Treatment
Pulmonary primary complex (hilar/mediastinal lymph node)	III	2RHZ / 4RH
Progressive primary like large consolidation/ cavitation	I	2RHZE/4RH
Pleural effusion	III	2RHZ / 4RH
Miliary/disseminated	I	2RHZE/7RH
Abdominal/peritoneal/ genitourinal	I	2RHZE/7RH
Meningeal and spinal	I	2RHZE/7RH
Osteo-articular except spinal	III	2RHZ / 7 RH
Isolated lymphadenopathy	III	2RHZ / 4 RH
Generalized lymphadenopathy	I	2RHZE/4RH

E. Monitoring of Treatment

1. *Monitoring of response to treatment*—In children monitoring of response to treatment needs to address the difficulties associated with obtaining sputum samples from children. A combination of the following is thus proposed:

    i. Wherever possible, follow-up sputum or gastric aspirate examinations should be performed at the end of initial phase and at the end of the treatment.

    ii. Clinical or symptomatic improvement should be assessed at the end of the initial or intensive phase of treatment and at the end of treatment. Improvement should be judged by lack of fever or cough, a decrease in the size of lymph node(s) and weight gain.

    iii. Radiological improvement should be assessed by chest X-ray examination in all smear-negative pulmonary TB cases at the end of treatment.

2. *Treatment adherence*—This must always be checked along with response to treatment. Monitoring of the drug intake could be undertaken by a pill count or prescription check.

3. *Monitoring for occurrence of side effects*— Monitoring of side effects like gastric intolerance, drug induced hepatitis, ocular or peripheral neurotoxicity and arthritis should also be done. As most side effects are usually mild ATT does not need to be stopped and symptomatic therapy alone may suffice in most cases. Commonest problem is pain abdomen and vomiting due to gastritis which responds well to anti-acids.

As the anti-TB drugs recommended are hepatic enzyme inducers, asymptomatic biochemical derangement without increase in bilirubin level may be tolerated till the enzymes remain up to 5 times the normal range. However if the patient has symptoms suggestive of hepatotoxicity particularly development of icterus on ATT, it is prudent to stop hepatotoxic drugs irrespective of the enzyme levels. The drugs are withheld till the serum bilirubin becomes normal and the enzymes also start touching the normal range. In most cases the regular four drugs treatment can be restarted after the liver enzymes have fallen and bilirubin has reverted back to normal[6]. Most pediatricians prefer to re-introduce drugs sequentially every 3–4 days, though some may add all together. In case the patient is seriously ill then using non-hepatotoxic drugs like streptomycin, ethambutol and flouroquinolones in the interim period is justified.

Arthralgia due to pyrazinamide is easily managed with non steroidal anti-inflammatory drugs. If the uric acid levels are very high and associated with gout like symptoms then drugs like allopurinol may be added. Severe skin reactions and oculotoxicity also require a review of therapy and exclusion of the offending drug. Pyridoxine is useful for INH induced paresthesias. Most children however, tolerate the treatment very well.

Management of Pediatric Tuberculosis Under the Revised National Tuberculosis Control Program

DOTS is the recommended strategy for treatment of TB and all pediatric TB patients should be registered under RNTCP. Inter-mittent short course chemotherapy given under direct observation, as advocated in the RNTCP, should be used in children. To assist in calculating required dosages and adminis-tration of anti-TB drugs for children, the medication are to be made available in the form of combipacks in patient-wise boxes, linked to the child's weight.

In patients with TBM on Category I treat-ment, the four drugs used during the intensive phase should be HRZS (instead of HRZE).

Continuation phase of treatment in TBM and spinal TB with neurological complications should be given for 6–7 months, extending the total duration of treatment to 8–9 months. Steroids should be used initially in hospitali-sed cases of TBM and TB pericarditis and reduced gradually over 6–8 weeks. In all instances before starting a child on Category II treatment he should be examined by a pediatrician or TB expert, wherever available. As recommended by WHO and in view of the growing evidence that the use of ethambutol in young children is safe, ethambutol is to be used as per RNTCP regimen for all age groups.

Chemoprophylaxis

Asymptomatic children under 5 years of age, exposed to an adult with infectious (smear-positive) tuberculosis from the same house-hold, will be given 6 months of isoniazid (5 mg per kg daily) chemoprophylaxis.

Management of Interruption of Treatment

Patient compliance is crucial factor in treat-ment failure and the development of acquired drug resistance. It is very important to realize that the emergence of MDR TB is always a man made problem and failure of the patient to complete the prescribed course completely and adequately is one of the reasons. In general, if it is certain that the patient was taking all medications correctly prior to interruption, then he can be managed as per the guidelines for treatment after interruption shown in Table 12.6. Whenever treatment is interrupted for more than 2 weeks, the child should be reassessed clinically and radio-logically, with bacteriological examination, wherever possible. In all such cases the resumption of treatment must be preceded by evaluation for activity and investigating the

Table 12.6: Managing patients with interruptions in treatment

Duration of therapy	Duration of interruption	Decision
Up to 4 weeks	<2 weeks	Resume original regime
	>2 weeks	Reassess and start treatment again
4–8 weeks	<2 weeks	Resume original regime
	2–8 weeks	Extend intensive phase by 1 month more
	>8 weeks	Consider Cat II if diagnosis is still TB
>8 weeks	<2 weeks	Resume original regime
	>2 weeks Review activity	• No active disease: Continue same treatment
		• Active disease: Category II therapy

causes for non-adherence. The pediatrician should not merely restart the treatment but also enable the completion of treatment by addressing issues related to non-adherence in the first instance. Addressing issues like side effects of the therapy (real or perceived), cost involved as well as educating about the need for a complete treatment even after the symptoms abate may help adherence. Both the child as well as the caregivers must be involved in decision making for re-initiating treatment.

References

1. American Thoracic Society. Treatment of tuberculosis in tuberculosis infection in adults and children. *Am J Respir Crit Care Med* 1994;149:1359-74.
2. IAP Working Group on the Treatment of Childhood Tuberculosis. Treatment of childhood tuberculosis. Recommendation. *Indian Pediatr* 1997;34:1093-96.
3. Arora VK, Gupta R. Directly observed treatment for tuberculosis. *Indian J Pediatr* 2003; 70: 885-9.
4. World Health Organisation. Treatment of Tuberculosis. Guidelines for National Programs. Geneva : WHO .(WHO/CDS/T B/2003.313).
5. RNTCP Statement. Management of pediatric tuberculosis under the revised national tuberculosis control program (RNTCP). *Indian Pediatr* 2004;41:901-5.
6. O'brien RJ. Hepatotoxic reaction to antituberculous drugs: adjustments to therapeutic regimen. *JAMA* 1991;265:3323.

13

Drug Resistant Tuberculosis in Children

Sangeeta Sharma

Ever since the introduction of anti-tuberculosis treatment (ATT) in 1952, *Mycobacterium tuberculosis* strains have acquired resistance to almost all anti-tuberculosis drugs (ATD)[1,2]. Overcrowding, immigration, poor drug prescription, use of substandard drugs, poor case management and in addition, human immunodeficiency virus (HIV) epidemic is contributing not only to the resurgence of TB but also leading to an increase in the incidence of resistant TB. Moreover, the occurrence of drug resistant *M. tuberculosis* strains is being reported not only in adults but in children also[3,4]. The emergence of drug resistant strains has thus reduced the efficacy of ATT to the pre treatment era[1], presenting an increasing threat to the global tuberculosis control and an added responsibility on the shoulders of all those involved in the management of these children.

East European countries have the highest incidence of MDR TB in the world[5]. Further reliable epidemiological data about the prevalence of drug resistant, multi-resistant and extreme drug resistant TB(XDR-TB) in children from endemic areas like Africa, East Europe and Asia is not known[1,2,5]. Overall, in India there are almost 20,000 new MDR infections in one year[6]. As per the recent estimates from the state representative drug resistance surveillance (DRS) survey held in Gujarat and various district level DRS studies, the prevalence of MDR TB in new smear positive pulmonary TB (PTB) cases (initial/primary resistance) is <3% and 12 to 17% amongst smear positive previously treated PTB cases (secondary or acquired resistance)[6,7]. Reviews of studies with representative samples do not indicate any increase in the prevalence of drug resistance over the years. Although isolated reports, both published and unpublished, do indicate the existence of resistance to multiple anti-tuberculosis drugs and even some second line anti-tuberculosis agents in our country, it is yet not possible to estimate its magnitude and distribution from the available data[5,7]. Nevertheless, documenting the level of drug-resistance in community is important in order to monitor the impact of national TB control programme over time and to ensure that the treatment regimens are appropriate[1].

Definitions (Case Registration, Bacteriology and Treatment Outcomes)[8,9]

1. *Drug resistant (DR) TB*

This is a patient of TB excreting bacilli resistant to one or more anti tuberculosis drugs.

Mono-resistance—A patient whose TB is due to tubercle bacilli that are resistant *in vitro* to exactly one anti-TB drug tested from an accredited laboratory.

Poly-resistance—A patient whose TB is due to tubercle bacilli that are resistant *in vitro* to more than one anti-TB drug, except not both isoniazid and rifampicin tested from an accredited laboratory.

2. *Multi-drug resistant (MDR) TB*

MDR TB is defined as *in-vitro* resistance to at least isoniazid and rifampicin, the two main AT drugs from an accredited laboratory. Therefore, it is an MDR TB suspect who is smear culture positive and has *M. tuberculosis* resistant to isoniazid and rifampicin, with or without resistance to other anti tuberculosis drugs.

3. *Extreme drug resistant (XDR) TB*[10]

XDR-TB is defined as resistance to at least isoniazid and rifampicin (i.e. MDR TB) plus resistance to any one of the fluoro-quinolones and any one of the three second-line injectable drugs (amikacin, kanamycin, or capreomycin) based on DST results from an accredited laboratory.

4. *MDR-TB suspect*

An MDR TB suspect is defined as:

A TB patient who fails an RNTCP category I or III treatment regimen

Any RNTCP category II patient who is sputum smear positive at the end of the fourth month of treatment or later.

After a TB patient has been declared as a failure of an RNTCP category I or III treatment, the initial priority is to ensure that the patient is initiated on an RNTCP Category II regimen and is re-registered in the appropriate TB Register as a Category II type "failure" patient[11]. Thus, MDR TB may be suspected in the following circumstances:

Failure of treatment—This is defined as a smear positive TB patient excreting bacilli at 5 months or more after starting category I WHO treatment regimen given under direct observation by a health worker. Failure also includes a patient who was initially smear/ culture negative but becomes smear/culture positive during category III treatment. These patients are placed under category II treatment afresh.

Failure of re-treatment: This is defined as a smear positive patient who remains smear positive at 4 months or more of category II WHO re-treatment regimen.

Chronic case—The failure of a fully supervised WHO re-treatment regimen given by health worker under direct observation. A chronic case must have received at least two or more courses of chemotherapy (complete or incomplete). These cases are usually but not always excretors of acquired resistant MDR bacilli.

Based on the history of prior ATT, resistance is classified as:

i. *Primary resistance*—In patients who have not had any prior treatment with anti-tuberculosis drugs, the bacterial resistance is called primary resistance.

ii. *Initial resistance*—In after clinical assessment, it is doubtful that the patient has received prior treatment, this is called initial resistance. Initial resistance is thus a mixture of primary resistance and undisclosed/unknown acquired resistance.

iii. *Acquired resistance*—In patients with some record of previous anti tuberculosis treatment, the bacterial resistance is called acquired resistance. In new patients, the WHO standard first line regimens (6 months) overcome the risk of failure due to primary resistance while majority of previously treated patients (taken ATD for >1 month), the WHO standard re-treatment regimen (8 months) reduces the risk of failure due to acquired resistance.

Microbiological Basis of Drug Resistance[5,8]

i. *Natural resistance (NR)*—This is a species specific resistance to a drug without the strain ever having been exposed to it. *M. tuberculosis, M. bovis* and *M. africanum* are naturally resistant to penicillin, pyrazinamide and thioacetazone respectively. Therefore, NR is used as a taxonomic marker for species identification.

ii. *Primary drug resistance*—This is observed in a patient without prior treatment. It follows an infection with:

a. A wild strain when the organism develops resistance usually to a single drug without ever coming in contact with it. Wild type resistance is the result of random spontaneous mutation in a naturally susceptible strain which has never been exposed to any anti-tuberculosis drug. These spontaneous mutations within the bacteria occur at a rather predictable rate. For example, isoniazid and streptomycin resistance develops at a frequency of 1 in 10^6 (1 million) organisms while for ethambutol at 10^4 and rifampicin at 10^8.

b. An infection with an isolate of *M. tuberculosis* that is already resistant to the given ATT when the patient comes in contact and acquires infection from an already drug resistant case.

iii. *Secondary (acquired) drug resistance*—This exists if the organisms with which the patient is infected were initially drug susceptible, but develop resistance during the course of ATT.

Primary and acquired resistance differ in terms of prevalence, severity and level of resistance. Primary resistance is less prevalent, less severe, more often to one drug and the level of resistance (i.e. minimum inhibitory concentration of the drug) is lower while acquired resistance is more severe and to two or more drugs, e.g. MDR and XDR. Primary resistance is natural, i.e. inherent resistance of bacillus while secondary resistance is entirely man-made (acquired).

Molecular Basis of Resistance[12-14]

Drug resistance (DR)—is caused by specific mutations in independent genes of *M. tuberculosis*. It is not transferable from one organism to another and is not interlinked between ATT drugs, however bacilli show cross-resistance to drugs of similar nature. Understanding the mechanisms underlying DR by gene mapping and recognising the specific gene mutations is being used for the development of molecular tests for rapid detection of DR bacilli and future anti-tubercular drugs[4].

Resistant to AT Drugs

1. *Rifampicin (R)*—Mis-sense mutation in gene *rpo B* encoding b unit RNA polymerase, 9 different types of codon mutations have been identified.

2. *Isoniazid (H)*—Complete absence or mutation of gene *Kat G, inh A* gene.

3. *Streptomycin (S)*—Mutation in 16 s ribosomal RNA gene.

4. *Ethambutol (E)*—Mis-sense mutation in gene *ernp B*.

5. *Pyrazinamide (Z)*—Mutation in gene *pnc A*[15].
6. *Ethionamide (Eth)*—Mutation in *Eth A* and *Eth R* genes[16].
7. *Quionolones*—Mis-sense mutation of *gyr A*[17].

Domino Effect or Serial Selection of Drug Resistance[8]

Basic mechanism of acquired drug resistance is gene mutation of *M. tuberculosis*, i.e. biological. A tubercular cavity as seen in adults, harbours 10^7–10^9 bacilli, which would contain a few hundred bacilli capable of dividing in the presence of isoniazid and a few bacilli resistant to rifampicin. A closed caseous lesion, as seen in children, contains 10^5–10^7 bacilli and a few resistant bacilli. Use of effective combination of AT drugs takes care of all these resistant forms, resulting in cure. But, if these resistant mutants are exposed to a single drug to which they are already resistant while the dominant mass of bacilli is susceptible, the resistant strain continues to grow and eventually becomes the dominant form in that particular patient. If this patient is further exposed to a second course of treatment with yet another single drug, naturally occurring mutants resistant to this new drug may be selected again and the patient may end up with bacilli resistant to 2 or more drugs, as further drugs or courses of ATT are used. This is called domino effect or serial selection of drug resistance.

This is the basis of using combination therapy and that too under direct observation so that the patient does not miss a dose. Also, the treating doctor should never add a single drug to a failing regimen.

As bacilliary load is less in children, they are less likely to develop secondary resistance than adults but children can have primary drug resistance if their source of infection has resistant TB[8,9].

Factors Contributing to DR (Table 13.1)[8,9,18]

It should be stressed that MDR-TB is entirely a man-made phenomenon—most important being the triad of 'poor treatment, poor drugs and poor adherence' leading to the development of MDR-TB. Thus the most common medical errors are shown in Table 13.1.

Prevention of MDR[19]

For the future, the top priority is not the management but the prevention of multi-drug resistant (MDR) TB[8,9] and for this, it is essential to administer standardized short course chemotherapy under direct observation (DOTS) for all smear positive cases (new and retreatment) to prevent the emergence of drug resistant strains[18,20]. In all countries that have adopted directly observed treatment-short course (DOTS) strategy under programme conditions, over the years, there will be a huge reduction in the source of infection, i.e. smear positive patients and in transmission.

In new cases

WHO recommended regimens are as effective in patients with bacilli initially resistant to isoniazid and/or streptomycin as in patients with susceptible bacilli. Theoretically infection with MDR bacilli will cause failure to respond to the initial regimen. Even when transmission of MDR bacilli from an "old" patient to a "new" patient is clearly demonstrated, it has still not been documented that primary MDR contributes significantly to treatment failure of WHO standard regimens for new cases in programme conditions[8].

Each new sputum positive pulmonary TB patient should be given 6 months category I (2HRZE/4HR) under direct observation, 4 drugs (isoniazid, rifampicin, pyrazinamide and ethambutol) during the first 2 months and 2 drugs (isoniazid, rifampicin) for further 4 months.

Table 13.1: Factors contributing to DR

Health-care providers: Inadequate regimens Physician related factors	Drugs	Patients: Inadequate drug intake
Absence of guidelines	Poor quality/substandard drugs	Poor adherence (or poor DOT) financial constraints
Poorly organized or funded TB control programmes	Use of fluoroquinolones as first-line AT drugs	Lack of information
Poor case management: • Failure to promptly diagnose MDR	Inappropriate regimens: • Use of drugs or drug combinations of unproven bioavailability	Adverse drug reactions Malabsorption Social barriers
• Inappropriate regimens – Only 2–3 drugs in multi-bacillary new smear positive patients – Addition of one extra drug to a failing regimen	• Wrong dose or treatment combination • Poor storage conditions • Unavailability of certain drugs (stock-outs or delivery disruptions)	Substance dependency disorders Chronic debilitating illness, Malnutrition HIV
• No monitoring of ATT • Noncompliance (when treatment is not directly observed) • Poor training of health-care providers		

In old cases

In TB patients treated with one or more courses of ATT and who remain sputum positive (by smear and/or culture) 3 subpopulations of bacilli are observed,

   i. Bacilli susceptible to all AT drugs.
   ii. Bacilli resistant to at least H, but still sensitive to R.
   iii. Bacilli resistant to at least H and R.

The respective proportion of these 3 subpopulations of bacilli varies in a particular patient and is dependent on:

   i. Chemotherapy taken by the patient in the past, including the drugs taken and the number of courses received.
   ii. Chemotherapy applied in the community.
       a. In patients, who have failed after the first course of chemotherapy (WHO recommended or any other) the proportion of patients excreting bacilli susceptible to all drugs is usually higher than the proportion of two other subpopulations. WHO guidelines recommend Cat-II retreatment regimen of 8 months (using 5 drugs for first 2 months, then 4 drugs for the third month and then 3 drugs for the remaining 5 months of treatment, i.e. 2SHRZE/1HRZE/5HRE given under direct observation. However, in some cases primary drug resistance remains a risk factor of failure and relapse and thus the standard re-treatment regimen appears inadequate for failure cases[21].
       b. Patients who have failed after 2 courses of chemotherapy, (second being the fully supervised directly

observed WHO retreatment regimen) known as chronic cases, the proportion of patients excreting resistant bacilli to R and H is the majority and a second application of the standard WHO retreatment regimen is likely to fail, i.e. approximately 80% have DR and 50% have MDR. Use of standardized short course chemotherapy in these patients diseased with multi-drug-resistant TB strains fails to cure this significant proportion of cases and can create even more resistance to the drugs in use. This has been termed the "amplifier effect of short course therapy" and it implies that the resistant strains in the bacterial population are selected repeatedly when a regimen is used continuously over a long period in a given community, and these become the dominant strains. Ongoing transmission of established drug-resistant strains in a population is also a significant source of new drug resistant cases[21].

Clinical Features

DR (drug resistant) can be pulmonary and extrapulmonary tuberculosis depending on site of involvement. The clinical picture of drug resistant and drug susceptible pulmonary and extrapulmonary tuberculosis usually does not differ. This is also true for HIV seropositive MDR patients[13]. The radiological patterns include hilar adenopathy, segmental lesions and collapse consolidation in infants and young children whereas adult type of disease with cavities and apical infiltrates are noted in older children and adolescents. In one study of 1098 PTB cases over 9 years, this trend is changing with more and more younger children having cavities and apical infiltrates[21].

Also suspect DR TB if patient has an acutely progressive lung lesion known as acutely progressive pulmonary TB (APPT). These patients have massive viable bacterial population of high virulence and almost half of these cases have drug resistance, which is one of the characteristics of APPT. In one study of APPT, 41.8% cases had DR and almost half cases of drug resistance were secondary MDR. The drug resistance and multi-drug resistance even progressed during APPT therapy[22]. These patients of APPT may have acute destructive TB, cheesy pneumonia, associated immune deficiency or X-ray involution in one lung and concomitant progression in the other which suggest the presence of *M. tuberculosis* strains showing different drug resistance patterns in the same patient[23]. Drug resistant and MDR extrapulmonary tuberculosis, tubercular lymphadenitis with increased incidence of infection with atypical mycobacteria is also on the rise[24,25]. There are reports of drug resistant tubercular meningitis (8.6%) which have higher morbidity and mortality than drug sensitive tubercular meningitis[26].

When to Suspect MDR (Case-finding Strategies)[8,9,27]

If a patient on prescribed antituberculosis treatment does not respond, multidrug resistant tuberculosis should be suspected if:

i. Child is in contact/ close exposure with:
  - A known case of DR TB.
  - An adult on chronic irregular treatment who continues to be sputum positive.

ii. History of irregular ATT in the past and remains sputum positive.

iii. Failure of ATT:
  - A known case of DR TB.
  - Smear AFB positive, at 4 months of category II treatment

Or at 5 months of starting category I WHO treatment regimen given under direct observation by a health worker Or initially smear/culture negative but becomes smear/culture positive during treatment (failure).

iv. Some initial improvement to ATT followed by deterioration in any one of these three parameters (sputum, radiological, clinical). Radiological deterioration may be due to intercurrent/persistent pneumonia or pulmonary embolism, so a repeat chest X-ray after 2–3 weeks of supportive management will probably show improvement. Apparent radiological deterioration, if not accompanied by bacteriological and clinical deterioration, is less likely to be tubercular. Clinical deterioration is the least reliable evidence of failure. Similarly, clinical deterioration, if not accompanied by radiological or bacteriological deterioration, is unlikely to be due to tuberculosis.

v. Fall and rise phenomenon, i.e. initially sputum smear becomes negative (or less positive) and later becomes persistently positive.

Special Considerations in Management of MDR[8,9,27]

Management of MDR is complex and to be successful, special attention needs to be paid for the following:

- Quality-assured laboratory capacity (smear, culture and DST);
- Treatment design;
- Adherence to difficult-to-take regimens for long periods;
- Monitoring and recording;
- Drug procurement;
- Side-effect management;
- Human and financial resource constraints.

Management of MDR[8,9,27]

Laboratory diagnosis of drug resistance—Diagnosis of drug-resistant TB is done through quality assurance, timely culture and DST.

Accurate and timely diagnosis is the backbone of management of MDR. MDR TB must be diagnosed correctly before commencement of treatment. Diagnosis is always bacteriological. Diagnosis in all suspected cases is confirmed by bacteriological studies which are mandatory on samples (sputum, induced concentrated sputum, gastric lavage or bronchoalveolar lavage, histopathology samples, fluid aspirates). Prompt diagnosis of drug resistance needs to be made by a reliable culture and drug sensitivity report from a standardized accredited laboratory[8,9,28]. Standardized laboratory is the one which is regularly checked by another reference laboratory at national or supranational level (WHO standards)[8,9,29,30]. However, diagnosis of pediatric MDR TB is often extremely delayed due to reliance on the adult case definitions and should be suspected early in cases of delayed response to prevent progressive, chronic illness. For this, programmatic changes could facilitate earlier diagnosis and treatment of paediatric MDR TB[7,11].

In tuberculosis bacteriology, an often-overlooked problem is that of obtaining adequate good quality specimens. The advantages of decontamination techniques, obtaining maximum yield by cultures, sensitive culture media and simple identification schemes will not be complete unless specimens are collected with care and promptly transported to the laboratory. For example, a good sputum specimen consists of recently discharged material from the bronchial tree, with minimum amounts of oral or nasopharyngeal material. Satisfactory quality implies the presence of mucoid or mucopurulent material. Ideally, a sputum specimen should have a volume of 3–5 ml. Specimens should be transported to the laboratory as soon as possible after collection. If delay is unavoidable, the specimens should be refrigerated to inhibit the growth of unwanted micro organisms. If refrigeration is not possible and a delay of more than 3 days is anticipated, a suitable preservative, viz. an equal volume of a mixture of 1% CPC, a quaternary ammonium compound, and 2% sodium chloride (NaCl) solution is recommended to be used to decontaminate the specimen while NaCl effects liquefaction. The use of this method not only decreases the number of cultures lost by contamination as a result of prolonged transit time but also decreases significantly the laboratory time required for processing the specimens.

Direct and Indirect Methods[8,9,29,31]

Both direct and indirect methods are available to diagnose drug resistance.

In the direct methods, the sample is inoculated into drug containing and drug-free culture media and the isolation for mycobacterium and drug susceptibility testing (DST) is done at the same time. It takes 3–6 weeks in liquid media and 6–8 weeks on solid media (conventional) for the organism to grow and further almost the same time for the susceptibility report.

Newer rapid techniques have been introduced to circumvent the delay in susceptibility results by conventional methods, like radiometric testing using BACTEC, mycobacterial growth indicator tube (MGIT) cultures, accelerated nitrate reductase test, luciferase reporter phages (LRP), PCR and other molecular genetic techniques like restricted fragment length polymorphism (RFLP) and single strand conformation polymorphism (SSCP), PCR based universal heteroduplex generator assay, DNA "micro-array", but these are costly and need to be made cost-effective[31].

Criteria of Resistance[8,9]

Resistance is defined as the growth of 1% (or more) on drug containing medium when compared with the amount of growth on drug-free medium. Any strain with 1% (the critical proportion) of bacilli resistant to a drug is classified as resistant to that drug. For calculating the proportion of resistant bacilli, the highest count obtained on the drug-free and on the drug-containing medium should be taken.

Radiometric assay using BACTEC[32]

The implementation of automated BACTEC-460 system helps in isolation of the organism in 1–2 weeks. Further 7–10 days are needed for susceptibility results. It also has the facilities for a detailed MIC analysis. Now, BACTEC is being replaced by MGIT in India.

Mycobacterial growth indicator tube (MGIT) cultures[33]

Live mycobacteria resistant to a particular drug in concentration 10^8/ml cause change in color and florescence under UV light. This is used for sensitivity testing for different drugs. It is of two types:

i. Manual MGIT.

ii. Automated BACTEC MGIT 960 system.

Sensitivity, ability to detect resistance, of MGIT system was 100% while specificity, ability to detect susceptibility, ranged 98.6 to 100% for all drugs tested as compared with the agar reference method[31]. Luciferase reporter phages can be used for identification and susceptibility testing for *M. tuberculosis* from MGIT cultures[32]. Both MGIT methods can be regarded as accurate and rapid alternatives to the BACTEC 460 method for detecting R and I resistance while BACTEC 460 is superior to MGIT for diagnosing S and E resistance. Average turn around time is 6–7 (6.4) days for both MGIT while 8–10 (8.7) days for BACTEC 460[33].

Accelerated nitrate reductase method (NRM)[33]

It is used to detect live *Mycobacterium tuberculosis* by recording their enzymatic activity using the Lowenstein-Jensen medium. NRM has been successfully used to determine the sensitivity of mycobacteria to the critical concentration of first line AT agents[14].

Luciferase reporter phages (LRP)

This is a biologic test, developed by Jacob *et al*[34]. The principle of the test is that when mycobacteria are infected with a phage carrying genetically altered fire fly luciferase gene, the product hydrolyses luciferin to produce light in the presence of ATP, which is found in all viable cells. The drug resistant bacilli produce ATP even in the presence of the drug and thus support the reactions and emit light. The results are available within two days after isolating the organism using the luminometer or Bronx box as compared to three weeks for photographic polaroid film detection. Bronx box is an inexpensive "low tech" alternative to polaroid film photographic detection[35]. LRP is comparably efficient as MCIT 960 system[37].

Polymerase chain reaction (PCR-SSCP)

PCR offers a rapid detection of resistance within 24 hours. This test involves 2 steps that combine an amplification step (PCR) of the DNA strands which then fold intra-molecularly to a characteristic single strand conformation. The presence of a single mutation will result in an altered conformation and lead to a different electrophoretic mobility of the separated and folded strands, or single strand conformation polymorphism. For identification of the mutant strains by this technique there should be at least 3–4 acid-fast organisms on microscopy and the resistant strains should represent > 15% of the total in the mixed bacterial populations.

Heteroduplex analysis

Direct heteroduplex analysis and a PCR-based universal heteroduplex generator assay is very useful to detect rifampin resistance rapidly by identifying specific mutations and resistance pattern and also cross resistance between rifampin derivatives, i.e. rifapentine, rifabutin, rifalazi[36].

DNA microarray "oligoarray TB"

It allows rapid detection of genes related to drug resistance to rifampicin (R), isoniazid (H), kanamycin (K), streptomycin (S), ethambutol (E) within 6 hours with DNA extracted directly from sputum or cultured cells using oligoarray TB. Also sequencing analysis of strains generating discrepant results can be done[37].

Problems with laboratory reports[8,9,38]

i. Non-viable cultures, culture contamination, and unreliable DST results.

ii. Laboratory report does not match with clinical scenario. This could be a lab error, can occur as elsewhere, e.g. mislabelling of sample, non-standarised lab. Answer is to check the reliability of the lab and get two culture susceptibility reports.

iii. Two different susceptibility reports from two different labs. In this case, assume the worst combination of resistance that has been found on susceptibility reports and design a new regimen accordingly.

iv. Drug susceptibility test results of the 1st line anti-TB drugs pyrazinamide, streptomycin, and ethambutol should be interpreted with caution due to the poor reproducibility of these results even under optimal laboratory conditions.

v. Drug susceptibility test (DST) results of 2nd line anti-TB drugs should be interpreted with great caution due to limited capacity of laboratories, absence of quality-assurance, and lack of standardized methodology. DST of kanamycin and fluoroquinolones is more reliable.

TREATMENT OF DR TUBERCULOSIS

Basic Principles

Specialized units

Treatment of MDR tuberculosis involves the use of "second line" reserve drugs, which are more expensive, less effective, more toxic and have more side effects than the standard drugs[39]. WHO recommends that these drugs should only be made available to a specialized unit and not in the free market. National health authorities should establish strong pharmaceutical regulations to limit the use of second line reserve drugs (Tables 13.2 and 13.3) in order to prevent the emergence of incurable tuberculosis.

Second-Line (Reserve) Anti tuberculosis Drugs[8,9,39]

Second line anti tuberculosis drugs are used in the treatment of apparent or proved MDR tuberculosis. Classes of second-line anti-tuberculosis drugs include the following. (refer Tables 13.2 and 13.3)

Aminoglycosides

When resistance to streptomycin is proved or highly suspected, one of the other aminoglycosides can be used as a bactericidal agent against actively multiplying organisms:

Kanamycin: The least expensive, but painful injection and largely used for indications other than tuberculosis in some countries.

Amikacin: As active as kanamycin and better tolerated, but much more expensive.

Capreomycin: Very expensive but very useful in cases with tubercle bacilli resistant to streptomycin, kanamycin and amikacin.

Thioamides

Ethionamide or prothionamide—These are two different presentations of the same active substance, with bacteriocidal activity. (WHO has recently classified it as static; although Indian evidence and RNTCP DOTS Plus Guidelines still consider it as bacteriocidal) Prothionamide may be better tolerated than ethionamide in some populations. Ethionamide may exacerbate adverse reactions (e.g. convulsions) due to cycloserine in some patients.

Fluoroquinolones

Currently, the most potent available fluoroquinolones in descending order based on in vitro activity and animal studies are: moxifloxacin = gatifloxacin > levofloxacin > ofloxacin> ciprofloxacin[8,9].

However, the long-term safety of the newer generation fluoroquinolones has not yet been fully evaluated. These drugs have almost complete cross-resistance within the group. These drugs have bactericidal activity and are useful in preventing emergence of further cross-resistance with other drugs. The microbiological and clinical improvement, greater short and long-term success rates, lower death rates are reported with regimen having fluoroquinolones[40,41].

Cycloserine (or terizidone)

It is a bacteriostatic agent, with two different formulations. It has no cross-resistance with other antitubercular agents. It might be valuable to prevent resistance to other active drugs, but its use is limited by its cost and high toxicity. Pyridoxine supplementation helps in preventing its adverse reactions.

Para-aminosalicylic acid (PAS)

This is a bacteriostatic agent, valuable for preventing resistance to isoniazid and strepto-

Table 13.2: Ranking of reserve antituberculosis drugs for treatment[8,9]

Rank drugs and type of antimyco-bacterial activity, availability	Average daily dosage and route	CSF permeabi-lity	Adverse effects	Toxicity	Acceptability	Tolerance
1. Aminoglycosides: (bactericidal against acitively multiply-ing organism outside macrophages) vial 0.5, 0.75 and 1 g	15mg/kg IM	Poor, unless TBM	Auditory and vesti-bular toxicity nephrotoxicity	Medium		
a. Streptomycin					Moderate	Moderate
b. Kanamycin or amikacin					Painful	Poor
c. Capreomycin					Painful	Moderate
2. Thioamides: (bactericidal) tab 250 mg Ethionamide, Prothionamide	10–20 mg/kg Oral	Good	Gastric intolerance hepatitis, hypothyroidism (especially if used with PAS)	Medium	Good	Moderate
3. Pyrazinamide (bactericidal at acid pH inside macro-phages) tab 250, 500, 750, 1000 mg	20–30 mg/kg oral	Good	Uric acid rise, gout, arthritis, hepatitis	Low	Good	Moderate
4. Ofloxacin (weakly bactericidal) 100, 200, 400 mg	7.5–15 mg/kg oral	Good	Can be given in children	Low	Good	Good
5. Ethambutol (bacteriostatic) tab 200, 400, 600, 800 mg	15–20 mg/kg oral	Good	Optic neuritis	Low	Good	Good
6. Cycloserine (bacteriostatic) cap 250 mg	10–20 mg/kg oral	Good	Acute psychosis, suicidal tendency, depression, seizures	High	Good	Moderate
7. PAS (bacteriostatic) tab 1 g granules 3.433 g (INA-PAS), 4g/Measure	200–400 mg/kg oral	Good	Reversible goiter, GI disturbances, hepatotoxicity	Low	Bad (bulk, taste), good for granules	Poor Moderate

Table 13.3: Anti-Tuberculosis agents
Alternative method of grouping anti-TB agents (WHO classification)[8]

Grouping	Drugs
Grouping	Drugs (abbreviation)
Group 1	First-line oral antituberculosis agents: isoniazid (H); rifampicin (R); ethambutol (E); pyrazinamide (Z)
Group 2	Injectable antituberculosis agents: streptomycin (S); kanamycin (Km); amikacin (Am); capreomycin (Cm); viomycin (Vi)
Group 3	Fluoroquinolones - ciprofloxacin (Cfx); ofloxacin (Ofx); levofloxacin (Lfx); moxifloxacin (Mfx)[a] gatifloxacin (Gfx)[a] pefloxacin
Group 4	Oral bacteriostatic second-line antituberculosis agents: Ethionamide (Eto); prothionamide (Pto); cycloserine (Cs); terizidone (Trd)a; *P*-aminosalicylic acid (PAS); Thioacetazone (Th)[b]
Group 5	Antituberculosis agents with unclear efficacy (not recommended by WHO for routine use in MDR TB patients) clofazimine (Cfz); amoxicillin/clavulanate (Amx/Clv); clarithromycin (Clr); linezolid (Lzd)

a The long-term safety and efficacy for MDR TB treatment have not yet been fully confirmed and therefore, use is not yet recommended for treatment of MDR TB.

b Thioacetazone should be used only in patients documented to be HIV-negative and should usually not be chosen over other drugs listed in Group 4.

mycin in the past and to other bactericidal drugs today.

Others

i. Macrolides (clarithromycin, azithromycin, roxithromycin)

ii. *Rifampicin derivatives:* Like rifabutin[42], rifapentine, rifalazil cannot be used since there is almost complete cross-resistance with rifampicin (especially when there is acquired resistance to rifampicin). Hetero-duplex analysis is useful in detecting rifampicin resistance and cross-resistance between newer rifampicin derivatives. Only rifabutin is available in India (as macbutin).

Beta-lactam and beta-lactamase inhibitors[43,44]

i. *Co-amoxyclav*—Amoxycillin-Clavulanic acid[43]

ii. *Cefazolin*—Clavulanic acid

iii. *Linezolid*—This has synergic activity with fluoroquinolones[44] and rifampicin.

iv. *Clofazimine*—This has some activity against *M, leprae* and *M. ulcerans*, but less activity against *M. tuberculosis.*

The dosage, type of anti-mycobacterial activity, CSF permeability, side-effects, acceptability and tolerance of some commonly used second-line anti-tuberculosis drugs are given in Table 13.2.

Cross-resistance[8,9]

As designing a regimen involves combining "reserve drugs", consideration of cross-resistance is important for selecting the drugs acceptable for treatment of MDR tuberculosis. It is ineffective to combine two drugs of the same group or to combine in the prescribed chemotherapy regimen, a drug rendered potentially ineffective because of cross-resistance.

Aminoglycosides—Strains resistant to streptomycin are susceptible to kanamycin-amikacin; resistance to kanamycin induces a complete cross-resistance to amakacin. They should be considered as the same drug. Resistance to kanamycin-amikacin also induces resistance to streptomycin. Strains resistant to streptomycin, kanamycin-amikacin are still susceptible to capreomycin.

Thionamide and prothionamide—Ethionamide induces complete cross-resistance with prothionainide. They should thus be considered as the same drug. Frequently, there is also cross-resistance between thionamides and thioacetazone; strains naturally resistant to thioacetazone are usually susceptible to ethionamide-prothionamide while strains resistant to ethionamide-prothionamide are usually resistant to thioacetazone in more than 70% of cases.

Fluoroquinolones—Ofloxacin, ciprofloxacin and sparfloxacin induce complete cross-resistance for all other fluoroquinolones and thus ciprofloxacin/ofloxacin must not be used in primary regimens–since complete cross-resistance with new more active quinolones (e.g. moxi/gati/levofloxacin) would render these ineffective. However, there is no cross-resistance of fluoroquinolones with other classes of drugs.

Cycloserine and terizidone—There is complete cross-resistance between these two drugs and they should be considered as the same drug. There is no cross-resistance with other classes of drugs.

Classification[8,9]

Several criteria are used for classifying antituberculosis drugs available for treatment of DR tuberculosis.

a. *According to their activity*

The main criteria are based on biological data, which determine 3 groups of antituberculosis drugs available according to their activity (Tables 13.2 and 13.3) and cross-resistance.

i. Drugs with bactericidal activity—Aminoglycosides, thioamides and pyrazinamide in conditions of acidic pH. Recently, thioamides are classified as bacteriostatic drugs by WHO .

ii. Drugs with low bactericidal activity—Fluoroquinolones.

iii. Drugs with bacteriostatic effect which prevent cross-resistance (when given at usual dosages in man): Ethambutol, cycloserine and PAS.

b. According to clinical criteria (Table 13.2)

i. Acceptability to the patient (linked to the bulk or total volume of drug to be injected or swallowed, painful injection, taste).

ii. Tolerance.

iii. Potential toxicity-Cycloserine-acute psychosis, depression, suicidal tendency, seizures. This may be exacerbated by ethionamide, prevented by pyridoxine supplementation. PAS -reversible goiter, requiring thyroxine supplementation.

c. According to their cost

The crucial criterion for the choice of second-line anti tuberculosis drugs is their cost (Table 13.4) which varies considerably from one country to another according to the suppliers, the market conditions and the size of the market. Information regarding suppliers of these drugs and their costs is available on request from WHO and IUATI.D.

With cycloserine the total approximate cost is Rs 72,184 and per month cost is Rs 2437.00. When cycloserine stopped after sputum conversion (approx 3 months)[14] the total cost is Rs 28,984 and monthly cost is Rs 1,380[8,9].

Table 13.4: Cost of some commonly used second line drugs

	Dose (for 30 kg child)	Duration (mths)	Cost (Rs/day)	Approx Total (Rs.)
Kanamycin	0.5 g	3	18.00	1.705
PZA	1000 mg	3	8.40	756
Ethionamide	500 mg	21	18.85	11,880
Cycloserine	500 mg	21	68.50	43,280
Ofloxacin	400 mg	21	6.65	4,185
PAS	6 g	21	2.40	9072
Ethambutol	600 mg	21	2.20	1,386

Regimens[8,9]

Important points

A number of recommendations for management of MDR TB have been made by the WHO[8] and RNTCP(DOTS Plus Guidelines)[9] and it is likely that future measures and modifications may be necessary[11,45-49].

1. Regimen should ideally be individualized (Individualized Treatment Regimen; ITR) depending upon the drug susceptibility report and taking into account the detail past drug history with proper charting of drugs including their duration, sputum results and X-ray report but to ensure compliance, WHO and RNTCP recommend category IV regimen used as DOTS- Plus (Standardized Treatment Regimen; STR-DOTS Plus) for management of MDR TB. (Tables 13.5 and 13.6)

2. It must be made amply clear to the patient, parents and the staff that meticulously taking the prescribed reserve regimen daily under direct observation, with each dose supervised, at least until sputum conversion, is all that stands between the patient and death. The entire course of treatment should preferably be directly observed. The only answer to prevent the major factor of non-adherence is the introduction of DOTS-plus whereby a health care worker is directly involved in the administration of Standardized Treatment Regimen of category IV reserve drugs to the patient (Table 13.5).

3. The patient must try to tolerate any unpleasant side effects in order to achieve conversion.

4. Reliable guaranteed supplies of expensive second-line drugs to successfully complete the entire course is a must.

5. It is mandatory to monitor bacteriological results (smear and culture) monthly from the third month until the seventh month and then quarterly until the end of treatment.

Table 13.5: Treatment strategies for MDR TB[8,9]

	Recommended treatment strategies for MDR TB
Standardized treatment (STR-DOTS Plus)	Representative DRS data in well-defined patient populations are used to design the regimen. All patients in a patient group or category receive the same regimen.
Standardized treatment followed by individualized treatment	Initially, all patients in a certain group receive the same regimen based on DST survey data from representative populations. The regimen is adjusted when DST results become available (often DST is only done to a limited number of drugs).
Individualized Treatment (ITR)	Each regimen is individually designed on the basis of patient history and then adjusted when DST results become available (often the DST is done for first and in suspected XDR cases to second-line drugs)

Individualized Treatment Regimen; ITR

In designing a regimen do not aim to keep drugs in reserve. This last battle must be won. Informed written consent is a must. As these drugs are costly, source of financial support also needs to be ascertained. Decision to start second-line (reserve) drugs should not be taken in a haste. Residual respiratory morbidity (e.g. destroyed lung, airflow obstruction, respiratory insufficiency) and prognosis that is only a limited number of patients have favourable response[42] needs to be explained. Repeated doctor-parent counselling and ongoing interaction is a must for monitoring, psychosocial and emotional support of the patient and the family.

The following applies to MDR patients with resistance at least to isoniazid and rifampicin, patients considered to have failed on the WHO standard retreatment category-II regimen, and other patients who have received a variety of bad regimens outside the national programmes.

Acceptable Regimen in Programme Conditions[8,9]

A. *Susceptability test not available at time of starting treatment*

It sometimes takes 2–4 months for susceptibility test results to be made available in a specialized unit with a reliable laboratory due to various reasons:

i. Initial culture negative or contaminated.

ii. Failure in logistics; transport of specimen, temporary shortage of reagents, etc.

A new chemotherapy regimen needs to be designed and initiated before the susceptibility test results are available only if representative DRS data indicates a very high probability of MDR TB, which can later be modified depending upon the laboratory report. Design a regimen with 5–6 drugs keeping the following in consideration:

- Site of drug-resistant tuberculosis disease (pulmonary and extrapulmonary): In general, recommended treatment regimens for drug-resistant forms of TB are similar, irrespective of site.

- Prescribe drugs, which the patient has not had previously. The bacilli are fairly certain to be sensitive to these. If most of the drugs have been used by the patient, add those drugs which have not been used in the recent past.

- At least 3 never used drugs, preferably bacteriocidal; aminoglycoside, ethionamide, or ofloxacin.

- Add pyrazinamide (even if previously used, because resistance is usually un-

likely). This combination aminoglycoside and pyrazinamide has a good bactericidal activity. Pyrazinamide can be used for the entire treatment if it is judged to be effective. Many MDR TB patients have chronically inflamed lungs, which theoretically produce the acidic environment in which pyrazinamide is active.

- The practice of adding isoniazid to these drugs confers no advantage.

- Add a bacteriostatic drug, ethambutol, cycloserine or PAS to prevent cross-resistance.

- Amikacin, rifabutin, clarithromycin and ethambutol seem to act best on atypical mycobacterial-MDR lymphadenitis[24,42].

B. *Susceptibility test results available*

Treatment strategies for mono and poly-resistant strains (drug-resistant tuberculosis other than MDR TB).

Third-line regimen if there is resistance to isoniazid, but rifampicin still active (Table 13.6).

i. *Resistance to isoniazid alone or in combination with resistance to streptomycin (and/or with thioacetazone):* It may be simplest to use the WHO standard retreatment (category II) regimen (2SHRZE/1HRZE/5HRE).

Combination with resistance to streptomycin—Though isoniazid and streptomycin are redundant and can be omitted, streptomycin can be replaced by kanamycin or amikacin, if resistance to streptomycin.

ii. *Resistance to isoniazid and ethambutol (with or without resistance to streptomycin)*—Use rifampicin and ethionamide for nine months at least, with pyrazinamide and one aminoglycoside (kanamycin or amikacin if resistance to streptomycin; capreomycin if resistance to streptomycin

Table 13.6: Acceptable "third line" regimens if there is resistance to
isoniazid but susceptibility to rifampicin

Resistance to	Initial phase		Continuation phase	
	Drugs	Minimum duration in months	Drug	Duration in months
Isoniazid	1. Aminoglycoside*	2–3	1. Rifampicin	6
(Steptomycin	2. Rifampicin	2–3	2. Ethambutol	6
thioacetazone)	3. Pyrazinamide	2–3		
	4. Ethambutol			
Isoniazid and	1. Aminoglycoside*	3	1. Rifampicin	6
ethambutol	2. Rifampicin	3	2. Ethionamide	6
(Streptomycin)	3. Pyrazinamide	3		
	4. Ethionamide**	3		

*S - If still active; if resistance to S, use kanamycin-amikacin, capreomycin.
** If ethionamide is not available or poorly tolerated, use ofloxacin.

and kanamycin) during the initial phase until smear conversion. If ethionamide is not available, ofloxacin can be used.

Resistance to at least isoniazid and rifampicin (MDR) (Table 13.7)

1. *Resistance to isoniazid and rifampicin (with or without resistance to streptomycin)*—When the two most important antitubercular drugs are not active, a five, preferably six, drug regimen is mandatory. During the initial phase, use ethionamide plus ofloxacin, ethambutol plus another bacteriostatic drug (cycloserine if possible) with pyrazinamide and an aminoglycoside available for a minimum of 6 months. Cycloserine should preferably be added and continued if tolerated by the patient.

   During the continuation phase, use ethionamide plus ofloxacin, ethambutol plus another bacteriostatic drug for atleast 18 months after smear conversion.

2. *Resistance to isoniazid, rifampicin, ethambutol (with or without resistance to streptomycin)* During the initial phase, use ethionamide plus ofloxacin plus another bacteriostatic drug (cycloserine or PAS) with pyrazina-

mide and an aminoglycoside available for a minimum of 6 months or until smear conversion. During the continuation phase, use ethionamide plus ofloxacin plus cycloserine (or PAS) for at least 18 months after smear conversion.

Usually resistance to pyrazinamide is rare, but if a reliable lab report shows resistance to pyrazinamide, it should be stopped and cycloserine or PAS included in the regimen. Cycloserine can also be stopped after sputum conversion, if it is too toxic or too costly for the patient.

Standardised Treatment Regimen (Category IV regimen)

RNTCP is using a standardised treatment regimen for the treatment of MDR TB cases under the programme.

RNTCP Category IV Regimen: 6(9) Km Ofx Eto Cs Z E / 18 Ofx Eto Cs E

Standardised treatment regimen (STR), comprising 6 drugs (kanamycin, ofloxacin, ethionamide, pyrazinamide, ethambutol and cycloserine) during 6–9 months of the intensive phase and 4 drugs (ofloxacin, ethionamide,

Table 13.7: Acceptable "third Line" regimens (category IV) for treatment of MDR tuberculosis

Resistance to	Initial phase		Continuation phase	
	Drugs	Minimum duration in months	Drug	Duration in months
Isoniazid, rifampicin and streptomycin	1. Aminoglycoside*	6	1. Ethionamide	18
	2. Ethionamide	6	2. Ofloxacin	18
	3. Pyrazinamide	6	3. Ethambutol	18
	4. Ofloxacin	6	4. Cycloserine/PAS	18
	5. Ethambutol	6		
	6. Cycloserine/PAS	6		
Isoniazid, rifampicin streptomycin and ethambutol	1. Aminoglycoside*	6	1. Ethionamide	18
	2. Rifampicin	6	2. Ofloxacin	18
	3. Pyrazinamide	6	3. Cycloserine/PAS	18
	4. Ofloxacin	6		
	5. Cycloserine/PAS'	6		

Maximum intensive (initial) phase duration – 9 months
*Kanamycin or amikacin or capreomycin.
'PAS, if cycloserine is not available or too toxic.

ethambutol and cycloserine) during the 18 months of the continuation phase. *p*-amino-salicylic acid (PAS) is included in the regimen as a substitute drug if any bactericidal drug (K, Ofl, Z and Eto) or any 2 bacteriostatic (E and Cs) drugs are not tolerated.

Monitoring[8,9,45-48]

Sputa are to be collected and examined by smear and culture at least 30 days apart from the 3rd to 7th month of treatment (i.e. at the end of the months 3, 4, 5, 6 and 7) and at 3 monthly intervals from the 9th month onwards till the completion of treatment (i.e. at the end of the months 9, 12, 15, 18, 21 and 24). The importance of the sputum examination during treatment needs to be emphasized, since the most important objective evidence of improvement is the conversion of sputum smear and culture to negative.

Chest radiograph is done during the pre-treatment evaluation, at the end of the intensive phase, end of treatment and when clinically indicated.

Serum creatinine is done every month for the first 3 months and every three months thereafter till the patient is receiving injection kanamycin.

Liver function tests and TSH are done as and when indicated.

Treatment Duration[8,9]

The treatment is given in two phases, the intensive phase (IP) and the continuation phase (CP). IP should be given for at least six months. After 6 months of treatment, the patient should be reviewed and the treatment changed to CP if the 4th month culture result is negative. If the 4th month culture result remains positive, the intensive treatment is extended by 1 month. Extension of IP beyond 1 month will be decided on the results of sputum culture of 5th and 6th months. If the 4th month culture is still awaited after 6 months of treatment, the IP is extended until the result is available, with further treatment being decided according to the culture result. The IP can be extended up to a maximum of 3 months after which the patient is initiated on the CP irrespective of the culture result. The recommended duration for CP is 18 months.

Patient is considered culture converted after having two consecutive negative cultures taken at least one month apart. Time to culture conversion is calculated as the interval between the date of MDR TB treatment initiation and the date of the first of these two negative consecutive cultures (the date that the sputum specimens are collected for culture should be used). Similarly patient is considered smear converted after having two consecutive negative smears taken at least one month apart. Two separate indicators, one based on sputum smears and the other on cultures should be calculated. Though smear conversion can be taken as an indicator, culture conversion which reflects viability of tubercle bacilli, is more sensitive and is necessary to monitor progress in MDR TB patients. Good quality sputum is essential to get proper results.

Patients who remain culture positive despite 9 months of regular treatment, are suspects of treatment failure to second-line drugs (suspected XDR) and DST for second line drugs, e.g. kanamycin, capreomycin and fluoroquinolones should be done at a National Reference Laboratory (NRL). At present, only Tuberculosis Research Institute(TRC), Chennai is accredited to perform DST for second-line drugs. It is planned that after training and proficiency testing by TRC, which is the WHO Supra-National Reference Laboratory (SNRL) for the WHO SEARO region, National Tuberculosis Institute(NTI), Bangalore: Lala Ram Sarup Institute (LRS), Delhi and JALMA Institute, Agra will be accredited for performing second-line DST.

Treatment Interruption and Default[8,9]

All efforts should be made to ensure that patients do not interrupt treatment or default.

Action should be taken to promptly retrieve patient. The following situations may be seen in case of treatment interruption:
- *Patients in IP/CP who miss doses*—All the missed doses during IP must be completed prior to switching the patient to CP. Similarly, all missed doses during CP must be completed prior to ending treatment.
- *Patients who interrupt treatment for less than 2 months during IP*—When the patient returns to resume treatment the IP will be continued, however, the duration of treatment will be extended to complete IP. The follow up cultures are done as per the revised date schedule.
- *Patients who interrupt treatment for less than 2 months during CP*—When the patient returns to resume treatment, the CP will be continued, however, the duration of treatment will be extended to complete the CP. The period of interruption shall not be included in the duration of treatment. The follow up cultures are done as per the revised date schedule.

Treatment Outcomes[8,9]

Standardised treatment outcome definitions are used following treatment of an MDR TB case and are as follows:

Cure—An MDR TB patient who has completed treatment and has been consistently culture negative (with at least 5 consecutive negative results in the last 12 to 15 months). If one follow-up positive culture is reported during the last three quarters, patient will still be considered cured, provided this positive culture is followed by at least 3 consecutive negative cultures, taken at least 30 days apart, provided that there is clinical evidence of improvement.

Treatment completed—An MDR TB patient who has completed treatment according to guidelines but does not meet the definition for cure or treatment failure due to lack of bacteriological results.

Death—An MDR TB patient who dies for any reason during the course of MDR TB treatment.

Treatment failure—Treatment will be considered to have failed if two or more of the five cultures recorded in the final 12–15 months are positive, or if any of the final three cultures are positive.

Treatment default—An MDR TB patient whose MDR-TB treatment was interrupted for two or more consecutive months for any reasons.

SUMMARY OF GENERAL PRINCIPLES FOR DESIGNING A REGIMEN[8,9]

Basic Principles Comments

1. *Use at least 4 highly likely drugs to be effective*—Effectiveness is supported by a number of factors (more the drugs certainly not used, more likely will be effective in the patient):
   A. DST results show susceptibility.
   B. No previous history of treatment failure with the drug.
   C. No known close contacts with resistance to the drug.
   D. Drug-resistance survey indicates resistance is rare in similar patients.
   E. The drug is not commonly used in the area.

   If at least 4 drugs are not certain to be effective, use 5–7 drugs depending on the specific drugs and level of uncertainty.

2. *Do not use*
   A. All rifamycin (rifampicin, rifabutin, rifapentene, rifalazil) drugs which have high levels of cross-resistance.
   B. Fluoroquinolones are believed to have variable crosses over cross-resistance, with in vitro data showing that some higher-generation fluoroquinolones remain susceptible when lower-generation fluoroquinolones are resistant. In

these cases, it is unknown whether the higher-generation fluoroquinolones remain clinically effective.
   C. Not all aminoglycosides and polypeptides crossresist; in general, only kanamycin and amikacin fully cross-resist.

3. *Eliminate drugs*
   A. Known severe allergy or unmanageable intolerance that are not safe.
   B. High risk of severe adverse effects including renal failure, in the patient with deafness, hepatitis, depression and/or psychosis.
   C. Quality of the drug is unknown or questionable.

4. *Include drugs from*
   A. Use any Group 1 (oral first-line) drugs that are likely to be effective (see table 13.3). Groups 1–5 are effective in a hierarchical order.
   B. Use an effective aminoglycoside or polypeptide by injection based on potency (Group 2 drugs).
   C. Use a fluoroquinolone (Group 3).
   D. Use the remaining Group 4 drugs to make a regimen of at least 4 effective drugs. For regimens with 4 effective drugs, add second-line drugs most likely to be effective, to give up to 5–7 drugs in total, on the basis that at least 4 are highly likely to be effective. The number of drugs will depend on the degree of uncertainty.
   E. Use Group 5 drugs as needed so that at least 4 drugs are likely to be effective.

5. *Be prepared to*
   A. Ensure laboratory services for hematology, biochemistry, monitor serology and audiometry should be done.
   B. Establish a clinical and laboratory baseline before starting each of the drugs.
   C. Initiate treatment gradually for a difficult-to-tolerate drug, split daily doses of Eto/Pto, Cs and PAS.

D. Ensure ancillary drugs are available to manage adverse effects.

E. Implement DOT for all doses.

Management of patients after MDR TB treatment failure[8-10]

Extensively drug-resistant TB (XDR TB) is a form of TB caused by bacilli resistant to all the most effective anti-TB drugs, and emerges through mismanagement of MDR TB treatment. According to WHO, there are 41 countries with XDR TB to date. Once created, XDR TB can spread from one person to another.

- XDR TB is resistance to at least isoniazid and rifampicin (i.e. multidrug-resistant TB or MDR TB), plus resistance to any fluoro-quinolones, and any one of the second-line anti-TB injectable drugs (amikacin, kanamycin or capreomycin).

- XDR TB raises concerns of a future TB epidemic with restricted treatment options, and jeopardizes the major gains made in TB control and progress on reducing TB deaths among people living with HIV/AIDS.

WHO Global Task Force on XDR TB plans to scale up the programmatic management of MDR TB and XDR TB and strengthen accredited laboratory services to diagnose XDR.

HIV and DR-TB[8-10,13,49]

HIV positivity does not increase the chances of drug-resistance by itself, against what was thought earlier, but only considerably accelerates the tuberculosis infection developing into the disease. Treatment of TB in HIV positive patients should always be under DOTS because of risk of non-compliance in these cases. There are reports of rifampicin mono-resistance in HIV co-infected patients. Treatment of DR and MDR is essentially the same but the doctor should be aware of interaction between rifamycin derivatives and protease inhibitors leading to increased rifamycin levels and resultant toxicity. Developing mutual TB control strategies between the National TB and AIDS Control Programmes will have an impact on growing HIV-1 epidemic and MDR TB[2,11].

The diagnosis of TB in HIV-positive persons can be more difficult and may be confused with other pulmonary or systemic infections. As the HIV disease progresses and the individual becomes more immunocompromised, the clinical presentation is proportionately more likely to be extrapulmonary or smear-negative than in HIV-uninfected TB patients. This can result in misdiagnosis or delays in diagnosis, and in turn, higher morbidity and mortality.

The treatment of HIV-positive individual with MDR TB is the same as for HIV-negative patients. However, treatment is more difficult and adverse events more common. Deaths during treatment, partly due to TB itself and partly due to other HIV-related diseases, are more frequent in HIV-infected patients, particularly in the advanced stages of immuno-deficiency. Due to the increased frequency of adverse drug events, rigorous monitoring in this particular group of patients is required in order to ensure adherence to treatment, early identification and treatment of adverse events and reduce default in general, it is recommended that patients who are already on highly active anti retroviral therapy (HAART) at the time of MDR TB diagnosis be continued on HAART when TB therapy is initiated. For patients not on HAART with severe immune-suppression (CD4 counts less than $200/\mu l$), TB therapy should be started followed by initiation of HAART except that nevirapine be replaced with efavirenez within two to four weeks. However, the potential drug interactions may result in ineffectiveness of antiretroviral drugs, ineffective treatment of TB, and an increase risk of drug toxicity.

Occasionally, patients with HIV-related TB may experience a temporary exacerbation of symptoms, signs or radiographic manifestations of TB after beginning TB treatment. This paradoxical reaction occurs in HIV-infected patients with active TB and is thought to be a result of immune restitution due to the simultaneous administration of antiretroviral and tuberculosis medication. Symptoms and signs may include high fever, lymphadenopathy, expanding central nervous system lesions and worsening of chest radiographic findings. The diagnosis of a paradoxical reaction should be made only after a thorough evaluation has excluded other aetiologies, particularly TB treatment failure. For severe paradoxical reactions prednisone (1–2 mg/kg for 1–2 weeks, then gradually decreasing doses) may be used.

MDR TB Requiring Surgery[8,9,50,51]

Indications for surgery

Surgery should be seriously considered in a patient who has a large localized cavity with little other disease, reasonable lung function and with bacilli resistant to all except two or three weak drugs[55]. Unfortunately, many such patients have too extensive a disease and poor lung function for surgery to be possible. To avoid serious and potentially fatal complications in a patient with drug resistant tuberculosis, operation must be done when the bacillary population is the lowest. If only a weak regimen is available, experience has shown that the most favorable time is after 6–9 months of treatment. After surgery the regimen should be continued for at least 18 months[52].

DOTS-Plus[8,9,11,48,53,54]

DOTS-Plus is a complementary DOTS-based strategy for treating MDR TB in context of RNTCP. It is, in fact, the best ray of hope for the MDR patients. It should only be imple-

mented in those areas where DOTS programme is already adequately functional. This strategy arose out of the constitution of Green Light Committee by WHO in 1999. The first WHO-endorsed DOTS-Plus programmes began in 2000. DOTS-Plus pilot projects have demonstrated the feasibility and effectiveness of MDR TB treatment in less affluent countries. In 2002, the Global Fund to fight AIDS, TB, and Malaria (GFATM) started financing TB control programmes, including MDR TB programmes, thus greatly reducing the economic barrier to MDR. Since then, DOTS-Plus projects have multiplied rapidly. By the end of 2007, 67 projects in 52 countries had been approved by the GLC, with a cumulative total of over 30,000 MDR TB patients, had been launched worldwide, many of them with financial support from the GFATM.

The task of Green Light Committee is to standardize the laboratories, supply quality assured reserved drugs at 50–80% cost cuts.

Management of Contacts of MDR TB[8,9]

Among contacts of patients with MDR TB, the use of INH may reasonably be questioned. Although alternative prophylaxis treatments have been suggested, there is no consensus regarding the choice of the drug(s) and the duration of treatment. Prompt treatment of MDR TB is the most effective way of preventing the spread of infection to others. The following measures should be taken to prevent spread of MDR TB disease:

1. Early diagnosis and appropriate treatment of MDR TB cases;
2. Screening of contacts as per RNTCP guidelines.

Newer Research Modalities

Clinical and operational research should be addressed to newer diagnostic and therapeutic modalities in resource-poor settings, where it is needed the most[1].

1. *Newer diagnostics*
    i. *PCR-based universal heteroduplex generator assay*—This is very useful for detecting DR, recognising specific mutations rapidly and also cross-resistance between rifampicin, rifapentine, rifabutin, rifalazil[36].
    ii. *DNA microarray*—This allows rapid detection of genes related to drug resistance to R, H, K, S, E within six hours[37].

2. *Newer drugs*
Research is going on for newer drugs/agents with antitubercular activity and initial reports show promising results.
    i. *Fluoroquinolones*—Win 57273, levofloxacin, lomefloxacin, gatifloxacin, pefloxacin[55,56].
    ii. *Beta-lactam and beta-lactamase inhibitors*— Cefazolin-clavulanic acid[43]
    iii. Linezolid[44].
    iv. *Riminophenazines:* B746, B4157, clofazimine.
    v. *Phenothiazines*—Thioridazine, chlorpromazine 3, 5 disubstituted thiadiazine thiones.
    vi. *Azole drugs*— Inhibitors of cytochrome p450 have shown potent anti-TB activity[57].
    vii. *Antimalarial agents*—Ethyl 5 phenyl-6-oxa-1-azabicyclohexane-2-carboxylate derivatives.
    viii. *Nitric oxide (NO)*—Use of NO donor DETA-NO[58].
    ix. *Extract from plants*—Hexane extracts from Lantana hispida[59].
    x. *Snake venom*—Small peptide vgf-1 from Naja-atra, a snake isolated from Yunnan province of China[60].

3. *Immune modulators*
    i. *Aerosoized interferon gamma inhalation therapy*— Given for six months was found to be effective in some cases of refractory MDR who do not respond to conventional therapy[61].
    ii. *Isofon*—Proved effective for DR and even MDR cases, but had significant adverse reactions as fever, weakness, dizziness, cardiac arrhythmias[62].

Conclusion

MDR TB presents an increasing threat to the global TB control with many crucial issues in the management remaining unanswered. Research should be addressed therapeutically in resource-poor settings. Suspecting, diagnosing and starting treatment early is crucial. Aggressive treatment regimens with high-end dosing are recommended given the lower potency of second-line ATD. Strategies to improve treatment adherence, such as directly observed therapy—DOTS Plus, should be used. Opportunities to treat MDR TB in developing countries are now possible through the Global Fund to fight AIDS, TB and Malaria and the Green Light Committee for access to second-line ATD. As the treatment of MDR TB becomes increasingly available in resource-poor areas, where it is needed the most, further clinical and operational research is urgently needed to guide clinicians in the management of this disease. Also programmatic changes to facilitate early diagnosis and treatment of paediatric MDR by modifications in adult case definitions for smear negative chronic progressive cases is suggested[30]. Only then this plague which threatens the mankind not only with MDR but with extreme drug resistant(XDR) or incurable TB (? XXDR ; in future), can be controlled.

References

1. World Health Organization. Global Tuberculosis Control: Surveillance, Planning, Financing. WHO Report 2008. (WHO/HTM/TB 2008. 362). Geneva, Switzerland:WHO 2008.
2. Antituberculosis drug resistance in the world. Third global report. The WHO/IUATLD global project on antituberculosis drug resistance

surveillance,1999–2002. Geneva, World Health Organization, 2004 (WHO/HTM/TB/2004.343)

3. Cox H, Flargreaves S, Ismailov C. Effect of multidrug resistance on global tuberculosis control. *Lancet* 2003;362:1858-9.

4. WHO Results from the largest survey on Drug-Resistant Tuberculosis Geneva, World Health Organi-zation 2008(WHO/HTM/TB/2008).

5. Blower SM, Chou T. Modeling the emergence of the "hot zones": Tuberculosis and the amplification dynamics of drug resistance. *Nature Medicine* 2004;10(10):1111–6.

6. Tuberculosis Research Centre, Indian Council of Medical Research, Chennai, India. Low rate of emergence of drug resistance in sputum positive patients treated with short course chemotherapy. *Int J Tuberc Lung Dis* 2001:5;40-5.

7. TB India 2008, RNTCP Status Report, p 46

8. WHO Guidelines for the Programmatic Manage-ment Of Drug-Resistant TB.WHO/HTM/TB/2008.402 Emergency Update 2008 Available, At Present, In English Only [Pdf 1.66Mb] 2006 Version Available In Other Languages Chinese (2006)[Pdf 7.9Mb] www.Who.Int/Tb/Publications /2008/Programmatic Guidelines For Mdrtb/En/Index.Html.

9. RNTCP DOTS-Plus Guidelines 2008, Central TB Division, Directorate General of Health Services, Ministry of Health and Family Welfare, NirmanBhavan, New Delhi–110011.

10. Tuberculosis, XDR-TB The Facts. Geneva, World Health Organization, 2007 (WHO/TB/2007).

11. Mukherjee JS, Rich ML, Socci AR, *et al*. Programmes and principles in treatment of multidrug-resistant tuberculosis. *Lancet* 2004; 363: 474-81.

12. Wade MM, Zhang Y. Mechanisms of drug resistance in *Mycobacterium tuberculosis*. *Front Bwsci* 2004;9:975-94.

13. Morozova I, Riekstina V, Sture G, Wells C, Leimane V. Impact of the growing HIV-1 epidemic on multidrug-resistant tuberculosis control in Latvia, *Int J Tuberc Lung Dis* 2003;7:903-6.

14. Ramaswamy SV, Dou SJ, Rendon A, Yang Z, Cave MD, Graviss EA. Genotypic analysis of multidrug-resistant Mycobacterium tuber-culosis isolates from Monterrey, Mexico. *J Med Microbiol* 2004;53:107-13.

15. Huang TS, Lee SS, Tu HZ, *et al*. Correlation between pyrazinamide activity and pnc A

mutations in Mycobacterium tuberculosis isolates in Taiwan. *Antimicrob Agents Chemother* 2003;47:3672-3.

16. Engohang-Ndong J, Baillat D, Aumercier M, *et al*. EthR, a repressor of theTetR/CamR family implicated in ethionamide resistance in mycobacteria, octamerizes cooperatively on its operator. *Mol Microbiol* 2004;51:175-88.

17. Johnnsen IS, Larson AR, Sandven L. Drug susceptibility testing of *Mycobacterium tuberculosis* to fluoroquinolones: First experience with a quality control panel in the Nordic-Baltic collaboration. *Int J Tuberc Lung Dis* 2003;7:899-902.

18. Nechaeva OB, Skachkova EL. Causes and factors of development of drug resistance in pulmonary tuberculosis. Probl Tuberk 2003;9:6-9.

19. Quy HT, Lan NT, Borgdorff MW, *et al*. Drug resistance among failure and relapse cases of tuberculosis: Is the standard re-treatment regimen adequate? *Int J Tuberc Lung Dis* 2003; 7:631-6.

20. Mitchison, D. How drug resistance emerges as a result of poor compliance during short course chemotherapy for tuberculosis. *Int J Tuberc Lung Dis* 1998;2:10-15.

21. Sharma S, Sarin R, Khalid UK, Singla N, Sharma PP, Behera D. The DOTS strategy for treatment of paediatric pulmonary tuberculosis in South Delhi, India. *Int J Tuberc Lung Dis* 2008;12:74-80

22. Davies PD. The role of DOTS in tuberculosis treatment and control. *AmJRespir Med* 2003; 2:203-9.

23. Kibrik BS, Chelnokova OG. Some specific features of drug resistance of *Mycobacteria tuberculosis* in patients with acutely progressive destructive forms of pulmonary tuberculosis. *Probl Tuberk* 2003;8:3-5.

24. Mukherjee S, Sarkar S. Treating tuberculous lymphadenitis–ifs and buts. *J Indian Mcd Assoc* 2003;101:16-7,23.

25. Sharma S. Menstrual dysfunction in nongenital tuberculosis. *Int J Gynecol Obstet* 2002;79:245-7

26. Patel VB, Padayatchi N, Bhigjee AL *et al*. Multidrug-resistant tuberculous meningitis in KwaZulu-Natal, South Africa. *Clin Infect Dis* 2004;38:851-6.

27. Mukherjee JS, Joseph JK, Rich ML, *et al*. Clinical and programmatic considerations in the treatment of MDR TB in children: a series of 16

patients from Lima, Peru, *Int J Tuberc Lung Dis* 2003;7:637-44.

28. Jensen, KA. Towards a standardisation of Laboratory methods. Second report of the Sub-Committee of Laboratory Methods of the IUAT. *Bull Int Union Tuberc* 1995, 25:89-1044.

29. IUATLD. The public health service National Tuberculosis Reference Laboratory and the National Laboratory Network, 1998.

30. Laboratory Services in Tuberculosis Control. Part I, II and III. WHO/ TB/98.258,1998.

31. Canetti G, Fox W, Khomenko A, Mahler, HT, Menon, NK, Mitchison DA *et al*. Advances in techniques of testing mycobacterial drug sensitivity and the use of sensitivity tests in tuberculosis control programmes.*Bull WHO*, 1969;41, 21-43.

32. Sulochana S, Paramasivan CN. Susceptibility of *Mycobacterium tuberculosis* strains to gatifloxacin and moxifloxacin by different methods. *Chemotherapy* 2006.

33. Golyshevskaia VI, Irtuganova OA, Smirnova NS, Domotenko LV. Comparison of nitrate reductase and automatic BACTEC MGIT 960 AST techniques for determining the drug sensitivity of *Mycobacteria tuberculosis*. *Probl Tuberk* 2003; 8:34-7.

34. Jacob WR Jr, Barletta RG, Udani R, *et al*. Rapid assessment of drug susceptibilities of *Mycobacterium tuberculosis* by means of luciferase reporter phager. *Science* 1993;260:819-22.

35. Hazbon MH, Guarin N, Ferro BH, *et al*. Photographic and luminometric detection of luciferase reporter phages for drug susceptibility testing of clinical *Mycobacterium tuberculosis* isolates. *Clin Microbiol* 2003;41:4865-9.

36. Saribas Z, Kocagoz T, Alp A, Gunalp A. Rapid detection of rifampin resistance in *Mycobacterium tuberculosis* isolates by heteroduplex analysis and determination of rifamycin cross-resistance in rifampin-resistant isolates. *Clin Microbiol* 2003;41:816-8.

37. Yoshikawa Y, Ichihara T, Suzuki Y. Detection of drug-resistant *Mycobacterium tuberculosis* isolates using DNA microarray. *Rinsho Bisei- butshu Jinsoku Shindan Kenkyukai Shi* 2003; 14:45-50.

38. Vareldzis BP, Grosset}, de Kantor 1, *et al*. Drug resistant tuberculosis: laboratory issues. World Health Organization recommendations, *Tuberc Lung Dis* 1994;75:1-7.

39. Iseman MD. Treatment of multidrug-resistant tuberculosis. *NEJM* 1993;329:784–91.

40. Cynamon MH, Sklaney M. Gatifloxacin and ethionamide as the foundation for therapy of tuberculosis. *Antimicrob Agents Chemother* 2003; 47:2442-4.

41. Yew WW, Chan CK, Chau CH, *et al*. Outcomes of patients with multidrug-resistant pulmonary tuberculosis treated with ofloxacin/levofloxacin-containing regimens. *Chest* 2000;117:744-51.

42. Preter S, l.ebeau A, Parrot R, *et al*. Combined chemotherapy including rifabutin for rifampicin and isoniazid resistant pulmonary tuberculosis. *Eur Resp* 1992;5:680-4.

43. Dincer 1, Ergin A, Kocagoz T. The vitro ellicacy of beta-lactam and beta-lactamase inhibitors against multidrug resistant clinical strains of *Mycobacterium tuberculosis*. *Int J Antimicrob Agents* 2004;23:408-11.

44. Rodriguez Diaz JC, Ruiz M, Lopez M, Royo G. Synergic activity of fluoroquinolones and linezolid against *Mycobacterium tuberculosis*. *Int J Antimicrob Agents* 2003;21:354-6.

45. Torun T, Gungor G, Ozmen Y, *et al*. Side effects associated with the treatment of multidrug-resistant tuberculosis. *Int J Tuberc Lung Dis* 2005; 9:1373-77.

46. Furin, JJ, Mitnick, CD, Shin, SS, *et al*. Occurrence of serious adverse effects in patients receiving community-based therapy for multidrug-resistant tuberculosis. *Int J Tuberc Lung Dis* 2001; 5:648-55

47. Chan ED, Laurel V, Strand MJ, *et al*. Treatment and outcome analysis of 205 patients with multidrug-resistant tuberculosis. *Am J Respir Crit Care Med* 2004;169:1103-9.

48. Espinal M, Dye, C, Raviglione, M, *et al*. A rational "DOTS-Plus" for the control of MDR TB. *Int J Tuberc Lung Dis* 1999;3(7):561-63.

49. Dlodlo RA, Fujiwara, Enarson DA. Controversial issues in tuberculosis: Should tuberculosis treatment and control be addressed differently in HIV-infected and -uninfected individuals? *Eur Respir J* 2005;25:751–57.

50. World Health Organization. Strategic framework to decrease the burden of TB/HIV. WHO/CDS/ TB/2002.296,WHO/HIV/AIDS/2002.2).

51. Pomerantz BJ, Cleveland JC, Olson HK, Pomerantz M. Pulmonary resection for multidrug resistant tuberculosis. *J Thorac Cardiovasc Surg* 2001;121:448-53.

52. Teasure RL, Seaworth B. Current role of surgery on *Mycobacterium tuberulosis Am Thorax Surg* 1995;59:1405-7.

53. Arora VK, Visalakshi P. Multi-drug resistant tuberculosis in context of RNTCP. *Indian J Chest Dis Allied Sci* 2003;45:215-9.

54. Leimane V, Riekstina V, Holtz TH, Zarovska E, Skripconoka V, Thorpe LE, *et al*. Clinical outcome of individualised treatment of multi-drug resistant tuberculosis in Latvia: a retrospective cohort study. *Lancet* 2005; 365:318-26.

55. Truffot-Pernot C, Ji B. Grosset J. Activities of pefloxacin and ofloxacin against mycobacteria: in vitro and mouse experiments. *Tubercle* 1991; 72:57-64.

56. Ji B, Truffot-Pernto C, Grosset J. In vitro and in vivo activities of sparfloxacin (AT 4140) against *Mycobacterium tuberculosis. Tubercle* 1991;72:181-6.

57. Munro AW, McLean KJ, Marshall KR, *et al*. Cytochromes P450: novel drug targets in the war against multidrug-resistant *Mycobacterium tuberculosis. Biochem Soc* Trans 2003; 31: 625-30.

58. Coban AY, Bayramoglu G, Ekinci B, Durupinar B. Antibacterial effect of nitric oxide. *Mikrobiyol Bui'* 2003;37:151-5.

59. Jimenez-Arellanes A, Meckes M, Ramirez R, *et al*. Activity against multidrug-resistant *Mycobacterium tuberculosis* in Mexican plants used to treat respiratory diseases. *Phytother Res* 2003; 17:903-8.

60. Xie JP, Yue J, Xiong YL, *et al*. In vitro activities of small peptides from snake venom against clinical isolates of drug-resistant *Mycobacterium tuberculosis. Int J Antimicrob Agents* 2003; 22:172 4.

61. Koh W Kwun O], Sub GY, *et al*. Six-month therapy with aerosolized interferon-gamma for refractory multidrug-resistant pulmonary tuberculosis. *J Korean Med Sci* 2004;19:167-71.

62. Chelnokova OG, Kibrik BS. Use of isofon in combined treatment of patients with acutely progressive forms of tuberculosis. *Probl Tubcrk* 2003;9:12-4.

14

HIV and Tuberculosis in Children

Indu Khosla, Tanu Singhal, Ira Shah, Joydeep Das

It is common knowledge that the two gigantic epidemics of human immuno-deficiency virus (HIV) and tuberculosis (TB) are inexorably linked and fuelling each other. HIV and TB are often referred to as "the cursed duet"[1]. According to UNAIDS and WHO Report on Global AIDS Epidemic published on July 2008, India has worlds 3rd largest burden of HIV infected patients (2.4 million) after South Africa (5.7 million) and Nigeria (2.6 million)[2]. One of every six new HIV infection occurs in India. Two Indians become HIV positive in every minutes.

According to RNTCP, status report 2008[3], India has the highest number of TB patients in the globe, bears one-fifth of global incidence, as a result India has highest number of HIV TB co-infected patients in the world. Two of every five Indians are infected with TB bacillus. Tuberculosis kills 1000 patients per day, most of them are in the age group of 15–45 years, a economically productive age group. So indirect cost of TB epidemic on India is approximately US$3 billion.

The impact of these deadly intersecting epidemics on children, though less well quantified is equally significant. With rising adult HIV seroprevalence and increasing perinatal HIV transmission a large number of HIV infected children are exposed to TB disease in their HIV infected parents. Children who escape perinatal HIV transmission and other HIV uninfected children in the community are at an increased risk of TB exposure due to increase in the adult TB pool. In a study from Zambia, TB accounted for 32% and 20% of deaths among HIV- infected children between the ages of 12–18 months and >18 months of age respectively[4]. Alternatively, HIV increased TB related mortality from 4% in HIV non-infected to 24% in HIV infected children in one African study[5].

This review attempts to deal with the manner in which these two infections impact each other, the magnitude of HIV and TB co infection in the Indian scenario, and the clinical presentation; diagnosis, management and prevention of TB in HIV infected children.

Impact of HIV on TB

Impact of HIV on risk of infection with TB—HIV increases the risk of exposure to TB indirectly by increasing the pool of TB cases in the community and not by increasing the infectivity of the cases. Several studies have shown that the risk of latent TB infection/TB disease in contacts of cases of pulmonary TB is same or lower for HIV infected as compared to HIV non-infected[6-9]. Lower risks of infection have been attributed in some studies to lower incidence of cavitation and consequently lower bacillary load in the sputum of HIV infected individuals[6].

Impact of HIV on risk of TB disease in those latently infected with TB

HIV increases the risk of TB infection progression to disease by depressing cell-mediated immunity, which is vital for TB immunity[10]. The annual risk of development of active TB following latent TB infection in HIV infected adults is estimated to be 5–10% which is 10–20 fold higher than the 5–10% lifetime risk of active TB in non HIV infected adults with latent infection[11]. In non HIV infected children, the risk of active disease following infection is 40% in infancy and 23% between the ages of 1 and 4 years[12]. Since this is much greater than the 5–10% life time risk of TB in non HIV infected adults with latent TB infection, the added impact of HIV on progression of latent childhood TB is difficult to determine but is likely to be substantial.

Impact of TB on HIV

It has been demonstrated by in vitro and in vivo studies that *Mycobacterium tuberculosis* (MTB) infection supports HIV-1 replication through its effect on host cytokines, chemokines, and their receptors[13]. Furthermore, concentrations of HIV-1 inhibitory chemokines are limited at sites of MTB infection[13]. As a clinical corollary, a retrospective cohort study among 106 HIV-infected patients with active TB and 106 HIV-infected patients without TB but with similar degrees of immunosuppression showed that the HIV TB co-infected group had greater frequency of opportunistic infections and significantly reduced survival rate, even after controlling for baseline differences and therapy for HIV infection[14].

WHO and its various HIV/AIDS and TB departments on April 2008, formulated three I's approach to decrease impact of TB on people living with HIV, these are:
1. Isoniazid preventive therapy (IPT).
2. Intensified case finding (ICF).
3. Infection (TB) control (IC).

Burden of HIV and TB Co-infection in India

Studies from Delhi and Mumbai in recent years have reported an HIV seroprevalence ranging from 6 to 8% in adult patients with TB[15,16]. Corresponding figures for children have ranged from 2% in Uttar Pradesh to 16% in Mumbai with higher prevalence in disseminated and extrapulmonary TB as compared to pulmonary TB[17-19]. These may be biased estimates due to poor selection of study population but nevertheless, TB is a sentinel infection for HIV, and HIV screening of all patients with TB particularly with disseminated TB is recommended[20].

The prevalence of TB in case series of HIV infected patients in India has been reported to range from 40–50% in adults and 30–40% in children[21-23]. The reasons for high prevalence of TB in HIV infected have already been alluded to, but over diagnosis of TB in HIV infected particularly children is not uncommon. This is because HIV, TB and some other HIV related illnesses such as lymphoid interstitial pneumonia(LIP), pneumocystis carinii pneumonia (PCP) share both clinical and radiographic features and are not easily distinguishable. An autopsy study from South

Africa revealed that whereas TB was diagnosed antemortem in 22% of the study children, postmortem studies could confirm it in only 4%[24]. TB may be underdiagnosed in HIV infected for the same reasons for which it may be overdiagnosed. Maintaining a high index of suspicion for TB in all HIV infected children is vital.

Clinical Presentation of TB in HIV Infected

TB should be considered as a differential diagnosis of any pulmonary (sometimes extra pulmonary) manifestation in HIV infected children of any age. In a case series of 87 culture confirmed TB in HIV infected children from South Africa, 11% were below the age of 3 months[25]. TB presenting as acute pneumonia in both HIV infected and uninfected children is being increasingly reported[26].

Clues to diagnosis of TB include history of contact with infectious case of TB, fever, weight loss, cough of greater than 2 weeks duration, non-response to antibiotics, pulmonary signs, generalized lymphadeno-pathy, hepatosplenomegaly, etc. Essentially the clinical manifestations of TB in HIV infected children have not been found to differ significantly from HIV non-infected children[5,10,27]. However, as mentioned earlier, the clinical features enumerated earlier are shared by HIV and HIV associated illnesses such as bronchiectasis, LIP, PCP, cytomegalo-virus pneumonia, etc.[10,24].

Unlike HIV infected adults, the prevalence of extrapulmonary disease has been reported to be similar in both HIV infected and HIV non-infected children[10].

Diagnosis of TB in HIV Infected Children

Problems

The diagnosis of TB in non-HIV infected has always been a problem owing to the pauci-bacillary nature of the disease and largely relies on history, clinical features, radiography and tuberculin test. HIV further exacerbates this problem by virtue of poor specificity of clinical and radiographic features and poor tuberculin sensitivity. Clinical scoring systems for diagnosis of TB fare poorly in areas of high HIV prevalence (specificity of only 25%) and cannot be relied upon[29].

Tuberculin skin test (TST)

HIV infected children, more so those with advanced disease are less likely to be tuber-culin positive as compared to HIV non-infected children due to poor cell mediated immunity[10]. An induration of 5 mm or more in response to 5 TU of PPD-S or 2 TU of PPD RT23 is considered as a positive tuberculin response in HIV infected children[30,31]. This has been extrapolated from adult data and its significance in HIV infected children is unknown[10]. In one study, 43% of children with culture proven TB had a TST of >10 mm. No child had an induration of 5–10 mm sugges-ting an "all or nothing" effect[28].

In spite of the poor sensitivity of the tuberculin test in HIV infected, it should still be ordered as part of investigative work up of an HIV infected child. Change in tuberculin test status due to antiretroviral therapy, nutritional rehabilitation and recent infection may occur and hence repeat testing should be done as and when indicated[32].

Radiography

The specificity of chest radiographs for diagnosis of pulmonary TB in HIV infected children is poor[5,10,33]. HIV associated bronchi-ectasis, PCP and bacterial pneumonia add to diagnostic confusion[10,24]. Miliary TB can commonly be confused with LIP. Compu-terized tomography of the chest can some-times help differentiate LIP from miliary TB[10].

Microbiology

Microbiologic yield in TB disease in HIV non-infected children is poor, the same applies to HIV infected[10]. Nevertheless all possible sites including gastric aspirates, lymph node aspirates, body fluids should be cultured. A recent study has reported sputum induction with hypertonic saline to be slightly superior to gastric aspirate for TB diagnosis in HIV infected children[34]. The yield from broncho alveolar lavage (BAL) is not superior to three gastric aspirates in non-HIV infected children with TB[35]. But in HIV infected children with non resolving/severe pneumonia, BAL may be useful in identifying unusual pathogens such as PCP and CMV.

Treatment of TB in HIV Infected Children

Treatment of HIV related TB is based on same principle as those used in non HIV related TB. In HIV-TB co-treatment, the pill burden is so high that a care giver should ensure that patient takes right drug in right doses, at right intervals, for right duration. DOTS strategy satisfy all these factors and it is practiced over 180 countries in controlling TB. It has been seen that treatment without observation achieves a success rate of 30–60%, whereas treatment with direct observation results in 85–95% success, thereby reducing emergence of drug resistance.

In DOTS strategy[37] an HIV infected patient with any kind of TB (pulmonary or extra-pulmonary) is always considered as seriously ill, so for treatment of pulmonary TB 4 drug intensive phase and 2 drug continuation phase for 2 and 4 months respectively are recommended. Actively growing bacilli are killed in intensive phase and the patient is rendered non-infective, subsequently semidormant bacilli are killed in continuation phase to prevent relapse. Duration of therapy may be extended up to 9 months for TB meningitis and TB spine.

Although there is no large scale randomized controlled pediatric trial available yet regarding daily therapy vs alternate day therapy but most of the expert are in the opinion that in extrapulmonary seriously ill TB, specially CNS TB, daily therapy is always preferred over intermittent therapy.

There are no formal efficacy studies in HIV infected children with TB. Extrapolating from adult studies and some observational pediatric studies, the American Academy of Pediatrics recommends 2 HRZE and 7 HR for treatment of TB in HIV infected children.

Interactions of antituberculosis therapy (ATT) with antiretroviral therapy (ARV)[20,36]

Many dually infected individuals are candidates for both ARV and ATT. Problems of instituting both ARV and ATT at the same time include drug interactions of the rifamycins with ARV's, a high pill burden, poor adherence, overlapping drug toxicities and a high incidence of paradoxical reactions. Rifamycins are potent inducers of the Cytochrome P450 pathway, rifampicin the most, rifapentine intermediate and rifabutin the least. Rifampicin causes significant lowering of levels and hence should not be co-administered with non-nucleoside reverse transcriptase inhibitors (NNRTI's) such as nevirapine and protease inhibitors (PI's) such as indinavir, saquinavir, nelfinavir, and amprenavir. However rifampicin may be used with boosted PI such as ritonavir/lopinavir and efavirenz. Rifabutin should not be used with hard gel saquinavir or delavirdine and cautiously with soft gel saquinavir. It may be administered at half its usual dose with indinavir, nelfinavir, amprenavir and one-fourth its usual dose with ritonavir, ritonavir/saquinavir, lopinavir/ritonavir. If used with indinavir as the sole protease inhibitor, the dose of indinavir should be increased. Rifabutin can be coadministered with nevirapine without any dose adjustment; with efavirenz the dose of rifabutin needs to be increased. In resource poor situation like ours nevirapine can be given with rifampicin by increasing the dose of nevirapine to 30%.

In view of the above mentioned problems concurrent institution of ATT and ARV is best avoided[20]. If there is no pressing reason to begin ARV, the complete course of ATT or at least the intensive phase of ATT should be completed[20]. However if the patient is in advanced stages of the illness (usually with CD4 counts >50–100/ml) and needs ARV urgently or if a patient develops TB while on ARV then concurrent ATT and ARV cannot be avoided. In such a scenario, modification of the ATT and/or ARV regimen is required. As efavirenz is contraindicated in children less than 3 years or 10 kg so options available are:

1. Increase the dose of nevirapine to 30%, so as to avoid enzyme induction effect of rifampicin and is freely available through NACO ART center.
2. Substitute rifampicin with rifabutin or rifapentin.
3. Instead of EFV or Nevirapine, add PI or boosted PI with 2NRTI which is a costly affair.

Monitoring is an important part of follow-up when ATT and ART is coadministered, child should be monitored for drug toxicity specially hepatotoxicity and occurrence of paradoxical reaction or IRIS.

Paradoxical reactions

The term paradoxical reaction refers to temporary exacerbation of symptoms, signs or radiographic manifestations of TB in patients started on antitubercular therapy[10,20]. Paradoxical reactions such as increase in size of lymph nodes and brain tuberculomas has been often reported in non-HIV patients. These phenomena are much commoner in HIV infected, more in those on ARV and even more in those who show rapid rise in CD4 counts from low baseline counts. Paradoxical reactions result from reconstitution of immune responsiveness following ARV or ATT and are also termed as immune reconstitution syndromes. Common paradoxical reactions in HIV infected patients with TB include high fevers, increase in size and inflammation of lymph nodes, new lymphadenopathy, expanding CNS lesions, worsening parenchymal infiltrates and pleural effusions. Before attributing these to paradoxical reactions, one should exclude alternative diagnosis/tubercular treatment failures. Mild reactions may be managed symptomatically. Severe reactions may necessitate use of short-term steroids. Rarely interruption of ARV is required[10].

Side effects of anti-tuberculosis drugs

Thioacetazone is contraindicated for use in HIV infected children due to high incidence of skin reactions and fatal Steven Johnson syndrome[38]. This is not of practical importance, as this drug is not used. Interestingly, Luo C *et al* reported a significant incidence of Steven Johnson's syndrome in a thioacetazone free regimen in HIV infected children with TB[39]. This observation has not been duplicated in other studies.

Prognosis of HIV infected with TB

Despite a satisfactory clinical and microbiological response in TB disease in HIV infected following initiation of ATT, most studies report increased mortality in HIV seropositive adults with TB despite ATT[10]. Early deaths during treatment may be related to TB, but deaths during the continuation phase are often related to advanced HIV disease. Studies in HIV infected children with TB have also reported high mortality on follow up (as high as 25% in one study)[5,33,40]. The poor final outcome is not due to inadequacy of ATT and cannot be altered with intensification or prolongation of ATT.

Multidrug Resistant (MDR) TB and HIV

HIV is not considered as an independent risk factor for MDR TB in adults and MDR rates do not differ significantly between HIV infected and non-infected adults in developing countries[10]. But HIV significantly worsens the outcome of MDR TB, with one series reporting 80% mortality in 4–19 weeks despite aggressive drug therapy[41]. In children, diagnosis of MDR TB is difficult as microbiologic confirmation is often not available. History of contact with an MDR adult patient is a helpful diagnostic clue. Non-response to ATT in HIV infected children should not be considered as evidence for MDR and institution of second line therapy. Other causes of therapeutic failure such as wrong diagnosis, poor adherence, drug interactions and paradoxical reactions should also be considered.

Prevention of TB in HIV Infected

Role of BCG

Studies prior to the advent of HIV have reported the protective effect of BCG to vary widely from 0–80%[42]. There is more agreement about the efficacy of BCG in protection against disseminated and meningeal disease in children[43].

There is insufficient evidence on the efficacy of BCG in HIV infected individuals. A study from Thailand reported a significantly higher incidence of non-reactivity to tuberculin, a negative tuberculin test and absence of BCG scar at 9 months in HIV infected children as compared to HIV non infected children. Longitudinal studies to indicate whether this low tuberculin conversion also predicts less

protection against natural infection are not available. Evidence for efficacy of the vaccine against clinical disease in children is limited to a single case control study from Zambia[45]. It reported an protective efficacy of 59% in HIV uninfected children as against no protection in HIV infected children. The results should be interpreted with caution since the diagnosis of HIV in infants <18 months was based on only a positive serology and the vaccination status was assessed by presence of a scar which may have lead to misclassification bias.

Complications arising from BCG vaccination include regional, extraregional localized, and disseminated disease. BCG causes local ulcers and regional lymphadenitis in normal hosts at rates varying from 4 to 30 per 1000 vaccinated infants[46]. Cases of regional lymphadenitis, poorly healing ulcers, and fistulae in HIV–infected infants have been frequently reported but at similar rates as in HIV–uninfected infants (lymphadenitis has been more severe in HIV–infected children)[47]. The risk of dissemination of BCG in the general population is estimated to be 3.4/ million babies vaccinated and 1% in children with congenital immunodeficiencies[46]. Only a handful of cases of disseminated BCG disease in HIV infected children and adults have been reported till date[47]. This is clearly an underestimate of the true problem owing to inadequate follow up and non-inclusion of mycobacterial blood cultures, biopsies and autopsies in most studies. Cross sectional studies have however failed to detect BCG bacteremia in severely immunosuppressed BCG vaccinated HIV infected children and adults[48,49].

On the strength of evidence available so far though the risk with BCG use appears to be low, its efficacy in HIV infected children is doubtful. Consequently the Advisory Committee for Immunization Practices (ACIP) and

American Academy of Pediatrics (AAP) recommend against routine BCG use in HIV infected in the United States where the risk of natural exposure to TB is low[50]. In developing nations however infants are at high risk of infection more so with high prevalence of TB in HIV infected adults often in the same household. The HIV serostatus of mothers is usually not known, even if known that of the newborn is not easy to establish till later in life. Moreover most of the infants born to seropositive mothers will be uninfected. Thus the WHO policy of continuing vaccination to all newborns makes sense from a population perspective as BCG will benefit infants uninfected with HIV and probably not alter the prognosis of the HIV- infected. The WHO however recommends against the use of the vaccine in children with symptomatic HIV[51].

Chemoprophylaxis[20,30,32,52]

It is fairly obvious that prevention of TB in HIV infected children is of utmost importance. Since efficacy of BCG is doubtful, chemoprophylaxis is the other alternative. In a meta analysis of randomized controlled trials in HIV-1 infected adults, INH prophylaxis in TST positive individuals was associated with a 48% reduction in cases of TB but no reduction in mortality[10]. Almost all recommendations pertaining to chemoprophylaxis for TB are based on adult studies as relevant studies in children are completely lacking[10].

Who merits chemoprophylaxis?[32]

i. Children with a TST reaction size of ≥5 mm following 5TU of PPD-S/ 2 TU of PPD RT23 who have not previously received treatment for *M. tuberculosis* infection/disease, regardless of their age.

ii. Children with recent contact with an infectious TB patient, regardless of their age, results of TSTs, or history of previous TB treatment.

iii. Children with a history of prior untreated or inadequately treated past TB that healed and no history of adequate treatment for TB, regardless of their age or results of TSTs.

In all the above instances, active tuberculosis should be ruled out by appropriate clinical evaluation and laboratory tests. The TST should be repeated yearly in all TST negative children to determine tuberculin conversion and hence need for TB preventive therapy. The TST should also be repeated in previously TST negative children if immune function has been restored with highly active antiretroviral therapy (HAART).

It had been proposed earlier that HIV infected individuals with advanced immunosupression may be anergic and thus be TST negative despite being infected with TB. Hence why rely on the TST for determining need for TB preventive therapy? However, studies have reported no reduction in incidence of TB disease following administration of chemoprophylaxis to TST negative HIV-1 infected adults[32].

What regime to use?

The preferred regime for treatment of latent TB infection in adult HIV patients is daily or twice weekly isoniazid for 9 months. Pyridoxine supplementation with isoniazid is required. Studies have clearly demonstrated superiority of a 9 month regime as compared to a 6 month regime for TB preventive therapy in HIV infected adults[52]. Alternative regimes in adults include 4 months of therapy daily with either rifampin or rifabutin; or 2 months of therapy with either rifampin and pyrazinamide or rifabutin and pyrazinamide. Since the 2 month regimen of rifampin and pyrazinamide has been associated with fatal and severe liver injury, it is better avoided.

The recommended regime for TB preventive therapy in HIV infected children is daily isoniazid at 5 mg/kg for 12 months[32].

There are a number of problems in extrapolating adult chemoprophylaxis studies to HIV-1 infected children. Adults usually acquire TB infection prior to HIV and thus are at risk for developing disease due to reactivation/ reinfection. Conversely, most children acquire HIV prior to TB and hence the focus should be on preventing or attenuating primary infection. Trials addressing these issues are currently underway[10].

Conclusions

HIV and TB intersect and potentiate each other at various levels. TB increases HIV replication, HIV related morbidity and mortality and is the commonest opportunistic infection in HIV infected individuals. HIV increases the risk of progression of TB infection to disease and TB related mortality. Over diagnosis and under diagnosis of TB in HIV infected children are common owing to sharing of clinical and radiographic features with HIV itself and other HIV related illnesses. Standard therapy for tuberculosis in HIV infected is 2 HRZE and 7 HR. The rifamycins have complex drug interactions with most ARV's. Concurrent ATT and ARV should be avoided as far as possible. The possibility of paradoxical reactions as a reason for clinical worsening in HIV infected children with TB should be considered. Chemoprophylaxis with 12 months of daily isoniazid is recommended for all children with a positive TST ($\geq$ 5 mm)/ recent contact with infectious TB/past history of inadequately treated tuberculosis. BCG administration to all asymptomatic HIV infected children should be continued and surveillance to detect BCG adverse effects strengthened.

References

1. Chretien J. Tuberculosis and HIV. The cursed duet. *Bull Int Union Tuberc Lung Dis* 1990;65:25-32.

2. UNAIDS/WHO. 2008 Report on Global AIDS epidemic,Executive Summery by UNAIDS / WHO published in July 2008.

3. TB INDIA 2008, RNTCP status report, published by Central TB division, Director General of Health Services, Ministry of Health and Family Welfare, Govt. of India. Sep. 2008. page 12.

4. Chintu C, Mudenda V, Lucas S, *et al.* Lung diseases at necropsy in African children dying from respiratory illnesses: a descriptive necropsy study. *Lancet* 2002;360:985-90.

5. Mukadi YD, Wiktor SZ, Coulibaly IM, *et al.* Impact of HIV infection on the development, clinical presentation, and outcome of tuberculosis among children in Abidjan, Cote d'Ivoire. *AIDS* 1997;11:1151-8.

6. Elliott AM, Hayes RJ, Halwiindi B, Luo N, Tembo G, Pobee JO *et al.* The impact of HIV on infectiousness of pulmonary tuberculosis: a community study in Zambia. *AIDS* 1993;7:981-7.

7. Klausner JD, Ryder RW, Baende E, *et al.* Mycobacterium tuberculosis in household contacts of human immunodeficiency virus type 1-seropositive patients with active pulmonary tuberculosis in Kinshasa, Zaire. *J Infect Dis* 1993; 168:106-11.

8. Espinal MA, Perez EN, Baez J, Henriquez L, Fernandez K, Lopez M, *et al.* Infectiousness of Mycobacterium tuberculosis in HIV-1-infected patients with tuberculosis: a prospective study. *Lancet.* 2000;355:275-80.

9. Cruciani M, Malena M, Bosco O, *et al.* The impact of human immunodeficiency virus type 1 on infectiousness of tuberculosis: a meta-analysis. *Clin Infect Dis* 2001;33:1922-30.

10. Cotton MF, Schaaf HS, Hesseling AC, Madhi SA. HIV and Childhood tuberculosis: the way forward. *Int J tuberc Lung Dis* 2004;8:675-682.

11. Dolin PJ, Raviglione MC, Kochi A. Global tuberculosis incidence and mortality during 1990-2000. *Bull WHO* 1994;72:213-20.

12. Miller FJW, Seale RME, Taylor MD. Tuberculosis in Children. Boston, MA: Little Brown, 1963.

13. Collins KR, Quinones-Mateu ME, Toossi Z, Arts EJ. Impact of tuberculosis on HIV-1 replication, diversity, and disease progression. *AIDS Rev* 2002;4:165-76.

14. Whalen C, Horsburgh CR Jr, Hom D, *et al.* Accelerated course of human immunodeficiency virus infection after tuberculosis. *Am J Respir Crit Care Med* 1995;151:129-35.

15. Sharma SK, Aggarwal G, Seth P, Saha PK. Increasing HIV seropositivity among adult tuberculosis patients in Delhi. *Indian J Med Res* 2003;117:239-42.

16. Gothi D, Joshi JM. Clinical and laboratory observations of tuberculosis at a Mumbai (India) clinic. *Postgrad Med J* 2004;80:97-100.

17. Shahab T, Zoha MS, Malik MA, Malik A, Afzal K. Prevalence of human immunodeficiency virus infection in children with tuberculosis. *Indian Pediatr* 2004;41:595-9.

18. Merchant RH, Shroff RC. HIV seroprevalence in disseminated tuberculosis and chronic diarrhoea. *Indian Pediatr* 1998;35:883-7.

19. Karande S, Bhalke S, Kelkar A, *et al.* Utility of clinically-directed selective screening to diagnose HIV infection in hospitalized children in Bombay. *Indian J Trop Pediatr* 2002;48:149-55.

20. Centers for Disease Control and Prevention. Treatment of Tuberculosis. American Thoracic Society, CDC, and Infectious Diseases Society of America. *MMWR* 2003;52(No RR-11):1-74.

21. Sircar AR, Tripathi AK, Choudhary SK, Misra R. Clinical profile of AIDS: a study at a referral hospital. *J Assoc Physicians India* 1998;46:775-8.

22. Madhivanan P, Mothi SN, Kumarasamy N, Yepthomi T, Venkatesan C, Lambert JS, Solomon S. Clinical manifestations of HIV infected children. *Indian J Pediatr* 2003;70:615-20.

23. Merchant RH, Oswal JS, Bhagwat RV, Karkare J. Clinical profile of HIV infection. *Indian Pediatr* 2001;38:239-46.

24. Rennert WP, Kilner D, Hale M, *et al.* Tuberculosis in children dying with HIV-related lung disease: clinical-pathological correlations. *Int J Tuberc Lung Dis* 2002;6:806-13.

25. Hesseling AC, Werschkul H, Westra A, *et al.* The clinical features and outcome of confirmed tuberculosis in HIV-infected children. *Int J Tuberc Lung Dis* 2002;6(Suppl 1):S181.

26. Zar HJ. Pneumonia in HIV-infected and HIV-uninfected children in developing countries: epidemiology, clinical features, and management. *Curr Opin Pulm Med* 2004;10:176-82.

27. Chintu C, Bhat G, Luo C, Raviglione M, Diwan V, Dupont HL, *et al.* Seroprevalence of human immunodeficiency virus type 1 infection in Zambian children with tuberculosis. *Pediatr Infect Dis J* 1993;12:499-504.

28. Schaaf HS, Geldenhuys A, Gie RP, Cotton MF. Culture-positive tuberculosis in human immunodeficiency virus type 1-infected children. *Pediatr Infect Dis J* 1998;17:599-604.

29. Van Rheenen P. The use of the paediatric tuberculosis score chart in an HIV-endemic area. *Trop Med Int Health* 2002;7:435-41.

30. Centers for Disease Control and Prevention. Targeted tuberculin testing and treatment of latent tuberculosis infection. *MMWR* 2000;49 (No. RR-6):1-43.

31. Lee E, Holzman RS. Evolution and current use of the tuberculin test. *Clin Infect Dis* 2002;34:365-70.

32. Kaplan JE, Masur H, Holmes KK; USPHS; Infectious Disease Society of America. Guidelines for preventing opportunistic infections among HIV-infected persons—2002. Recommendations of the U.S. Public Health Service and the Infectious Diseases Society of America. *MMWR Recomm Rep* 2002;51(RR-8):1-52.

33. Palme IB, Gudetta B, Bruchfeld J, Muhe L, Giesecke J. Impact of human immunodeficiency virus 1 infection on clinical presentation, treatment outcome and survival in a cohort of Ethiopian children with tuberculosis. *Pediatr Infect Dis J* 2002;21:1053-61.

34. Zar HJ, Tannenbaum E, Hanslo D, Hussey G. Sputum induction as a diagnostic tool for community-acquired pneumonia in infants and young children from a high HIV prevalence area. *Pediatr Pulmonol* 2003;36:58-62.

35. Chan S, Abadco D, Steiner P. Role of flexible fibreoptic bronchoscopy in the diagnosis of childhood endobronchial tuberculosis. *Pediatr Infect Dis J* 1994;13:506-9.

36. Panel on Clinical Practices for Treatment of HIV Infection. Guidelines for the Use of Antiretroviral Agents in HIV-1 Infected Adults and Adolescents, 2004. Available from: URL: http:/\ AIDSinfo.nih.gov

37. Daley P. Distance Learning Module 12, HIV & TB, Fellowship in HIV Medicine, 2007. page 54-55.

38. Chintu C, Luo C, Bhat G, *et al.* Cutaneous hypersensitivity reactions due to thiacetazone in the treatment of tuberculosis in Zambian children infected with HIV-I. *Arch Dis Child* 1993;68:665-8.

39. Luo C, Chintu C, Bhat G, *et al.* Human immunodeficiency virus type-1 infection in Zambian children with tuberculosis: changing seroprevalence and evaluation of a thioacetazone free regimen. *Tuber Lung Dis* 1994;75:110-5.

40. Jeena PM, Mitha T, Bamber S, *et al*. Effects of the human immunodeficiency virus on tuberculosis in children. *Tuber Lung Dis*. 1996;77:437-43.

41. Iseman MD. Treatment of Multidrug-Resistant Tuberculosis. *N Engl J Med* 1993;329:784-91.

42. Colditz GA, Brewer TF, Berkey CS, *et al*. Efficacy of BCG vaccine in the prevention of tuberculosis. Meta–analysis of the published literature. *JAMA* 1994;271:698–702.

43. Thilothammal N, Krishnamurthy PV, Runyan DK, Banu K. Does BCG vaccine prevent tuberculous meningitis? *Arch Dis Child* 1996;74: 144-7.

44. Thaithumyanon P, Thisyakorn U, Punnahita-nanda S, Praisuwanna P, Ruxrungtham K. Safety and immunogenicity of Bacillus Calmette-Guérin vaccine in children born to HIV-1 infected women. *Southeast Asian J Trop Med Pub Hlth* 2000; 31:482-6.

45. Bhat GJ, Diwan VK, Chintu C, *et al*. HIV, BCG and TB in children: A case control study in Lusaka, Zambia. *J Trop Pediatr* 1993;39:219–22.

46. Lotte A, Wasz - Hockert P, Poisson N, Dumitrescu N, Verron M, Couvet E. BCG complications: Estimates of the risks among vaccinated subjects and statistical analysis of their main characteristics. *AdvTuber Res* 1984;21: 107-93.

47. Moss WJ, Clements CJ, Halsey NA. Immuniza-tion of children at risk of infection with human immunodeficiency virus. *Bull WHO* 2003;81:61-70.

48. Marsh BJ, von Reyn CF, Edwards J, Ristola MA, Bartholomew C, Brindle RJ, *et al*. The risks and benefits of childhood bacille Calmette–Guérin immunization among adults with AIDS. *AIDS* 1997;11:669–72.

49. Archibald LK, Kazembe PN, Nwanyanwu O, Mwansambo C, Reller LB, Jarvis WR. Epidemiology of bloodstream infections in a bacille Calmette-Guérin-vaccinated pediatric population in Malawi. *J Infect Dis* 2003;188:202-8.

50. Evaluation and medical treatment of the HIV-exposed infant. American Academy of Pediatrics. Committee on Pediatric AIDS. *Pediatr* 1997;99: 909-17.

51. World Health Organization. Immunization policy. Geneva: World Health Organization; 1996. WHO document WHO/EPI/GEN/95.03.p. 25–7). Available from: URL: http://whqlibdoc.who.int/hq/1995/WHO-EPI- GEN-95.03-ev.1.pdf

52. Prevention and treatment of tuberculosis among patients infected with human immunodeficiency virus: principles of therapy and revised recommendations. Centers for Disease Control and Prevention. *MMWR Recomm Rep* 1998; 47(RR-20):1-58.

15

BCG Vaccine and Other New Vaccines to Prevent Tuberculosis in Children

Digant D Shastri

Introduction

Infectious diseases are the largest cause of death in the world, and tuberculosis is the second largest cause of death in the world from any single infectious disease, behind only HIV/AIDS. In the year 2006 more than 2 billion people, equal to one-third of the world's population, were infected with TB bacill, there were 9.2 million new TB cases and 1.7 million people died from TB in 2006 including 231,000 people with HIV. This is equal to 4,500 deaths a day. Every year an estimated 490,000 new MDR TB cases occurs. The WHO estimates that between 2000 and 2020 tuberculosis will cause 200 million people to get sick and will kill 35 million people.[1-3]. Despite the availability of cheap and effective curative and preventive therapy and with more than 4–5 billion persons across the world have received the BCG vaccine still tuberculosis remains the "Captain of Death of Men".

Composition

Vaccine is supplied as multi-dose (10 dose) vial plus diluent (1 ml of sodium chloride). Each dose of the vaccine (0.1ml) contains 1×10^5 and 33×10^5 colony forming units.

Storage and Stability

The undiluted vaccine should be stored in dark between 2° and 8°C. Reconstituted vaccine should be used immediately and any not used by the end of the day should be destroyed. The reconstituted vaccine should be stored at 4°C. Vaccine should not be exposed to sunlight. Exposure to artificial light should be kept to a minimum[4].

Route of Administration

Different routes/techniques for the BCG vaccination has been tried with advantages and disadvantages associated with that particular route. Most current BCG vaccines are given by the intradermal route, generally by injection with a 25 or 26 gauge needle, in the deltoid insertion region of the upper arm.

    i. *Intradermal route*—It is the most commonly accepted route of BCG vaccination Advantage: This is the most accurate method because the dose can be controlled. Although many body sites can be used for vaccination, the most commonly used site is the deltoid insertion region of the upper arm. Disadvantage:

1. Intradermal injection can be difficult in newborns, especially if a large number of infants require vaccine fairly rapidly.
2. The rate of local reactions, including ulcers and lymphadenitis, is higher with the intradermal method than with any other method.
3. The intradermal method is relatively expensive. Despite these problems, the intradermal method remains widely used throughout the world.

ii. *Subcutaneous route:*

Advantage: This technique is easier to learn. It gives adequate results in terms of induced tuberculin sensitivity. In one study, just under 16% of infants immunized in this way were found to be tuberculin negative on skin testing three months later.

Disadvantage: Frequently produces abscesses and unsightly, retracted scars.

iii. *Multiple puncture:* This technique has been developed in 1940s with good early success. In Japan this technique has been used for more than 40 years with very low rate of adverse reaction.

iv *Other techniques:* Many different techniques are tried for BCG immunization such as scarification, jet injection, and use of bifurcated needles.

Advantage: These techniques are associated with lower incidence of local complications. In this method only single dose vaccine is used, there is no risk of cross contamination among vaccine recipients.

Disadvantage: These different techniques have yielded highly variable and, in some case, inaccurate results.

Dosage

Dosages of BCG vaccine differs by vaccine strain and age of the recipient. For each strain, the dosage is adjusted to maximize the protective effect and minimizing the local complications. In general newborns are given half of the standard dose. Dose in adults and children over 1 year of age is 0.1 ml (100 µg) and children under 1 year of age are given 0.05 ml (50 µg) intradermally.

Timing for Immunization

There is wide disparity among nations concerning vaccine schedules. The official recommendation of the WHO is a single dose given in infancy[5,6]. However, only three prospective community trials have evaluated the efficacy of BCG vaccine given at birth. Studies of lymphocyte blastogenesis in response to PPD have shown much higher rates of immunogenic sensitization in children when BCG vaccination is delayed from the first week to 9 months of life[7,8]. However, even low-birth-weight newborns develop lymphocyte proliferation and interleukin-2 production in response to a BCG vaccine[9]. In the United Kingdom, a single dose of BCG is administered during adolescence. Many countries give the first dose of BCG in infancy then give repeated vaccinations throughout childhood. Absence of a scar after BCG vaccination does not correlate with lack of tuberculin sensitivity or any specific immunological parameter. It is reasonable that the recommended schedules would vary with the local epidemiology of tuberculosis; age groups at highest risk of disease (young children versus adolescents or young adults). It must be concluded that the optimal age for administration and schedule (single versus multiple doses) has not been firmly established because adequate comparative trials have not been reported.

Indications

BCG vaccine is indicated for the vaccination of tuberculin negative individuals against tuberculosis. BCG vaccine is recommended to administer only to individuals who have not been infected by the tubercle bacillus and who are negative to the tuberculin PPD (Mantoux) test. In neonates prior tuberculin testing before BCG vaccination is usually not deemed necessary. BCG vaccination policies differ greatly between different countries.

BCG only at birth (or first contact with health services)

This is the current recommendation of the EPI and the Global Tuberculosis Programme (GTB), and is the policy in most of the world today, in particular in developing countries. WHO has emphasized this policy , because of consistent evidence that BCG protects against serious childhood forms of tuberculosis, even where it may not protect to a high degree against adult pulmonary forms of the disease[10].

BCG in symptomatic HIV positive/immunocompromised children

There is considerable debate about giving the BCG vaccine to newborn infants who are known to be at risk of HIV infection.

In most developing and some industrialized countries where both diseases are significantly more common. It is recommended that where the risk of childhood TB is high, BCG should be given to infants as early as possible, even if mothers are known to have HIVinfection[11-13]. It would be difficult, in any case, to identify and subsequently exclude those infants who are already HIV infected. WHO currently recommends BCG vaccination for asymptomatic HIV-infected children who are at high risk for infection with *M. tuberculosis*. A recent review has concluded that there may be a slight increase in minor adverse reactions after the administration of BCG to infants with asymptomatic HIV infection and that the benefits of immunization outweigh the risk of complications[14] (i.e. in countries in which the prevalence of TB is high). WHO does not recommend BCG vaccination for children who have symptomatic HIV infection or for persons known or suspected to be infected with HIV if they are at minimal risk for infection with *M. tuberculosis*.

BCG Vaccination for Prevention and Control of TB among HIV-Infected Persons

Several studies have been conducted to determine the safety of BCG vaccination in HIV-infected children and adults. The results of these studies were inconsistent. The protective efficacy of BCG vaccination in HIV-infected persons is unknown. Therefore, the use of BCG vaccine in HIV-infected persons is not recommended. In high risk individual TB preventive therapy should be administered, unless contraindicated, to HIV-infected persons who might be co-infected with *M. tuberculosis*. In Uganda, the preliminary results of a study indicate that preventive therapy with isoniazid in HIV-infected persons was associated with few side effects and a 61% reduction in the risk for active TB disease[15] (after a median length of follow-up of 351 days) .

Contraindications

i. Individuals suffering from conditions which have lead to immunosuppression such as measles, whooping cough, exudative or inflammatory dermatologic conditions.

ii. Until the risks and benefits of BCG vaccination in immunocompromised populations are clearly defined, BCG vaccination should not be administered to persons (a) with impaired immunologic responses because of HIV infection, congenital immunodeficiency, leukemia, lymphoma, or generalized malignancy or (b) whose immunologic responses have been suppressed by steroids, alkylating agents, antimetabolites, or radiation[16,17].

Skin reaction at BCG vaccination site

Normal reactions to the vaccine are characterized by the formation of a bluish-red papule within 1–3 weeks after vaccination. After approximately 6 weeks, the pustule ulcerates, forming a lesion approximately 5 mm in diameter. Draining lesions resulting from vaccination should be kept clean and bandaged. Scabs form and heal usually within 3 months after vaccination. BCG vaccination generally results in a permanent scar at the puncture site (typically round and slightly depressed). The probability that BCG vaccination leaves a lasting scar is lower after vaccination in early infancy than at older ages. Individuals with dormant tuberculosis infection often have an accelerated response to BCG vaccine characterized by induration within 1 to 2 days and scab formation and healing within 10 to 15 days.

Adverse Effects

BCG is considered to be a safe vaccine with a low incidence of adverse effects. Although BCG vaccination often results in local adverse effects, serious or long-term complications are rare. Complications are more likely to occur in infants, where large doses of BCG are inadvertently given or with faulty technique. Higher rates of local reactions may result from using subcutaneous injection in comparison with reactions from intradermal injection. Suppurative adenitis has been reported in 4% of infants who have received intradermal BCG

and 0.3% of older children; osteomyelitis is an uncommon complication and disseminated BCG infection is extremely rare in normal children, occurring in about one to three cases per million doses[18].

BCG vaccination often results in permanent scarring at the injection site. Hypertrophic scars occur in an estimated 28–33% of vaccinated persons, and keloid scars occur in approximately 2–4%[19,20]. Keloid formation on the scar site appears to be more common in African and Asian populations than in others.

More severe local reactions include ulceration at the vaccination site, regional suppurative lymphadenitis with draining sinuses, and caseous lesions or purulent drainage at the puncture site; these manifestations might occur within the 5 months after vaccination and could persist for several weeks. If small cold abscesses should appear, spontaneous resorption usually occurs. In a few instances, the abscess may soften and may open spontaneously producing an ulcer. If an abscess forms, it may be punctured with a syringe and a fine needle in order to avoid ulceration and scar formation[21,22].

The opinion vary regarding the management of BCG adenitis, majority resolves with time but some cases may be indolent and may form fistulas tract. A course of 2 weeks of erythromycin have shown benefit in some cases[23]. Some recommend total surgical excision to prevent chronic suppuration and fistula formation.

The most serious complication of BCG vaccination is disseminated BCG infection[24-27]. BCG osteitis affecting the epiphyses of the long bones, particularly the epiphyses of the leg, can occur from 4 months to 2 years after vaccination. The risk for developing osteitis after BCG vaccination varies by country; in one review, this risk ranged from 0.01 cases per million vaccinees in Japan to 32.5 and 43.4 cases per million vaccinees in Sweden and

Finland, respectively[27]. Regional increases in the incidence of BCG osteitis have been noted following changes in either the vaccine strain or the method of production. The skeletal lesions can be treated effectively with anti-TB medications, although surgery also has been necessary in some cases.

Case reports of other severe adverse reactions in adults have included erythema multiforme, pulmonary TB, and meningitis[28-29]. Fatal disseminated BCG disease has occurred at a rate of 0.06–1.56 cases per million doses of vaccine administered. Anti-TB therapy is recommended for treatment of disseminated BCG infection.

In summary, millions of persons worldwide have been vaccinated with BCG vaccine, and serious or long-term complications after vaccination were infrequent. Possible factors affecting the rate of adverse reactions include the BCG dose, vaccine strain, and method of vaccine administration.

Tuberculin skin testing and interpretation of results after BCG vaccination post vaccination BCG-induced tuberculin reactivity ranges from no induration to an induration of 19 mm at the skin-test site[30,31]. Tuberculin reactivity caused by BCG vaccination wanes with the passage of time and is unlikely to persist >10 years after vaccination in the absence of repeated *M. tuberculosis* exposure and infection[32,33]. The presence or size of a post vaccination tuberculin skin-test reaction does not predict whether BCG will provide any protection against TB disease. Moreover, the size of a tuberculin skin-test reaction in a BCG-vaccinated person is not a factor in determining whether the reaction is caused by *M. tuberculosis* infection or the prior BCG vaccination[34,35].

Duration of Immunity

Since there is no serological test to measure immunity to tuberculosis and the immune response after BCG vaccination estimates are based on data from clinical trials and case-control studies the exact duration of immunity after BCG vaccination is not known. Kassimi and colleagues in their case control study compared BCG vaccine status in 537 cases of tuberculosis with 5756 normal control subjects. All subjects were vaccinated in the neonatal period, and protection was estimated by age group of years after vaccination. The study found decreasing protection with increasing age, demonstrating a waning immunity 20 years after vaccination[36]. Experts speculate that protection declines over time and is probably nonexistent 10 to 20 years after vaccination.

BCG Vaccine Efficacy

Since its introduction in 1921 over 4 billion doses of the vaccine have been given world wide. Although BCG remains the world's most popular vaccine with over 80% coverage of the world's population, there is considerable debate with respect to its effectiveness in the control of TB. The true effectiveness of BCG has been debated for decades.

A meta-analysis of more than 1200 articles from international publications has concluded that the overall protective value of BCG against all forms of TB was of the order of just 50%, but that protection against more serious infection was greater, being 64% and 78% against tuberculous meningitis and disseminated infection, respectively[37,38].

Reported rates of the protective efficacy of BCG vaccines might have been affected by:

i. Variation in study validity.

ii. Use of differing BCG preparations.

iii. Diverse population genetics and levels of nutrition.

iv. Environmental factors such as exposure to environmental (atypical) mycobacteria, climate, socioeconomic issues, and sunlight.

v. The methods and routes of vaccine administration.

Since 1975, case-control studies using different BCG strains indicated that vaccine efficacies ranged from 0 to 80%[39,40]. In young children, the estimated protective efficacy rates of the vaccine have ranged from 52% to 100% for prevention of tuberculous meningitis and miliary TB and from 2% to 80% for prevention of pulmonary TB[41,42]. Most vaccine studies have been restricted to newborns and young children; few studies have assessed vaccine efficacy in persons who received initial vaccination as adults. The largest community-based controlled trial of BCG vaccination was conducted from 1968 to 1971 in Chingelput-southern India. Although two different vaccine strains that were considered the most potent available were used in this study, no protective efficacy in either adults or children was demonstrated 5 years after vaccination. These vaccine recipients were re-evaluated 15 years after BCG vaccination, at which time the protective efficacy in persons who had been vaccinated as children was 17%; no protective effect was demonstrated in persons who had been vaccinated as adolescents or adults.

In summary, the recently conducted meta-analyses of BCG protective efficacy have confirmed that the vaccine efficacy for preventing serious forms of tuberculosis in children is high (i.e. >80%).

Simultaneous Administration with Other Vaccines

BCG vaccine can be administered safely with other childhood vaccines. It is impossible to measure whether simultaneous adminis-tration reduces the efficacy of BCG, because there is no serological test for the immune response.

BCG Vaccination during Pregnancy

Although no harmful effects on the fetus have been observed, use of BCG is not recommen-ded during pregnancy unless there is an excessive risk or unavoidable exposure to infective tuberculosis.

Other Uses of BCG Vaccine

Freeze Dried Therapeutic BCG Vaccine

For the management of superficial bladder cancer intravesical bacillus Calmette-Guérin (BCG) immunotherapy is found to be highly effective in high-grade tumors and provides long-term protection from tumor recurrence and reduces disease progression.

Future Developments[43-45]

Tuberculosis will be eliminated only if new, more effective vaccines are developed. Modern molecular genetics and biotechnology techniques should be applied rapidly to this problem. Recent research has described the role of Th1 and Th2 cells as well as the possible regulatory function of certain adrenal steroid metabolites. One experimental adjunct to treatment, based on immunotherapy, attempts to alter the immune response from one of tissue damage to that of bactericidal activity. *Mycobacterium vaccae* is a relatively harmless environmental species that has been used in immunotherapy, with some encouraging results in patients with active tuberculosis.

Future Vaccines for Tuberculosis[46-48]

Today, most of the world's population is vaccinated with BCG. It is generally accepted that BCG protects against childhood TB but this immunity wanes with age, resulting in no or insufficient protection against TB. Several laboratories are pursuing the development of new tuberculosis vaccines in an international collaborative research effort coordinated by WHO's Immunology of Mycobacteria (IMMYC) task force. Different approaches are attracting attention.

1. One is based on the identification and evaluation of subunit antigens of the tubercle bacillus. There is particular interest in secretory antigens, such as "ESAT-6" and the "antigen 85" complex, which are thought to be released by tubercle bacilli early in the infection process. It is thus argued that an immune response to these antigens might affect tubercle bacilli early in the course of an infection[49,50].

   Advantages: Fewer adverse reactions and are easier to manufacture reproducibly than whole cell vaccines.

   Disadvantages: Relatively expensive purification of material, short-lived duration of immunity (would likely require booster shots and complex adjuvant or delivery systems).

2. Another approach is based upon the development of mutant or auxotropic strains of BCG or other mycobacteria in order to set up time-limited infections in the host but still induce protective immune responses[51].

   Advantages: Potential ability to engender immunological memory that persists for long periods of time, induces immune responses at mucosal surfaces, and be relatively inexpensive.

   Disadvantages: Risk of adverse effects since it is a live attenuated vaccine - particularly in immunodeficient hosts.

3. Yet another approach involves the delivery of DNA, encoding various specific mycobacterial antigens within plasmid carriers. This DNA is taken-up by host muscle cells, where it is translated into foreign proteins that induce specific antibody and T cell responses[51-53].

Advantages: Simplicity, possibility of introducing multiple antigens at low cost. *Disadvantages:* Long-term efficacy and safety of naked DNA vaccines have not been established in humans.

Public Health Considerations

For most infectious diseases, the expectation is that the availability of potent vaccine can lead to the elimination of disease from human populations. Clearly, the BCG vaccines have not led to the elimination of tuberculosis from any country in the world. The distribution of these vaccines to 4 billion people has had almost no effect on the worldwide epidemiology of tuberculosis.

In most developing countries, BCG was introduced as an emergency measure because it was the only inexpensive tuberculosis control measure that could be applied on a national scale. With the advent of effective and inexpensive chemotherapy, a two-pronged approach:

a. Case finding and treatment of the case.

b. BCG vaccination, tuberculosis control became possible. In developing countries early effective vaccination can be the only effective measure to reduce the development of disease in children because[54,55].

   i. Current health care facility is not up to level were the case finding and case treatment can have significant impact on the tuberculosis control.

   ii. In most of the cases the transmission of the tuberculosis in children occurs before the adult source can be identified.

   iii. Lack of sensitive diagnostic technique for confirming the diagnosis of tuberculosis in children precludes early effective treatment.

   iv. In developing countries source of the tuberculosis transmission to children is usually within their house hold, where early vaccination with the BCG vaccine is the only effective public measure to prevent cases of childhood TB.

As the protection offered by BCG vaccination is of limited duration the BCG vaccination in children will not be able to prevent infectious pulmonary tuberculosis among adult population. In developed countries protecting high risk adults – specially those working with patients who have multidrug resistant TB is becoming a critical need as the chemotherapy is not effective in such situation[56]. Also it is not clear whether "booster" immunization with BCG can maintain or even enhance protection against tuberculosis. The WHO has recommended that a single dose of BCG vaccine should be given to all newborns in developing countries. This dose will have economic impact and short term impact on the mortality without significant contribution to the control of tuberculosis.

Conclusions

An improved vaccine that would provide greater protection against *M tuberculosis*, although technically feasible, is still far from being an achievable goal. In the meantime, BCG remains an effective and safe vaccine when given[57]. Local BCG immunization program should be defined in accordance with local need, coordinated and implemented by multidisciplinary groups, and evaluated by means of clinical audit. It must also be remembered that the use of BCG is just one important aspect of the overall process of tuberculosis control. Vigilance, early detection of children who have been infected with *M tuberculosis,* and effective treatment for those with active disease is also required. Pediatricians who are relatively unfamiliar with childhood TB may need to re-educate themselves in this area.

References

1. Ravoglione MC, *et al* Global epidemiology of tuberculosis: morbidity and mortality of a worldwide epidemic. *JAMA* 1995;273:220-26.
2. Kochi A. The global tuberculosis situation and the new control strategy of the World Health Organization. *Tubercle* 1991;72:1-6.
3. http://www.who.int/tb-Factsheet April 2008.
4. Stainer Dw, Landi S. Stability of BCG vaccines. *Tubercle* 1986;58:119-25.
5. World Health Organization. BCG Vaccination of the Newborn: Rationale and Guidelines for Country Programs. Geneva, World Health Organization, 1986.
6. Brewer TF, Wilson ME. BCG immunization: review of past experience, current use, and future prospects. *Current Clinical Topics in Infectious Diseases* 1995;15:253-270.
7. Orefici G, Scopetti F, *et al.* A Study of a BCG vaccine: Influence of dose and time. *Boll Ist Sieroter Milan* 1982;61:24-8.
8. Ildirim I, *et al.* Comparison of BCG vaccination at birth and at third month of life. *Arch Dis Child* 1992;67:80-82.
9. Ferreira AA, *et al.* BCG vaccination in low birth weight newborns: Analysis of lymphocyte proliferation, II-2 generation and intradermal reaction to PPD. *Tuberc Lung Dis* 1996;77:476-81.
10. WHO Global Tuberculosis Programme and Global Programme on Vaccines. Statement on BCG revaccination for the prevention of tuberculosis. *WHO Wkly Epidem Rec* 1995;70: 229-31.
11. O'Brien KL, Ruff AJ, Louis MA, *et al.* Bacillus Calmette-Guérin complications in children born to HIV-1-infected women with a review of the literature. *Pediatrics* 1995;95:414-18.
12. Lallemant-Le Coeur S. Bacillus Calmette-Guerin immunization in infants born to HIV-1-seropositive mothers. *AIDS* 1991;5:195-9.
13. Carswell M. BCG immunization in the children of HIV-positive mothers. *AIDS* 1987;1:258.
14. Trevnen CL, Pagtakhan RD. Disseminated tuberculoid lesions in infants following BCG. *Canad Med J* 1982;15:502-04.
15. Whalen C, Nsubuga P, Johnson J, Mugerwa R, Ellner J. Preventive therapy for tuberculosis in HIV-infected Ugandans. *The Lancet* 1995.
16. WHO Global Programme for Vaccines and Immuni-zation. Immunization Policy. Geneva: WHO, 1996;1-51.

17. Galazka AM, Lauer BA, Henderson RH, Keja J. Indications and contraindications for vaccines used in the Expanded Programme on Immunization. *Bull WHO* 1984;62:357-66.

18. Lotte A, Wasz-Hockert O, Poisson N, *et al.* Second IUATLD study on complications induced by intradermal BCG-vaccination. *Bull Int Union Tuberc* 1988;63:47-59.

19. Fang JW, KO BM, Wilson JA. BCG vaccination scars: incidence and acceptance amongst British high-school children. *Child Care Health Dev* 1993;19:37-43.

20. Chao CW. Post-vaccination keloid. *Bull Int Union Tuberc* 1972;47.

21. Expanded Program on immunization/BIologicals Unit. BCG associated lymphadenitis in infants. *Wkly Epidemiol Rec* 1989;30:231-2.

22. Oguz F, Mujgan S, Alper G, *et al.* Treatment of bacillus Calmette-Guerin-associated lymphadentis. *Pediatr Infect Dis J* 1992;11:887-88.

23. Power JT, Stewert IC, Ross JD, Erythromycin in the management of troublesome BCG lesions. *Br J Dis Chest* 1984;78:94.

24. Ninane J, *et al.* Disseminated BCG in HIV infection. *Arch Dis. Child,* 1988;63:1268-9.

25. Smith E. Infection with Mycobacterium bovis in a patient with AIDS: a late complication of BCG vaccination. *Scand J Infect Dis* 1992;24:109-10.

26. Armbruster C, Junker W, *et al.* Disseminated BCG infection in an AIDS patient 30 years after BCG vaccination . *J Infect Dis* 1990;162:1216.

27. Kroger L, Korppi M, Brander E, *et al.* Osteitis caused by bacillus Calmette-Guerin vaccination: A retrospective analysis of 222 cases. *J Infect Dis* 1995;172:574-76.

28. Dogliotti M. Erythema multiforme — an unusual reaction to BCG vaccination. *S Afr Med J* 1980; 57:332-4.

29. Morrison WL, Webb WJS, Aldred J, Rubenstein D. Meningitis after BCG vaccination. *Lancet* 1988;1:654-5.

30. Orefici G, Scopetti F, Grandolfo ME, Annesi I, Kissopoulos A. Study of a BCG vaccine: influence of dose and time. *Boll Ist Sieroter Milan* 1982;61:24-8.

31. Menzies R, Vissandjee B. Effect of BCG vaccination on tuberculin reactivity. *Am Rev Respir Dis* 1992;145:621-25.

32. Horwitz O, Bunch-Christensen K. Correlation between tuberculin sensitivity after 2 months and 5 years among BCG vaccinated subjects. *Bull World Health Organ* 1972;47:49-58.

33. Comstock GW, Edwards LB. Tuberculin sensitivity eight to fifteen years after BCG vaccination. *Am Rev Respir Dis* 1971;103:572-5.

34. Fine PEM, Sterne JAC, Ponnighaus JM, Rees RJW. Delayed-type hypersensitivity, mycobacterial vaccines and protective immunity. *Lancet* 1994;344:1245-9.

35. Fine PEM, Ponnighaus JM, Maine NP. The relationship between delayed type hypersensitivity and protective immunity induced by mycobacterial vaccines in man. *Lepr Rev* 1986;57 (suppl 2):275-83.

36. Kassimi Fa, al-Hajjaj MS, al-Orainey IO, *et al.* Does the protective effect of neonatal BCG correlate with vaccine-induced tuberculin reaction? *Am J Respir Crit Care Med* 1995;152: 1575-78.

37. Colditz GA, Berkey CS, Mosteller F, *et al.* The efficacy of bacillus Calmette-Guérin vaccination of newborns and infants in the prevention of tuberculosis: Meta-analyses of the published literature. *Pediatrics* 1995;96:29-35.

38. Colditz GA, Brewer TF, Berkey CS, *et al.* Efficacy of BCG vaccine in the prevention of tuberculosis: meta-analysis of the published literature. *JAMA* 1994;271:698-702.

39. Smith PG. Case-control studies of the efficacy of BCG against tuberculosis. In: International Union against Tuberculosis, ed. Proceedings of the XXVIth IUAT World Conference on TB and Respiratory Diseases. Singapore: 1987:73-9.

40. Tripathy SP. Fifteen-year follow-up of the Indian BCG prevention trial. In: International Union Against Tuberculosis, ed. Proceedings of the XXVIth IUAT World Conference on Tuberculosis and Respiratory Diseases. Singapore: Professional Postgraduate Services International, 1987:69-72.

41. Thilothammal N, Krishnamurthy PV, Runyan DK *et al.* Does BCG vaccine prevent tuberculous meningitis? *Arch Dis Child* 1996;74:144-47.

42. Rodrigues LC, Diwan VK, Wheeler JG. Protective effect of BCG against tuberculous meningitis and miliary tuberculosis: a meta-analysis. *Int J Epidemiol* 1993;22:1154-8.

43. Schurr E, Bushman E, Gros P, *et al.* Genetic aspects of mycobacterial infection in mouse and man. In Melchers F (ed). Progress in Immunology Vol. VII. New York: Springer-Verlag, 1990:994-1001.

44. Kaufmann SHE. Vaccines against tuberculosis. The impact of modern biotechnology. *Scand J infect Dis* 1990;75(suppl):54-9.

44a. Stanford JL, Grange JM. New concepts for the control of tuberculosis in the twenty first century. *J R Coll Physicians* 1993;27:218-23.

45. Stanford JL *et al*. New concepts for the control of TB in twenty first century. *JR Coll Physicians* 1993;27:218-23.

46. Blueprint for Tuberculosis Vaccine Development. By the US Dept. of Health. Workshop. March 1998;5-6.

47. Fine PEM, Rodrigues LC. Modern vaccines: Mycobacterial diseases. *Lancet* 1990;335:1016-20.

48. Orme IM. Progress in the development of new vaccines against tuberculosis. *Int J Tuberc Lung Dis* 1997;1:95-100.

49. Morris ON *et al. Curr Opin Infect Dis* 2005 Jun;18(3):211-5

50. Andersen P. Host responses and antigens involved in protective immunity to mycobacterium tuberculosis. *Scand J Immunol* 1997;45:115-31:102.

51. Sorensen AL, Andersen P, Andersen AB. Purification and characterization of a low-molecular mass T cell antigen secreted by Mycobacterium tuberculosis. *Infect Immun* 1995; 63:1710-17.

52. Guleria I, Teitelbaum R, Kalpana G, Bloom BR. Auxotrophic vaccines for tuberculosis. *Nature Med* 1996;2:334-37.

53. Lowrie DB, Silva CL, Tascon RE. Protection against tuberculosis by a plasmid DNA vaccine. *Vaccine* 1997;15:834-38.

54. Rouillon A, Waaler H. BCG vaccination and epidemiological situation: A decision making approach to the use of BCG. *Adv Tuberc Res* 1976;19:64-126.

55. Styblo K. Overview and epidemiologic assessment of the current global tuberculosis situation with an emphasis on control in developing countries. *Rev Infect Dis 1989;11(suppl 2)*:S339-S346,1989

56. Banta. International Group of Health Experts Issues Global 'Declaration to Stop TB", *JAMA Medical News and Perspectives*, 2000;8:283.

57. Gheorghiu M. The present and future role of BCG vaccine in tuberculosis control. *Biologicals* 1990;18:135-41.

Section 3
Malaria

16

Life Cycle of Malaria Parasites and Clinical Features of Malaria

Baldev S Prajapati, Rajal B Prajapati

LIFE CYCLE OF MALARIA PARASITES

Malarial parasite passes its life cycle in two hosts, man and mosquito. Man represents the intermediate host in which the parasite resides in hepatic cells and RBCs and reproduce by asexual method. It is called as schizogony (Schizo means to split and goni means generation). Female anopheline mosquito represents the definitive host in which sexual forms (male and female gametocytes) are transferred from human host during blood meal. Maturation and fertilization occurs in the mosquito, giving rise to a large number of sporozoites (Sporo means seed) which are infective to man. This sexual method of reproduction is called sporogony.

HUMAN CYCLE (FIG. 16.1)

Inoculation

When an infected female anopheline mosquito bites a man, sporozoites present in the salivary glands of mosquito enter the bloodstream of man.

Pre-erythrocytic Stage

Sporozoites leave the circulation within half an hour and enter the liver cells. The elongated spindle-shaped sporozoites become rounded in the liver. They enlarge in size and undergo repeated nuclear division followed by cytoplasmic division. Each daughter nucleus is surrounded by cytoplasm. This stage of parasite is called pre-erythrocytic schizont. A pre-erythrocytic schizont of *P. vivax* measures about 45 μm in diameter and contains about 10,000 merozoites. The merozoites are released into the circulation when the infected liver cells rupture. This pre-erythrocytic schizogony takes about 6 to 16 days depending on the plasmodium species and determines the incubation period of malaria.

The duration of pre-erythrocytic phase in the liver, number of merozoites produced by different species and other differential characters are shown in Table 16.1.

Relapse

All of the sporozoites do not develop directly into pre-erythrocytic schizonts in the liver

139

Table 16.1: Salient features of pre-erythrocytic schizogony of malarial parasites in man

	P.vivax	*P.falciparum*	*P.malariae*	*P.ovale*
Duration of PE schizogony	7 days	5 to 7 days	14 to 16 days	9 days
Mean diameter of mature PE schizogony	45 µm	60 µm	56 µm	60 µm
No merozoites in PE schizogony	10,000	30,000	15,000	15,000

cells. In case of *P.vivax* and *P.ovale* infections, some sporozoites develop into hypnozoites. Hypnozoites are uninucleate forms with 4 to 6 µm diameter. They remain dormant in the liver for sometime and cause relapse. Relapse may occur after 24 weeks to 5 years after initial infection. This stage is absent in *P.falciparum* and *P.malariae*. Reactivation of hypnozoites leads to initiations of erythrocyte cycles and new malarial attacks.

Erythrocytic Stage

The infected liver cells rupture and merozoites released by pre-erythrocytic schizonts invade red cells (Fig. 16.1).

P.vivax primarily infects young erythrocytes. *P. malariae* primarily infects old erythrocytes and falciparum infects erythrocytes of all ages. The merozoites released from hepatic cells are pear-shaped bodies with an apical complex and measures 1.5 µm in length. The receptors for merozoites on RBCs are glycophorin, a major glycoprotein which is species specific for malarial parasites. The merozoites attach to the erythrocytes by their apex, which possess organelles that secrete a substance producing pit on the red cell membrane. The red cell membrane becomes indented and the merozoites enter the cells by endocytosis. The merozoite contained within a parasito-phorous vacuole formed by the vagination of red cell membrane, becomes a trophozoite. The process of entry into RBC takes about 30 seconds. Once merozoite is inside the cell, it rounds up and looses its internal organelles. Most of the merozoites released by hepatic cells enter the RBCs in the sinusoids of liver and a portion are destroyed by phagocytosis.

Trophozoite

Once the RBCs and reticulocytes have been invaded, the parasites grows and feed on haemoglobin. Within the RBC, the merozoite or young trophozoite appears as a rounded body having a vacuole in the center with the cytoplasm pushed to the periphery and the nucleus situated at one pole. In Leishman or other Romanowsky stained smears of blood, they appear to consist of a blue cytoplasmic ring, a red nucleus and an unstained central vacuole. This gives the parasite an annular or signet ring appearance, hence these young forms of parasites are known as ring form. The diameter of the ring is approximately one third of that of an erythrocyte except *P. falciparum* in which it is 1/5th of RBC. The nucleus is usually seen as a single chromatin dot except in *P. falciparum* in which it is double chromatin dot.

The parasites feed on hemoglobin. They do not metabolize hemoglobin completely. The excess protein, an iron porphyrin and hematin left over by the parasites after metabolism of hemoglobin combine to form malarial pigment formerly known as hemozoin pigment. After release from the ruptured parasitized red cells, malarial pigment is taken up by the reticulo-endothelial cells. Presence of pigment laden macrophages, in histological sections is an evidence of past malarial infection.

As the young trophozoite (ring-form) grows its size is enlarged and the shape becomes more irregular due to ameboid movement. It is called late trophozoite or ameboid form. The ameboid movement gives rise to diverse shape. During ameboidal growth of trophozoite bits of membrane from the developing parasite accumulate on the surface of RBC which appear as stippling clefts on the surface of RBC, called Schüffner's dots. The parasite within RBC till the time its nucleus starts dividing is known as the trophozoites.

Schizont

When the trophozoite is fully developed, it becomes compact, vacuole disappears and malarial pigments are scattered throughout the cytoplasm. The nucleus is large and lies at the periphery. From the time the nucleus starts dividing, the parasite within the red cell is now called sporozoite. It is larger in size than a RBC (10 μm diameter).

The nucleus first divides into a variable number of small nuclei. Depending upon the species, about 8 to 32 divisions of nucleus occur. Then, the cytoplasm divides into the same number as the nucleus masses, forming same number of daughter cells. These are called merozoites, which arrange themselves in the form of rosette, usually two rows.

Mature schizonts rupture from the red cells, releasing merozoites, malarial pigment and toxins into the circulation which gives rise to malarial paroxysm of fever. The merozoites invade the fresh RBCs and the cycle is repeated. This erythrocytic cycle takes 48 hours in *P. falciparum, P. ovale, P. vivax* and 72 hours in *P. malariae* infections. The interval between the entry of sporozoite into the host and the earliest manifestations of clinical disease is the incubation time.

Gametogony

After several erythrocytic cycles, some of the merozoites enter RBCs and instead of developing into trophozoites and schizonts, they follow a sexual development and become gametocytes. They grow in size till they almost fill the RBC and the nucleus remains undivided. Gametocytes generally develop in RBCs of the capillaries of internal organs such as spleen and bone marrow and only the mature gametocytes appear in peripheral blood. It takes 96 hours for maturation of gametocytes.

Mature gametocytes are round in shape except in *P. falciparum* in which they are crescent shaped. RBCs increase in size during gametocyte development. The female gametocytes are macrogametocytes and they have a dark blue cytoplasm with a small compact deep red nucleus. The male gametocytes are microgametocytes and they stain pale blue or pink and the nucleus is larger, pale stained and diffuse. Pigment granules are prominent. Female gametocytes generally outnumber the male.

The time of appearance of gametocytes into circulation, from the first appearance of asexual forms in blood differs with different species, e.g. 4 to 5 days in *P. vivax* and 10 to 12 days in *P. falciparum*. Gametocytes do not give rise to any febrile reactions and individual harbouring gametocytes is called carrier. Children are more effective carrier than adults. It has been estimated that in order to infect a mosquito, the blood of a human carrier must contain at least 12 gametocytes per cmm of blood and the number of female gametocytes must be in excess.

MOSQUITO CYCLE (FIG. 16.1)

A female anopheles mosquito during its blood meal ingests both the sexual and asexual forms of the parasite. The asexual forms are digested. The sexual forms, gametocytes are set free in the stomach where they undergo further development.

Within 15 minutes of entry into the stomach of the mosquito, the nucleus of each male gametocyte divides into 8 long flagellated

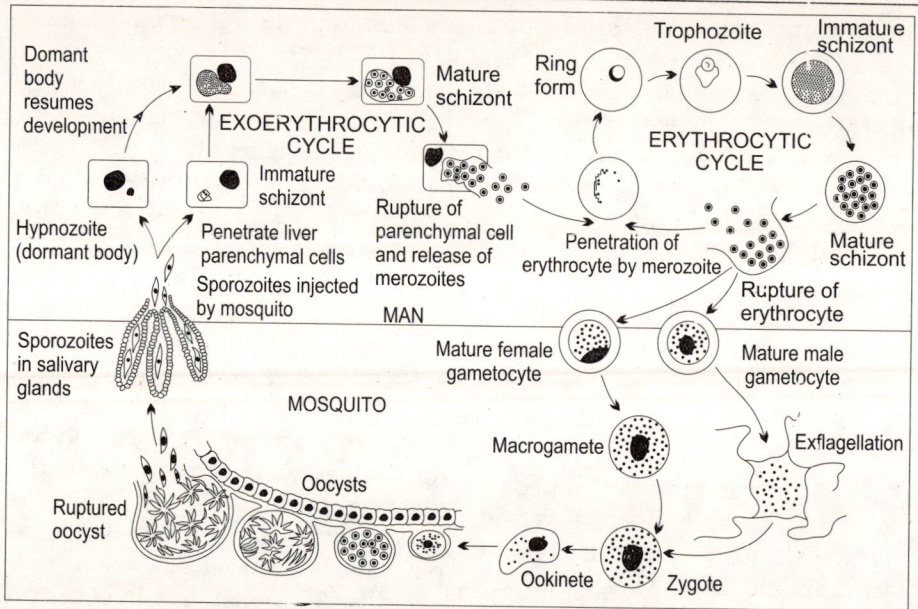

Fig. 16.1: Life cycle of malarial parasites

bodies (microgametes) each of which is 20–30 μm long. These flagellated bodies are thread like filaments and lash out for some time and then break out of the RBC. These free microgametes are highly motile. It increases in size and its nucleus shifts to the surface. Since this process of development can also be observed outside the mosquito host in a moist thick film preparation of blood, it is also known as exflagellation.

The female gametocyte does not divide but undergoes a process of maturation to become the female gamete. The male microgametes fertilizes the female macrogamete by fusion of two pronuclei and a zygote is formed. Zygote develops in 20 min. to 2 hours after the mosquito's blood meal.

Initially the zygote is a motionless round body. In the next 18 to 24 hours, the zygote becomes mature, elongate and motile and is called ookinete (traveling vermicule). The ookinete migrates to the stomach wall of the mosquito and comes to lie just beneath its basement membrane, secretes a thin wall and

grows into oocyst. Large number of sporozoites are formed in oocyte. When fully mature, on or about 10th day of ingestion, the oocyte ruptures liberating the sporozoites in the body cavity of the mosquito that spread to all parts of the mosquito, particularly to the salivary glands, ready to transmit when the mosquito takes a blood meal.

The time taken for completion of sporogony at 28°C is 8 to 10 days in *P.vivax* and 9 to 10 days in *P.falciparum*, 14–16 days in *P.malariae* and 12 to 14 days in *P.ovale*.

In the same mosquito, different species of plasmodia can develop and the bite of such an infected mosquito to a man can give rise to mixed infection, the commonest being *P.vivax* and *P.falciparum*. Once a mosquito becomes infective, it remains so throughout the life.

References

1. Chakraborty P. *Plasmodium* and Babesia. Textbook of Medical Parasitology, 2nd ed. Kolkata: New Central Book Agency (P) Ltd., 2005; 84-104.

2. Krause PJ.Malaria (Plasmodium) In : Kliegman RM, Jenson HB, Behrman RE, Stanton BF eds Nelson Textbook of Pediatrics 18th edn. New Delhi: Elsevier, 2008,1477-78.
3. Chatterjee KD. Parasitology 12th edn. Calcutta. Chatterjee Medical Publishers 1980,74-76.

CLINICAL FEATURES OF UNCOMPLICATED AND COMPLICATED MALARIA

Introduction

Malaria continues to be a major global health problem, with over 40% of the world's population exposed to varying degree of malaria risk in some 100 countries[1-3]. Malaria is endemic in India. A recent upsurge in the incidence of falciparum malaria has been noted in our country[4]. As delay in institution of appropriate therapy can result in a fatality, prompt diagnosis of malaria is very crucial for a tropical pediatrician[4]. Although demonstration of the parasite in the blood film is the cornerstone for diagnosis of malaria, it has a failure rate of a high magnitude due to several practical reasons[5]. Recently some sophisticated serodiagnostic tests are introduced, but they are expensive, need expertise and are time consuming for routine diagnosis.[5] Ultimately, the clinician has to rely upon his clinical diagnosis. Malaria presents with marked clinical heterogenicity. Presentation may vary from severe and fatal illness to symptomless parasite circulation in the blood. Its clinical picture mimics with many other common illnesses in children. In fact, it is a sound policy to exclude malaria in all cases of pyrexia of doubtful origin in the tropical countries[5]. High degree of suspicion is of paramount importance in the diagnosis, especially at our set up.

Paroxysmal bouts of fever associated with chills and rigors considered as typical feature of malaria in adults, is hardly seen in children. In fact, intermittent pattern of fever is invariably absent in children and instead an irregular fever with respiratory, gastro-intestinal and symptoms involving other systems mark the onset of the disease[5,6]. For clinicotherapeutic purposes malaria could be divided as uncomplicated malaria and severe complicated malaria. This chapter includes the details of clinical features of both these groups as well as some rare presentations reported in the literature.

Uncomplicated Malaria

No age is exempted from development of malaria specifically in endemic areas like our country. It can affect from the time of conception to any age with varied presentations. The following arbitrary groups are identifiable for their diverse clinical presentations.

 i. Effect on the fetus of maternal malaria during pregnancy.
 ii. Neonates.
 iii. Early infancy (infants under six months).
 iv. Late infancy and early childhood (six months to five years).
 v. Late childhood.

Effect on the fetus of maternal malaria during pregnancy

Maternal malaria is an important cause of abortions, stillbirths and low birth weight babies[6]. Several studies undertaken in our country have shown that antimalarial prophylaxis to the pregnant women decreases the incidence of complications like still births, prematurity and small for date babies[6].

Neonatal Malaria[8-12]

Neonatal malaria in endemic areas is uncommon due to number of mechanisms that suppress malarial infection including:

1. Passively transferred maternal malarial specific IgG antibodies which may act as opsonizing agents or block the merozoitic invasion of erythrocytes.

2. Fetal hemoglobin which retards maturation of plasmodia.
3. An exclusive breast milk which deprives the parasite of para-amnio benzoic acid, required for growth of the parasites[5,7].

Neonatal malaria is of three types:
1. Congenital,
2. Transfusion malaria,
3. Naturally acquired malaria[7].

Congenital malaria[7,13,14]

It is due to transplacental transmission of the malarial parasite and is rare since placenta is supposed to act as a barrier to such a transfer. The incidence of placental malaria in endemic areas may be as high as 30% while incidence of congenital malaria in infants of immune mothers is estimated to be as low as 0.3% (up to 10% in the non-immune mothers). Placental malaria is symptomless and it silently causes fetal wasting. The difference between the birth weight of an infant born with a negative and positive placenta for malarial parasite is around 150 to 300 grams. The blood film of the mother is often negative. Confirmation of diagnosis relies on detection of parasites in peripheral blood along with detection of specific IgM antibodies in neonate's blood. Presence of IgM antibodies in the neonate indicates prenatal reaction to the infection. The disease manifests around 2 to 8 weeks of age with fever, jaundice, hemolytic anemia, thrombocytopenia and hepatosplenomegaly. Maternal history of fever with rigors and positive smear for malarial parasites during late pregnancy may be available.

Transfusion malaria[12,13]

It develops following transfusion of infected blood. The diagnosis of post transfusion malaria is more difficult due to overlapping of symptoms with the existing disease[12,13]. Malaria during neonatal period most commonly occurs due to administration of infected blood[15]. Monoclonal antibody test of the patient as well as its blood donor will ascertain the diagnosis[13].

Naturally acquired malaria

Differentiation between malarial infection acquired very early in the neonatal period and transplacental infection acquired very late in pregnancy is virtually impossible. Still following points favour the diagnosis of congenital malaria[7,15].

- History of malaria in the mother during pregnancy.
- Manifestations occurring before the minimal incubation period (12 to 16 days for *P.vivax* and 10 to 13 days for *P. falciparum*).
- Presence of IgM antibodies against plasmodium in the neonate's blood.
- Absence of history of blood transfusion.

Clinical Features[5-11,14,15]

In endemic areas, malaria is invariably mild in neonates. Hepatosplenomegaly, anemia and jaundice with or without fever are usual presentations. It is quite mimicking septicemia. Non-immune neonate may present with severe anemia as seen in erythroblastosis fetalis. Congenital malaria and transfusion associated malaria do not have exoerythrocytic phase.

Early Infancy (infants under six months)[5,6]

In this group some of the infants are partially immune to malaria due to their transplacentally received immunity in form of IgG antibodies from the mother, while others are non immune and they are very susceptible to the disease.

Partially immune infants suffer from mild disease. They have mild fever, pallor and just enlarged spleen. There may not be history of significant fever. Peripheral smear may not show presence of parasites, but they respond very well to antimalarials. Non immune infants become very sick following malaria. They present with huge splenohepatomegaly, severe anemia and occasionally jaundice. There is indirect hyperbilirubinemia indicating hemolytic process. Very often it is mistaken for thalassemia major. Peripheral smear shows presence of malarial parasites in many children from this group.

Late Infancy and Early Childhood (six months to five years)[5,6]

With waning of all the factors offering protection from malaria, this group becomes the most susceptible for disease. Not only does the disease is more frequent in this group, but very often it gets complicated. The clinical picture varies greatly due to several factors. Classical cold and hot stages are exception rather than the rule. A child with malaria initially appears listless, irritable or drowsy. Refusal of food is very common. Vomiting is also significant complaint in this group. The temperature may shoot upto 105° to 106°F. It may precipitate febrile convulsions in susceptible children. The fever may subside within a short period or may last up to few hours. It may subside by its own or in response to antipyretic therapy. It may recur on alternate day or at the fixed interval. During afebrile stage, the child appears well and is found playful. This type of clinical picture is more common with *Plasmodium vivax*.

Development of sudden pallor, headache and bodyache are also common manifestations of malaria in this group. Sudden drop in hemoglobin in any child in endemic area for malaria, malaria should be considered unless proved otherwise.

Various manifestations involving different systems are known in this group.

Respiratory Symptoms[5,6]

This is the most common form of presentation. The child suffers from fever, cough and even breathlessness. Chest signs like wheezing and crepitations may be detected on auscultation. Mild hepatosplenomegaly is also evident.

School going children from malarious area, may present with dry cough of 3 to 4 weeks duration. Other causes of cough like tuberculosis should be ruled out by Mantoux test and chest X-ray. Peripheral smear may be positive for *P.vivax* or *P.falciparum*. There may be history of fever. They do respond very well to antimalarials[16].

Gastrointestinal Symptoms[5,6]

Marked vomiting and loose stools characterize this form of malaria. Stools are usually mucoid and may rarely contain blood and pus giving rise to a clinical picture of dysentery. Abdominal colick and tenesmus may be associated with it.

Febrile Convulsions[5,6]

In endemic area, malaria is the common cause for febrile convulsions. If there is no any other evident cause for fever, look for malaria.

Urticaria[17-19]

In a child presenting with high grade fever and urticaria, after exclusion of viral etiology and drug therapy known to cause urticaria, one should think of malaria.

Late Childhood[5,6]

By late childhood, the presentation of malaria becomes classical paroxysmal pattern. Malarial paroxysm comprises of three successive stages namely cold storage, hot stage and sweating stage. Depending on infective species, paroxysms tends to recur on tertian or quotidian frequencies. In between the two paroxysms, the child is afebrile, playing, doing routine activities and appetite remains normal.

Malarial Paroxysm[5,16,20]

Cold stage—The patient feels intense cold with vigorous shivering or rigors lasting for 15 to 60 minutes.

Hot stage—Cold stage is followed by hot stage. There is abrupt rise in temperature with maximum spike. Body temperature may reach upto 105° and 106°F or occasionally more than that. The skin becomes dry and burning. Throbbing headache is very characteristic.

Sweating stage: There is profuse sweating after hot stage and body temperature declines. Sometimes it may reach to subnormal level. Patient feels exhausted and weak. There is significant fluid loss. It may last for few hours.

Anemia and hepatosplenomegaly are constant features with all forms of malarial presentations. Splenic enlargement occurs 4 to 10 days after fever. A faster and greater enlargement of spleen than the liver is commonly seen in *P.vivax* malaria. Conversely, enlargement of liver precedes splenic enlargement with *P.falciparum* infection. Perisplenitis may lead to tenderness.

Severe and Complicated Malaria

Severe and complicated malaria is commonly caused by *Plasmodium falciparum* infection[3]. It involves multiorgan systems. It occurs in most cases as a result of delay in treating an uncomplicated attack, because of misdiagnosis or for other reasons[3]. Sometimes it develops very fast or patient may present with multiple complications without any notice. It mimics many other serious conditions and at times it is very difficult to diagnose. It requires high index of suspicion and experience regarding various presentations of the condition.

It is important to note that these severe manifestations can occur singly or in combi-

Table 16.2: Severe malaria is defined as one or more of following plus asexual parasitemia[1-3,21-23]

A. *Specific manifestations*
I. Cerebral malaria
Generalized, repeated convulsions
Severe anemia
Hypoglycemia
Fluid, electrolyte and acid-base disturbances
Renal failure
Pulmonary edema
Algid malaria
Hematological complications
Black water fever (hemoglobinuria)
Hyperparasitemia
II. Autopsy diagnosis of *P.falciparum*
B. *Non specific manifestations*
Impairment of consciousness
Hyperpyrexia
Jaundice
Too weak to walk

nation in the same patient. Children and non immune adults are at more risk in endemic areas.

The following differences between adult and children in severe malaria should be noted as in Table 16.3[3].

Cerebral Malaria

Definition[2,16,24,25]

The strict scientific definition of cerebral malaria should be fulfilled by following criteria:

i. Deep coma persisting for 30 minutes following generalized convulsions.

ii. Confirmation by finding asexual forms of *P.falciparum* on peripheral smear or bone marrow examination.

iii. Other causes of encephalopathies are ruled out.

iv. In fatal cases histopathology of brain confirms the diagnosis.

Table 16.3: Differences between adults and children in severe malaria

Sign/Symptom	Children	Adults
Cough	Common	Uncommon
Convulsions	Very common	Common
Duration of illness	1–2 days	5–7 days
Resolution of coma	1–2 days	2–4 days
Neurological sequelae	> 10%	< 5%
Jaundice	Uncommon	Common
Pre treatment hypoglycemia	Common	Uncommon
Pulmonary edema	Rare	Common
Renal failure	Rare	Common
CSF opening pressure	Variable often, raised	Usually normal
Bleeding/clotting disturbances	Rare	Upto 10%
Abnormality of brain stem reflexes	More common	Rare

Most clinicians regard any manifestation of cerebral dysfunction in a patient of malaria as an evidence of cerebral malaria. It is most accepted working definition.

Cerebral malaria is the most common clinical presentation and cause of death amongst the severe form of malaria. In most of studies, it has been reported as 70% of total cases from severe and complicated malaria. Though cerebral malaria due to *P.falciparum* is a well documented entity, some reports mention *P.vivax* as a causative agent[5,26-29]. Mixed infection, *P.falciparum* as well as *P.vivax* has also been reported in cases of cerebral malaria[30,31].

The following are salient clinical features of cerebral malaria in children.

- The earliest symptom of cerebral malaria in children is usually fever, refusal of feeds and vomiting[6].
- All patients of cerebral malaria present with altered sensorium. It includes impaired consciousness, delirium, abnormal neurological signs and focal or generalized convulsions. Some patients show gradual progress from altered sensorium to unconsciousness while others may directly present in coma. The depth of coma should be assessed as per Modified Glasgow Coma Scale (Blantyre Coma Scale)[32].

- Convulsions are common in both adults and children. Convulsions may be in a subtle form such as deviation of eyes to one side, stereotyped movements of limbs and/or minor twitchings. To make a distinction between cerebral malaria and transient postictal unconsciousness, altered sensorium should persist for at least 30 minutes after an episode of seizures to classify the child as having cerebral malaria[32].
- A variety of transient abnormalities of eye movement especially disconjugate gaze, have been reported[3].
- Fixed jaw closure and tooth grinding are common.
- Mild neck stiffness occurs, but neck rigidity is absent[3].
- Motor abnormalities such as decerebrate rigidity, decorticate rigidity and opisthotonos occur in severely ill children[3].
- Monoplegia and hemiplegia are other manifestations of cerebral malaria[26,33,34].
- Tremors, ataxia and other cerebellar signs have been reported by several workers[34-37].
- Signs of raised intracranial pressure has been reported in some series[3].
- Cranial nerve lesions have been reported[3].
- Neuropsychiatric behavior has also been reported.
- Acute transverse myelitis, Guillain Barré syndrome and acute flaccid paralysis like manifestations have been reported rarely in cases of cerebral malaria.
- Retinal hemorrhages are associated with poor prognosis[3].
- Papilledema is rare[3].
- Photophobia is absent[3].

Neurological deficits are seen in 12% children. Common sequelae of cerebral malaria are hemiplegia, cortical blindness, aphasia and ataxia. Many of them make full recovery within period of 6 months[16].

Anemia[1-6,16,20]

Anemia is common clinical feature in severe malaria. Anemia in falciparum malaria is attributed to a combination of hemolysis of both parasitized and non parasitized red cells as well as ineffective erythropoiesis. The rate of development and degree of anemia depend on the severity and duration of parasitemia. In some children, repeated untreated episodes of otherwise non complicated malaria may lead to normochromic anemia in which dyserythropoietic changes in the bone marrow are prominent. Parasitemia is often scanty, although numerous pigmented monocytes can be seen in the peripheral blood. In other children, severe anemia may develop rapidly in association with heavy parasitemia. In these cases, acute destruction of parasitized red cells is responsible.

Children with severe anemia may present with tachycardia, dyspnea and signs of cardiac failure. Anemia may contribute to cerebral signs – confusion, restlessness and coma.

Other hematological disturbances[1-6,16,20-26]

Clinically significant thrombocytopenia and disseminated intravascular coagulation are other known hematological disturbances in falciparum malaria. They are rapidly reversible with appropriate antimalarial therapy.

Hypoglycemia[1-6,16,20-26]

Hypoglycemia is an important complication of severe falciparum infection and can be present in 20 to 30% of children with severe complicated malaria. It is more common in young children (under 3 years) and in those with hyperparasitemia. It is also common in patients treated with quinine as a result of quinine induced hyperinsulinemia. Sweating, cold extremities and unconsciousness are important signs of hypoglycemia. Patient may develop convulsions. It is easily overlooked clinically because the manifestations may be similar to those of cerebral malaria. Signs of hypoglycemia are indistinguishable from signs of malaria. Therefore, estimation of blood sugar level is mandatory in all patients with severe and complicated malaria. It should be monitored at certain intervals during the therapy.

Fluid, Electrolytes and Acid-base Disturbances[1-5,16,20,23-26]

Patients with severe falciparum malaria often present with hypovolemia, low volume pulse, tachycardia, hypotension and oliguria.

Anerobic glycolysis occurring in tissues where sequestrated and parasitized red cells interfere with microcirculation and failure of hepatic lactate clearance contribute to the development of lactic acidosis. Lactic acidosis may accompany hypoglycemia and both the complications are associated with increased mortality. Any child with falciparum malaria presenting with tachypnea and deep shallow breathing, acidosis should be suspected.

Hyponatremia may also be observed in severe malaria due to volume expansion.

Acute Renal Failure[1-3,5,16,20,24,25,26,32]

Renal dysfunction seen in severe malaria is usually due to acute tubular necrosis and is characterized clinically by prolonged oliguria leading to anuria. But it is less common in children than in adults. Black water fever and hemoglobinuria result from severe and sudden intravascular hemolysis which may lead to anuria.

Pulmonary Edema[1-3,5,16,32]

Pulmonary edema is a grave complication of severe malaria with a very high mortality (over 50%). It is rare in children. It may appear several days after chemotherapy has been started and at a time when the patient's general condition is improving and the peripheral parasitemia is diminishing. It must be differentiated from iatrogenically produced pulmonary edema due to fluid overload. Hyperparasitemia, renal failure, hypoglycemia and metabolic acidosis are often associated. The first indication of impending pulmonary edema is an increase in respiratory rate which precedes the development of other chest signs. Hypoxia may cause convulsions and deterioration in the level of consciousness. X-ray chest shows heterogenous or homogenous opacities on both sides. Acute lung injury, aspiration pneumonia and nosocomial pneumonia are other causes of respiratory distress which should be differentiated from pulmonary edema.

Pulmonary edema in malaria results from increased capillary leak, oliguric renal failure and increased TNF-alpha levels. Mortality is around 80% and patient may die within a few hours.

Circulatory Collapse (Algid Malaria)[1-3,16,32]

Some patients present in a state of collapse; a cold, clammy, cyanotic skin; collapsed peripheral veins, rapid feeble pulse and hypotension. In some patients it may be associated with complicating gram-negative septicemia.

Circulatory collapse is also seen in patients with pulmonary edema, metabolic acidosis and following massive gastrointestinal hemorrhage. Dehydration with hypovolemia may also contribute to hypotension.

Hemoglobinuria[1-3,16,32]

It presents with brown red urine (Coca-Cola urine) with or without acute renal failure. It may be associated with black water fever even in the absence of malaria. It typically develops in non-immune patients taking prophylactic or presumptive treatment in form of quinine, accompanied by mild or absent fever, scanty or absent parasitemia. It carries a poor prognosis. It is now very rare.

Hyperparasitemia[1-3,16,32]

Generally, high parasite densities (above 5%) and peripheral schizotemia are associated with severe disease in non immune subjects. However, in highly endemic malarious areas, partially immune children can tolerate surprisingly high densities (20–30%) often without clinical symptoms.

Hyperpyrexia[1-3,16,25,32]

Hyperpyrexia is more common in children associated with convulsions, delirium and coma. High body temperature (>105°F) may cause permanent severe neurological sequelae.

References

1. World Health Organization. Division of Control of tropical diseases: Severe and Complicated Malaria. *Trans R Soc Trop Med Hyg* 1990;84 (Supp 2);1-65.
2. WHO Guidelines for the treatment of malaria. Geneva: WHO, 2006.
3. Gills HM, ed. Management of Severe and Complicated Malaria. A Practical Hand Book Gilles HM (ed.) WHO Geneva 1991;11-34.
4. Thapa BR, Marwaha RK, Walia BNS *et al.* Falciparum Malaria. *Indian Pediatr* 1987;24:221-25.
5. Kapse A Malaria in Children In: Parthasarthy A, Menon PSN, Nair MKC (Eds.): IAP Textbook of Pediatrics, 2nd ed. New Delhi, Jaypee Brothers 2002;243-48.
6. Desai AB. Symposium: Clinical presentation and treatment of malaria in children. *Gujarat Medical Journal* 1989;35:31-34.
7. Congenital malaria: *Ann Trop Med Parasitol* 1987;81:499-509.

8. Singh T. Neonatal malaria. *Indian Pediatr* 1985; 22:785-86.

9. Chaudhari SP, Dabi DR, Singh RN, *et al.*: Malaria in the newborns *Indian Pediatr* 1983;20:41-43.

10. Lal H, Singh N, Ram Kumar L. Neonatal malaria. *Indian J Pediatr* 1981;48:191-93.

11. Sammuel HS. Clinical features of Malaria in neonates *Indian J Pediatr* 1981;48:193-94.

12. Choudhury N, Jolly JG, Ganguly NK, *et al.* Transfusion associated malaria in endemic areas. *Indian pediatr* 1981;28:554-57.

13. Wells L, Ala FA. Malaria and blood transfusion. *Lancet* 1985; i:1317-19.

14. Cole FS. Protozoal Infections: Congenital toxoplasmosis and Malaria In: Taeusch HW, Ballard RA, eds.: Avery's Diseases of the Newborn. 7th ed. Philadelphia W.B. Saunders Company 2000:532-34.

15. Singh M. Congenital Malaria Care of the Newborn, 5th ed New Delhi: Sagar Publications. 1999;204.

16. Gujar PN, Gujar KN, Parale M. Falciparum malaria. Quarterly Medical Review Raptakos, Brett and Co. Ltd. Mumbai, 1998;49:18-31.

17. Mitra A. Malaria presenting with urticaria as the initial feature. *Indian pediatr* 1989;26:728.

18. Maheshwari RK, Gupta BD. Urticaria in malaria *Indian Pediatr* 1984;21:663.

19. Singh RP, Mittal SP, Chib P. *et al*: Occurrence of Urticaria as a manifestation of Falciparum malaria. *J Assoc Phys India* 1988;36:261-62.

20. Dani VS. Malaria In: Gupte S (ed): Recent Advances *In Pediatrics*. New Delhi, Jaypee Brothers 2004;14:19-32.

21. Bag S, Samal GC, Deep N *et al.*: Complicated malaria. *Indian Pediatr* 1994;31:821-25.

22. Chandra V, Mehta SR, Sharma PP, *et al.* Falciparum Malaria. *Indian J Pediatr* 1989;56: 365-69.

23. Mehta SR, Naidur G, Chander V, *et al.*: Falciparum Malaria. Present day problem. An experience with 424 cases. *J Assoc Physicians India* 1989;37:264-66.

24. Kushwaha KP, Singh YD, Rathi AIC, *et al.* Severe malaria In : Gupte S ed.: Recent Advances In Pediatrics (Sp Vol 3). New Delhi, Jaypee Brothers 1999;127-42.

25. Gandhi DJ, Nayak US, Shendurnikar N, Shah AR. Cerebral Malaria – A diagnostic and therapeutic approach. *Indian Pediatr* 1990;27:651-57.

26. Sachdev HPS, Man Mohan. Vivax cerebral malaria. *J Trop Pediatr* 1985;31:213-15.

27. Verma KC, Magotra ML. Vivax cerebral malaria in Jammu. *Indian Pediatr* 1976;13:229-31.

28. Valecha N, Bagga A, Chandra J, Sharma D. Cerebral symptoms with P.Vivax. *Indian Pediatr* 1992;9:1176-78.

29. Sanklecha MU, Raghavan K, Mehta MN. Cerebral malaria Vivax or mixed? *Indian Pediatr* 1994;31: 1133.

30. Brown AE. Demonstration by the polymerase chain reaction of mixed *P.Falciparum* and *P.Vivax* infections undetected by conventional microscopy. Trans 12 Soc Trop Med Hyg 1992;6: 609.

31. Shendurnikar N, Agrawal M. Severe falciparum malaria In: Sachdev HPS, Choudhury P, Bagga a *et al*. Principles of Pediatric and Neonatal Emergencies, 2nd edn. New Delhi, Jaypee Brothers 2004;326-32.

32. Mathur GP, Kushwaha KP, Mathur S. Cerebral malaria In: Gupte S (ed.): Recent Advances In Pediatrics New Delhi: Jaypee Brothers.

33. Jhal DR, Parmar IB, Sharma JR. Cerebellar syndrome in malaria. *Indian Pediatr* 1992;29: 1053-55.

34. Mehta AA, Shah AR. A study of cerebral malaria in children ; 50 cases. Dissertation for the degree MD Pediatrics, MS University, Baroda, 1989.

35. Chitakara AJ, Anand NK, Sainin L. Cerebellar syndrome in malaria. *Indian Pediatr* 1989;21:908-10.

36. Bhandari K, Bhandari P. Cerebellar Syndrome in malaria *Indian Pediatr* 1989;26:1037.

37. Shendurnikar N, Gandhi DJ. Cerebellar ataxia in malaria *Indian Pediatr* 1989;26:1060-61.

17

Laboratory Diagnosis of Malaria

Ritabrata Kundu, Nupur Ganguly

Malaria diagnosis still remains a challenge in most of the countries. Lack of infrastructure and expertise leads to presumptive diagnosis based exclusively on the clinical symptoms. Various clinical algorithms have both poor specificity and positive predictive value. They invariably lead to over treatment of malaria in endemic areas and missing the diagnosis in low transmission areas. Indiscriminate use of antimalarials leads to increased drug pressure which results in widespread resistance to antimalarials. Hence every effort should be given for a parasitological diagnosis of malaria before commencing treatment. However, in severe life threatening malaria presumptive treatment may be started before confirmation after collecting blood for examination.

Parasitological diagnosis include light microscopy and rapid diagnostic tests (RDTs). As treatment of malaria has become expensive due to use of artemisinin based combination therapy (ACT) parasitological diagnosis beside saving cost has the following advantages[1]:

i. Improved care owing to certainty of diagnosis.
ii. Search for alternative diagnosis in parasitological negative cases.
iii. Reducing unnecessary use of antimalarials.
iv. Confirmation of treatment failure.
v. Improved health information.

Microscopic Diagnosis

Conventional light microscopy by an expert microscopist of a well prepared and stained blood film remains the "gold standard" for detecting and identifying malaria parasite[2].

Collection of blood sample—Blood should be collected as soon as malaria is suspected irrespective of fever and not necessarily only at the height of fever but definitely before administration of antimalarials which alter the morphology of parasites[3]. Blood should be obtained from finger tip or earlobe as these capillary rich areas contain greater density of developing parasites[4]. Blood obtained by venipuncture should preferably, collected in EDTA vials and films should be prepared within 2 hours for best result[5].

151

Staining

For quicker diagnosis Fields stain is used whereas longer methods like Giemsa stain provide best staining for successful indication of species.

Examination of blood film—Both thick and thin films should be prepared. Smears should be prepared soon after blood collection which ensures better adherence of the films to the slide and causes minimal distortion of parasites and red cells. A minimum of 100 fields should be examined before concluding the slide to be negative. Once negative, samples may be examined for at least three consecutive days where clinical suspicion of malaria persists.

Both thin and thick smear should be prepared. Thickness of the thick film should be uniform and correct which may be ascertained by the legibility of printed text seen through the slide. Thick film are nearly 10 times more sensitive for diagnosis of malaria as larger amount of blood are there in a given area as compared to thin film[5]. As in thick film RBCs are lysed which alters the morphology of the parasites making it a good screening test for diagnosis of malaria. They are much better than thin film for detection of low levels of parasitemia and reappearance of circulating parasites during recrudescence or relapse. In thin film as fixed monolayer of RBC are available, morphological identification of the parasite to the species level and stage of parasite can be determined.

Performance characteristic of microscopy

i. Skilled microscopist with proper infrastructure can pick up parasites as low as 5–10 parasite/µl of blood[6]. However in actual practice most diagnostic laboratories generally achieve detection when parasite level is 100–500 parasite/µl of blood[7,8].

ii. Species identification can be done which is vital where treatment differs with different species. Stage of parasite can also be ascertained in the peripheral blood. In general prognosis worsens with predominance of more mature parasite stage. In general if more than 50% of the peripheral blood parasite are at the tiny ring stage (diameter of the nucleus <50% of the diameter of the rim of cytoplasm) the prognosis is relatively good. Presence of pigment containing asexual parasite of *P. falciparum* indicates bad prognosis if more than 20% of the parasite shows it. It indicates mature trophozoites or schizonts which has been released in the peripheral blood from parasites sequestered in the capillaries of internal organs[9].

iii. Determination of the number of circulating parasite (parasite density) is exceedingly important to monitor the severity of malaria, evolution of the disease and assessing therapeutic efficacy. Parasite density can be calculated from both thick and thin film and expressed either as number of parasite present in per microliter of blood or percentage of parasitized RBC. There in no uniform agreed definition of hyperparasitemia but parasite count of more than 250,000/µl of blood or more than 5% parasitized red blood cells carry poor prognosis[9]. It is important that every positive blood film should have parasite density assessed exactly in the same way on post treatment specimens as on the initial specimen to judge therapeutic efficacy. Counting parasite in a limited area of thick film is acceptable when large number of parasite are encountered whereas percentage infection of RBC in thin film are method of choice with low parasitemia.

iv. The presence of malaria pigment in polymorphonuclear leukocyte are diagnostic of malaria. It is particularly useful in anemic children with severe malaria associated with low parasitemia. If more than 5% of polymorphonuclear leukocyte contain visible pigment prognosis worsens[9].

Disadvantages of microscopy

i. It is time consuming often requiring more than 60 minutes from blood collection to result[2].

ii. It is labor intensive, needs significant technical skill and proper infrastructure which are often unavailable at peripheral health centers.

iii. There is often long delay in providing the results of microscopy leading to treatment without the benefit of the results.

iv. It cannot detect parasite sequestered deep in the vascular compartment which often requires repeated blood examination.

Rapid Diagnostic Tests (RDTs)

These tests were developed with the hope that it would offer accurate, cheap and rapid results as compared to traditional diagnosis. Tests are sensitive at parasite level of more than 100–500 parasite/µl of blood. However they have shown limitation in sensitivity in low parasite count, ability to differentiate between species and robustness under field condition in the tropics. It was expected they would give information on parasite densities, distinguish between viable parasite from parasite products not associated with viable parasite and prediction of treatment outcome.

They employ monoclonal antibodies targeted against the parasite antigens. The test kit contains specific antibody that is labeled with a visually detectable marker. If the antigen under investigation is present then antigen-antibody complex is formed. The labeled antigen-antibody complex will be immobilized at the pre-deposited line of capture antibody and will be visually detectable. Whether the blood contains antigen or not, the control line will become visible as labeled antibody is captured by the pre-deposited line of antibody directed against it. The test time varies from 5 to 15 minutes.

Targeted antigens in currently available RDTs

1. *Histidine-rich protein II (HRP-II)*—This is a water soluble protein produced by asexual stage and young gamatocytes of *P falciparum*[10].

2. *Parasite lactate dehydrogenase (pLDH)*—pLDH is an enzyme located in the glycolytic pathway of the malaria parasite produced by both sexual and asexual stages of the parasite. It is found in all the four species of malaria namely *P. falciparum, P. vivax, P. malarie* and *P. ovale* and is known as pan specific.
   Distinct isomers of pLDH for each of the four plasmodium species infecting humans exist and they can be detected.
   The next antigen is *P. falciparum* specific, pLDH[11].
   Some newer kits target *P. vivax* specific pLDH for detection of vivax malaria[11].

3. *Certain new antigens like plasmodium aldolase*—Plasmodium aldolase is also an enzyme of the glycolytic pathway produced by all four species has been recently developed[12].

Performance characteristics of RDTs

It is an important consideration before choosing an RDT which should include:

The test should be able to distinguish between malaria species at least falciparum and vivax. Falciparum and vivax malaria occurs in nearly equal number as single species infection in our country. Differentiation is essential as treatment of these two malaria differs hence accurate diagnosis is essential.

In our country where falciparum and vivax malaria parasite cocirculate, typically occurring as a single species infection an RDT which can detect both falciparum and vivax malaria and distinguishing between them is warranted[13].There are some commercially avaible kits which detects falciparum specific LDH and panspecific LDH. So they can distinguish between falciparum from non falciparum malaria. Problem with these kits are two fold, firstly they cannot distinguish falciparum malaria from mixed infection, secondly as vivax malaria is almost the only non falciparum malaria in our country so often they equate non falciparum malaria with vivax malaria.

1. The sensitivity and specificity for detection of each of the species should be noted. The World Health Organization (WHO) has recommended a minimum standard of 95% sensitivity for *P. falciparum* densities of 100 parasite/μl of blood and a specificity of 95%[14].

2. RDTs using HRPII are generally more sensitive than RDTs detecting *P. falciparum* specific PLDH. *P. vivax* specific monoclonal antibodies have undergone limited evaluation. Unfortunately independent peer reviewed evaluation for most commercially available RDTs are not available. In general with high parasite density these tests are fairly sensitive but with low parasite load sensitivity decreases often yielding false negative results. False positive result may also develop when gametocytes are present but asexual stage parasites are eradicated by therapy. One of the US FDA approved RTD was extensively investigated for its performance in tropical country[15]. The trial showed for detection of any plasmodium species overall sensitivity of the test was 82%. The overall sensitivity for detection of *P. falciparum* was 95%, with a sensitivity of 99% for parasitemia in excess of 1000 parasite/μl, dropping to 89% for parasitemia of 100 to 500 parasite/μl of blood. The overall specificity of *P. falciparum* was 94%. There are some reports of occasional failure of RDTs to detect high parasite densities. Reports of failure to defect both *P. falciparum* and *P. vivax* has been demonstrated even when parasite densities exceeded 5000/μl of blood[16].

3. HRPII antigen persist at detectable levels for more than 28 days even after successful therapy[17].

Aldolase and PLDH rapidly fall to undetectable levels after initiation of effective therapy but these antigens are expressed in gametocytes which may appear after clinical infection is cleared[18]. So none of the RDTs are useful for monitoring the response to treatment for which microscopy is the investigation of choice.

4. Test are usually simple without much training requirement, easy to interpret, does not need electricity and results are available rapidly. The stability of the kit in high environmental temperature and humidity of tropics should be taken into account.

Disadvantages of RDTs

1. RDTs are not quantitative but qualitative gives a yes or no answer. Hence they are not suitable for prognostication and cannot be used for assessment of therapeutic efficacy of antimalarial drugs.

2. Persistance of antigenemia after parasite clearance preludes using the test to monitor response to therapy.

3. RDTs have decreased sensitivity at lower levels of parasitemia yielding false negative results in non immune patients with low levels of parasitemia.

4. False positive results when gametocytes are present but asexual stage parasite are eradicated by therapy may lead to unnecessary treatment.

5. RDTs cannot determine the stage of parasite, i.e. early ring form or late schizonts and thus does not help is prognostication.

Advantages of RDTs

1. Relatively easy with minimal training and results are available quickly.

2. They are able to detect falciparum infection even when the parasite are sequestered in the deep vascular compartment and thus undetectable by microscopic examination of a peripheral blood smear.

Role of RDTs in the diagnosis of malaria in our country

In comparison to high transmission areas, malaria in our country occurs less frequently, in all age groups and almost always symptomatic. Drug resistance including multi drug resistance has started developing in our country so laboratory confirmation of malaria is an essential component of disease management. Expert microscopic diagnosis is available in central levels of health care system like metro cities but it is often unreliable or unavailable in areas with poor health facilities. So RDTs will be useful in following situations in our country:

i. In far away communities with poor health care facilities where microscopic diagnosis is not available. Also in areas where laboratory service is inadequate, of an unacceptable standard or not available at odd hours.

ii. In places where quality microscopy is available, RDTs and microscopy can run in parallel. RDTs will provide rapid or screening diagnosis whereas microscopy reserved for resolution of confusing cases, confirmation of negative result in RDTs with high clinical suspicion of malaria.

iii. US FDA has approved RDT with a note that negative results by the RDT be confirmed by microscopy[19].

iv. In some cases of severe and complicated malaria, peripheral parasitemia may be negative due to sequestration but RDTs are expected to provide evidence of antigenemia.

v. According to the new national Drug Policy of Malaria (2008) that any fever case clinically suspected of malaria should preferably be investigated for confirmation of malaria by microscopy or RDT so as to ensure full therapeutic dose with appropriate drug to all confirmed cases[20].

So in conclusion RDTSs permit on the spot confirmation of malaria even at the peripheral health care system, by unskilled health worker with minimal training. Rational use of RDTs as a complement to microscopy might offer following benefits:

i. Early treatment will reduce mortality and morbidity.

ii. In multi drug resistance areas expensive drugs and drug combination will be given to only to those who need them.

iii. Aviodance of unnecessary treatment will reduce drug pressure and delay progress of drug resistance.

Other Methods of Malaria Diagnosis

Fluorescent microscopy

The test is based on the ability of fluorescent dyes to detect RNA and DNA of the parasite. As mature red blood cells have no nucleus anything which binds the dye is presumed to be the parasite.

Quantitative buffy coat assay

A modification of fluorescent microscopy in which blood is first centrifused to separate the parasite below the grannulocyte layer. Subsequently the parasites are detected by fluorescent microscopy and are suitable for screening a large number of samples. Again this method is not useful for routine practice.

Polymerase chain reaction (PCR)

They are able to identify genetic material of the parasite. The test is highly sensitive which enables to detect even negligible amount of parasite DNA. It can also identify different species and mutations co-relating to resistance. However their use is limited to only research laboratories.

References

1. WHO Guidelines for the Treatment of Malaria, 2006. WHO/HTM/MAL/2006;1108:8-10.
2. World Health Organization. Approaches to the Diagnosis Malaria, In : New Perspectives Malaria Diagnosis. Report of a Joint WHO/USAID Informal Consultation 2000;10-18.
3. Nandy A. National Antimalarial Drug Policy and its implications in the malaria control in India. In: Ganguly N, Kundu R, Ghosh TK, eds. Common MDR Infections in Children. Typhoid, Tuberculosis Malaria. New Delhi : CBS Publication, 2005:197-207.
4. Gilles H. Diagnostic methods in malaria. In: Gilles HM, Warrekk DA, eds. Essential Malariology, 3rd ed. London: Arnold 1998;78.
5. Houwen B. Blood film preparation and staining procedure. *Clin Lab Med* 2002;22:1-14.
6. WHO. Severe and complicated Malaria. *Trans R Soc Med Hyg* 1990; 84(Suppl. 2):23-5.
7. WHO. Malaria diagnosis: Memorandum from a WHO meeting. *Bull WHO* 1988;66:575-94.
8. Milne LM, Chiodini PL, Warhurst DC. Accuracy of routine laboratory diagnosis of malaria in the United Kingdom. *J Clin Pathol* 1994;47:740-2.
9. World Health Organization. Control of tropical disease. Severe and complicated malaria. *Trans R Soc Trop Med Hyg* 1990;84(Suppl 2):1-65.
10. Hayward RE, Sullivan DJ, Day KP. *Plasmodium falciparum*: Histidne – rich protein II is expressed during gametocyte development. *Exp. Parasitol* 2000;96:139-46.
11. Makler MT, Piper RC, Milhous WK. Lactate dehydrogenase and the diagnosis of malaria. *Parasitol Today* 1998;14:376-77.
12. Meier B, Dobeli H, Certa U. Stage specific expression of aldolase isoenzyme in the rodent malaria parasite *Plasmodium bergei*. *Mol Biochem Parasitol* 1992;52:15-27.
13. WHO. The role of laboratory diagnosis to support malaria disease management: Focus on the use of rapid diagnostic tests in areas of high transmission. Geneva: WHO, 2006.
14. WHO, Western Pacific Region. Towards quality testing of malaria rapid diagnostic tests : evidence and methods. Manila WHO: Western Pacific Region, 2006.
15. Gasser RA Jr. Magill AJ, Ruebush T, Miller RS, Sirichaisinthop J, Forney JR, *et al.* Malarial diagnosis : performance of NOW ICT Malaria in a large scale field trial. Abstr 54th Annu. Meet. Am Soc Trop Med Hyg. Abstr 2338.
16. Iqbal J, Khalid N, Hira PR. Comparison of two commercial assays with expert microscopy for confirmation of symptomatically diagnosed malaria. *J Clin Microbial* 2002;40:4675-78.
17. Karbwang J, Tasanor O, Kanda T, Wattanagoon Y, Ibrahim M, Na-Bangchang K, *et al.* ParaSight – F test for the detection of treatment failure in multidrug resistant *Plasmodium falciparum* malaria. *Trans R Soc Trop Med Hyg* 1996;90:513-15.
18. Mueller L, Betuela I, Ginny M, Reeder JC, Genton B. The sensitivity of the OptiMAL rapid diagnostic test to the presence of *Plasmodium falciparum* gametocytes compromises its ability to monitor treatment outcomes in an area of Papua New Guinea in which malaria is endemic. *J Clin Microbial* 2007;45:627-30.
19. http://www.fda.gov/edrh/pdf6/K061542 pdf. Access on 27.01.2009.
20. National Drug Policy on Malaria. Directorate of National Vector Borne Disease Control Program. Directorate General of Health Services. Ministry of Health and Family Welfare, 22 Shamnath Marg, Delhi 110054, 2008.

18

Treatment of Uncomplicated Malaria

Ritabrata Kundu

Malaria is a major public health problem of our country and one of the leading causes of mortality and morbidity. It is heartening to note that the total number of laboratory confirmed malaria cases have declined from 3 million reported in 1997 to 1.84 million in early 2000[1]. At the same time it is of concern that the number of falciparum cases is constantly on the rise and in recent years they contribute nearly 50% of the total cases[2]. Chloroquine (CQ) resistant falciparum malaria was identified first in the districts of north eastern India along the international borders. Subsequently CQ resistance has spread widely throughout the country. Treatment failure to CQ resulted in the use of second line drug like sulphadoxine- pyrimethamine (SP) for resistant falciparum malaria. Unfortunately resistance to SP combination at a various levels has also been reported in the district of seven north eastern states of India. This multidrug resistance to conventional antimalarials like CQ and SP is the result of their inappropriate use. Antimalarial drug was used in the past on a large scale often without a confirmed diagnosis. They were used as monotherapies, introduced in sequence and were continued despite unacceptably high level of resistance.

Malaria parasite develops resistance to drugs randomly due to *de novo* genetic mutations. As non immune patients of our country are infected with large number of parasites, if they receive inadequate treatment are a potent source of *de novo* resistance. Here lies the importance of prescribing highly effective treatment regimen in hyper parasitaemic patients and ensuring good adherence to prescribed drugs[3].

It has been noted that monotherapy of case of resistant falciparum malaria invariably results in failure. SP introduced following CQ resistance fell rapidly to resistance in the early 1980s[4]. Whereas mefloquine introduced as monotherapy for falciparum malaria took only 4–5 years to report resistance[4].

So to counter the threat of resistance of falciparum to monotherapies WHO recommends combinations of antimalarials for the treatment of falciparum malaria.

Status of Drug Resistance in India

In India first reports of resistance of *P. falciparum* to CQ came from Diphu of Karbi Anglong district in Assam state. Thereafter it started spreading throughout the country. The Directorate of national vector borne diseases control program is monitoring the response of antimalarial drugs in falciparum malaria since 1978 according to new WHO protocol on therapeutic efficacy of anti-malarial drugs in uncomplicated *P. falciparum* malaria"[5]. The list of areas showing high treatment failure to chloroquine is given and depicted in map in Fig. 18.1 and Table 18.1[6].

Reports of resistance to SP at various levels in district of seven north eastern states of our country are there[7]. Five therapeutic efficacy studies with SP were undertaken in Assam, West Bengal, Meghalaya and Orissa. Of these, three states namely Assam, West Bengal, and Meghalaya reported treatment failure in more than 10% cases[8]. Studies in Arunachal Pradesh also observed treatment failure with SP in falciparum malaria[9].

Though few reports of emergence of chloroquine resistant *P. vivax* are there yet the drug still retains its affectivity against vivax malaria in our country[6].

Antimalarial Combination Therapy

To improve treatment outcome and halt the threat of resistance to monotherapy WHO recommends combination of antimalarials for the treatment of falciparum malaria. Anti-malarial combination therapy is the simul-taneous use of two or more blood schizonto-cidal drugs with independent mode of action and thus unrelated biochemical target in the parasite[3].

If two drugs with different modes of action and hence different resistance mechanisms are used in combination, the probability of developing resistance to both drugs is the product of their individual per parasite is there. To site an example, say 1 out of every 10^{12} parasites has a probability to develop resistance to drug X. Similarly chance of developing resistance to another drugs Y is also 1 out of 10^{12} parasites. Then the chance of a mutant parasite resistant to both drugs X and Y will be 1 out of every 10^{24} parasites ($10^{12} \times 10^{12}$). Fortunately this amount of parasite is usually not present in an individual infection. To simplify the matter if a mutant parasite arises *de novo* during the course of infection to one drug it will be killed by the other drug. However, to reap the benefit of combination therapy the partners in the combination should be individually effective. This mutual protection will prevent or at least delay emergence of resistance to individual drugs. The only disadvantage of combination therapy is increased risk of adverse effect and increased cost of therapy.

According to WHO one of the partners in combination therapy will be artemisinin and its derivatives hence known as artemisinin-based combination therapy (ACT) The reason for choosing artemisinin is its rapid clearance of parasitemia and resolution of symptoms. They reduce the parasite number by approxi-mately 10,000 fold (10^4) in each asexual cycle. The second important reason is its rapid elimination from the body so that the residual concentration of the drug does not provide a selective filter for resistant parasites. The other reasons being its lack of serious adverse effects and absence of significant resistance till date[10].

If artemisinin are combined with other rapidly eliminated antimalarials like tetracycline or clindamycin, a 7 days course of treatment is required. This long course invariably results in poor adherence. But when combined with slowly eliminated anti-malarials like SP, mefloquine (MQ) or lumifantrine shorter courses of treatment (3 days) will be effective and also ensure adherence.

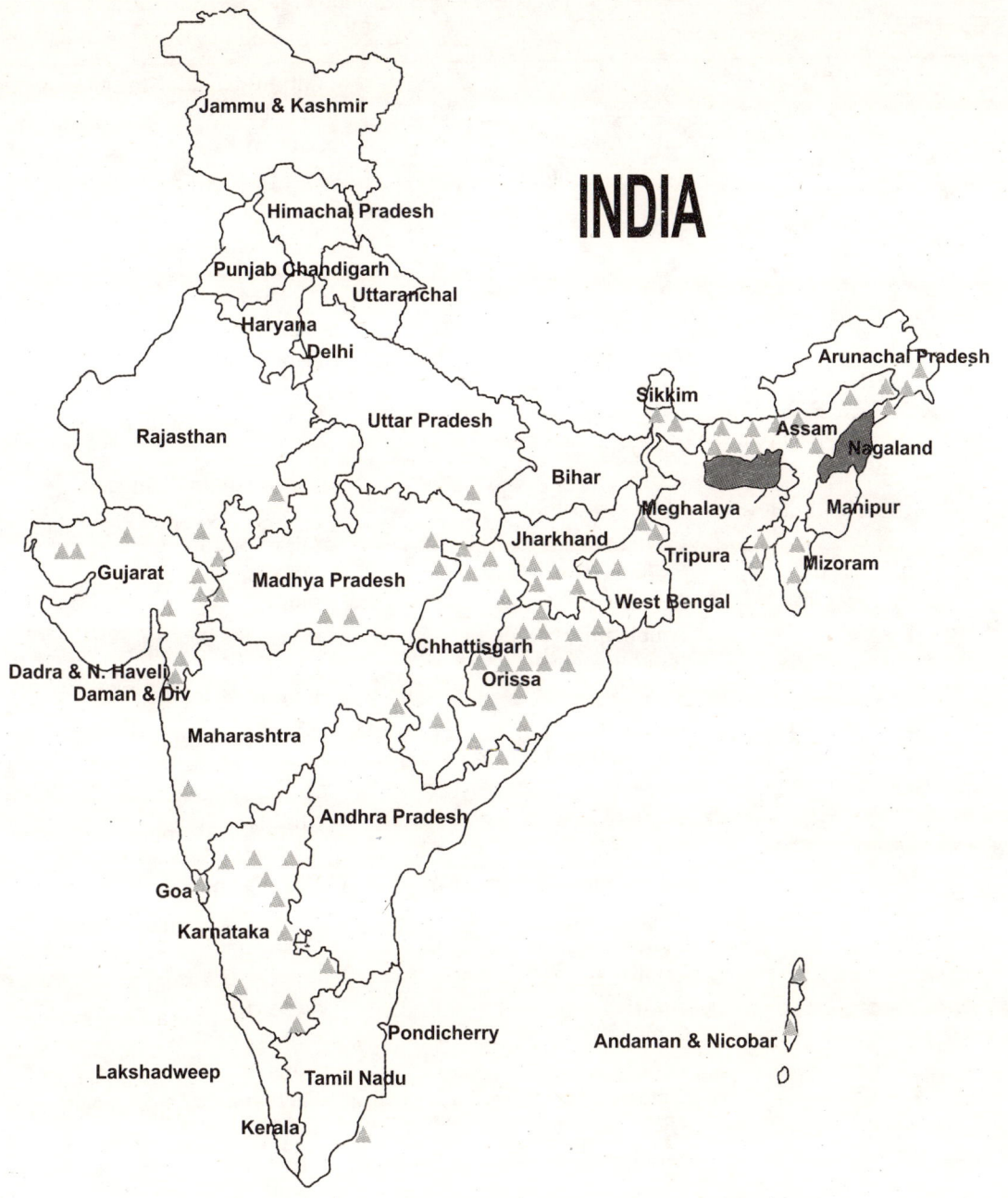

Fig. 18.1: Chloroquine resistant areas (1978-2008 updated to August)

Table 18.1: List of chloroquine resistant areas

S.no.	State/UT	District	No. of PHCs	Name of PHCs
1.	Andhra Pradesh	Vizianagaram	2	Modumkhalu, Kurupam
2.	A and N Islands	Great Nicobar	1	Cambel Bay
		Little Andaman	1	Hutbay
3.	Assam	Karbi Anglong	2	Manja and Bokajan
		Nagaon	2	Simonbasti and STE
		Darrang	1	Orang
		Kamrup	1	Sonapur
		Nalbari	1	Tamalpur
		Sonitpur	1	Behali
		Tinsukhia	1	Samdang TE
		Lakhimpur	1	Nowboicha
		Kokrajhar	2	Balajan and Gossaigaon
		Chirang	1	Balamguri
		Baksa	2	Musalpur and Naukata
4.	Arunachal Pradesh	Lohit	2	Namsai and Chowkham
		Changlang	2	Jairampur and Miao
5.	Chhattisgarh	Jagdalpur	1	DNK project area
		Korba	1	Pondiuprora
		Ambikapur	1	Wadrafnagar
		Raigarh	1	Lailunga
		Korea	1	Khadgawal
6.	Dadra and Nagar Havell	UT Dadra and Nagara Haveli	1	Khanvel
7.	Goa	North Goa	3	Aldoma, Panjim and Candolim
		South Goa	1	Mudgaon
8.	Gujarat	Panchmahal	1	Kadana
		Kutch Bhuj	2	Kavada and Gorewali
		Anand	1	Pansora
		Dahod	1	Degawada
		Patan	1	Lolada
		Surat	1	Surat city
9.	Jharkhand	Gumla	1	Palkot
		Ranchi	1	Angada
		Simdega	3	Thethaitanagar, Simdega and Jaldega
		Saraikela	1	Chandil
10.	Karnataka	Kolar	1	Gulur
		Raichur	3	Echanal, Ramdurga and Nagarala
		Bellary	1	Kamalpura
		Mandya	1	DK halli
		Bagalkot	2	Kamatagi and Nandikeshwar

Contd...

Contd...

S.no.	State/UT	District	No. of PHCs	Name of PHCs
		D Kannada	1	Mangalore
		Chemarajanagar	1	Sathegala
		Gadag	1	Bellatti
		Chitradurga	1	Ranganathapura
		Belgaun	1	AK Hall
11.	Madhya Pradesh	Jhabua	1	Kalyanpura
		Dindori	1	Banjag
		Shahdol	1	Jaisinghnagar
		Chhindwara	1	Harrai
12.	Maharashtra	Raigarh	1	Washi
		Gadchiroli	2	Dhanora and Yetapalli
13.	Meghalaya	W Garo Hills	3	Zikzak, Darengiri, Chokpot
14.	Mizoram	Aizwal	1	Sairang
		Lunglei	1	Hnanthial
15.	Nagaland	Dimapur	1	Dimapur
		Mokokchung	1	Mokokchung
16.	Orissa	Keonjhar	3	Keonjhar town, Telkoi and Banspal
		Kandhamal	2	Daringabari and Phiringia
		Sundergarh	3	Kuarmundu, Bisra and Guruindia
		Angul	1	Bantala
		Dhenkanal	1	Khajurikata
		Deogarh	1	Tileibbani
		Mayurbhanj	2	Badanpaher and Kaptipada
		Bolangir	1	Khaprakhol
		Kalahandi	2	M Rampur and Kokasara
		Boudh	2	Adenigarh and Manmmunda
		Nuapada	3	Khariar, Bhella and Sinpali
		Koraput	1	Borigumma
		Sambalpur	1	Charmal
		Gajapati	1	Mohana
17.	Rajasthan	Dungarpur	1	Bicchiwara
		Banswara	1	Kushalgarh
		Baran	2	Kishanganj and Shahbad
18.	Tamil Nadu	Rameshwaram Island	1	Rameshwaram Island
19.	Tripura	South Tripura	1	Santibazar
		Dhalai	1	Kulai
20.	Uttar Pradesh	Mirzapur	1	NTPC Shaktinagar
21.	West Bengal	Purulia	3	Bagmundi, Bandhwan and Sirkabad
		Jalpaiguri	2	Uttar Latabari, Mal
		Bankura	1	Ranibandh
		Darjeeling	2	Naxalbari, Sukna
	Total	**82 districts**	**113 PHCs**	

In 3 days ACT regimen artemisinin is present in the body during the two asexual parasite life cycles each lasting for 2 days. This treatment reduces the number of parasites in the body by a factor of approximately one hundred million ($10^4 \times 10^4 = 10^8$). The complete clearance of the parasites is dependent on the partner medicine being effective and persisting at parasiticidal concentration until all the infecting parasites have been killed. Thus the partner compound is to be relatively slowly eliminated.

As a result of combination therapy the artemisinin component is protected from resistance by the partner medicine, provided it is efficacious and partner medicine is in turn protected by the artemisinin derivative.

The only significant adverse effect from clinical trials with artemisinin is rare type I hypersensitive reaction manifested by urticaria. It has also the advantage of reducing gametocyte carriage and thus transmission of malaria which is particularly important in malaria control. The following ACTs are currently available in our country:

1. Artesunate (AS) + SP
2. Artesunate + MQ
3. Artesunate-lumefantrine

Of these artesunate-lumefantrine is available as co-formulated tablets and lumifantrine is not available as monotherapy. So it has been never used alone for the treatment of malaria. Other combinations are available separately.

Basis of Antimalarial Therapy

Malaria in children has some unique features. Young children whose passive immunity from mother wanes and as yet to develop sufficient immunity on their own are most vulnerable. Falciparum malaria can show rapid deterioration in children hence constant monitoring is essential.

Children can tolerate antimalarials better than adults and also their symptoms resolve more quickly following successful therapy.

According to the national drug policy on malaria 2008 presumptive treatment with incomplete dose of chloroquine in fever cases has been stopped[11].

All efforts should be given to treat malaria after diagnosis by microscopic examination, rapid diagnostic tests or both as facilities and circumstances dictate. In situations where such facilities are not available one should make at least clinical diagnosis of malaria following clinical algorithmic approach. If decision to treat is made, a full effective treatment is to be given whether or not the diagnosis is confirmed by a test[10].

Some patients cannot tolerate oral treatment and may require parenteral therapy for few days until they can swallow and retain oral medications. Such patients even if they show no signs of severe malaria should receive same antimalarial dose regimes meant for severe malaria[10].

Patients with hyperparasitemia but without signs of severity are at increased risk of developing severe malaria. They can be treated with oral medications recommended for uncomplicated malaria but need close monitoring and may require longer courses of treatment[10].

In symptomatic treatment of fever in indicated particularly in small children where fever can induce vomiting and may result in seizures, paracetamol or ibuprofen may be used. Tepid sponging may also be done.

One should ensure proper adherence to treatment as medicine is taken at home without supervision. According to the national drug policy on malaria 2008 resistance should be suspected if in spite of full treatment with no history of vomiting or diarrhea, patient does not respond within 72 hours parasitologically[11].

Treatment Regimen in Uncomplicated Malaria

Treatment regimens are to be tailored specifically according to the resistance pattern of the region under consideration. According to the Directorate General of Health Services, National Vector Borne Disease Control Programme ACT (AS + SP combination) in faciparum malaria is being implemented in 117 districts (i.e. 50 highly endemic districts of states namely Andhra Pradesh, Chhattisgarh, Jharkhand, Madhya Pradesh and Orissa + 67 in North Eastern States) in addition to 253 PHCs of 46 districts included on the basis of chloroquine resistance status and its surrounding clusters of blocks as shown in Table 18.2. However, in view of gradually increasing resistance it has been suggested that all falciparum cases may be treated with ACT both in public or private health care system to win the war against ongoing drug resistance[8]. Tables 18.2a, 18.2b and 18.2c show the recommended therapy of malaria.

Table 18.2a: Recommended treatment in chloroquine sensitive malaria

Drug sensitivity	Recommended treatment
P. vivax and chloroquine sensitive	Chloroquine 10 mg base/kg stat orally followed by 5 mg/kg at 6, 24 and 48 hours (total dose 25 mg/kg) OR
P. falciparum	Chloroquine 10 mg base/kg stat orally followed by 10 mg/kg at 24 hours and 5 mg/kg at 48 hours (total dose 25 mg base/kg). In case of vivax malaria to prevent relapse primaquine should be given in a dose of 0.25 mg/kg once daily for 14 days. In case of falciparum malaria a single dose of primaquine (0.75 mg/kg) is given for gametocytocidal action.

i. Chloroquine should not be given in empty stomach and in high fever. Bring down the temperature first. If vomiting occurs within 45 minutes of a dose of chloroquine that particular dose is to be repeated after taking care of vomiting by using antiemitic (Domperidone/Ondansetron).

ii. As primaquine can cause hemolytic anemia in children with G6PD deficiency they should be preferably screened for the same prior to starting treatment. As infants are relatively G6PD deficient it is not recommended in this age group and children with 14 days regimen should be under close supervision to detect any complication. In cases of borderline G6PD deficiency once weekly dose of primaquine 0.6 – 0.8 mg/kg is given for 6 weeks.

Table 18.2b: Recommended treatment in chloroquine resistant *P. falciparum*

Drug sensitivity	Recommended treatment
Chloroquine resitant *P. falciparum*	Artesunate 4 mg/kg of body weight orally once daily for 3 days and a single administration of SP as 25 mg/kg of sulfadoxine and 1.25 mg/kg of pyrimethamine on day 1 OR
	Artesunate as above and mefloquine 25 mg/kg of body weight in two divided doses (15 mg/kg and 10 mg/kg) on day 2 and day 3. OR
	Co-formulated tablets containing 20 mg of artemether and 120 mg of lumefantrine can be used as a six dose regimen orally twice a day for 3 days. For 5–14 kg body weight 1 tablet at diagnosis, again after

Contd...

Contd...

8–12 hours and then twice daily on day 2 and day 3. For 15 to 24 kg body weight same schedule with 2 tablets. For 25–35 kg body weight and above same schedule with 3 and 4 tablets respectively.

A single dose of primaquine (0.75 mg/kg) is given for gametocytocidal action.

i. Currently there are insufficient safety and tolerability data on mefloquine at its recommended dosage of 25 mg/kg body weight in children. Mefloquine shares cross resistance with quinine which is still an effective drug in our country. Health planners of our country do not advocate use of mefloquine.

ii. Advantage of artemether lumefantrine combination is that lumefantrine is not available as monotherapy and has never been used alone for the treatment of malaria. Lumefantrine absorption is enhanced by coadministration with fatty food like milk.

Table 18.2c: Recommended treatment of multidrug resistant *P. falciparum* (Both to CQ and SP)

Drug sensitivity	Recommended treatment
Multidrug resistant	• Quinine, 10 mg salt/kg/ dose orally 3 times daily for 7 days.
P. falciparum, i.e. both to CQ and SP	+ Tetracycline (above 8 years) 4 mg/kg/dose 4 times daily for 7 days OR Doxycycline (above 8 years) 3.5 mg/kg once a day for 7 days OR Clindamycin 20 mg/kg/day in 2 divided doses for 7 days.

Contd...

Contd...

• In case of developing cinchonism, quinine, 10 mg salt/kg/dose orally 3 times daily for 3–5 days

+

Tetracycline (above 8 years) 4 mg/kg/dose 4 times daily for 7 days

OR

Doxycycline (above 8 years) 3.5 mg/kg once a day for 7 days

OR

Clindamycin 20 mg/kg/day in 2 divided doses for 7 days.

OR

• Artemether lumefantrine combination orally as in table 18.2b.

OR

• Artemether mefloquine combination orally as in table 18.2b.

A single dose of primaquine above 1 year age (0.75 mg/ kg) is given for gametocytocidal action.

i. Doxycycline is preferred to tetracycline as it can be given once daily and does not accumulate in renal failure.

ii. One of the drawbacks of quinine therapy is its long course. Unsupervised and ambulatory setting may decrease patients compliance and many patients might not complete the full course of prescribed therapy.

iii. Fortunately children tolerate quinine better than adults.

Management of Treatment Failure with ACT

Failure within 14 days

This is very unusual as reported by the various trials conducted throughout the world[10].

Recurrence may be due to either reinfection or recrudescence, which in individual patient are virtually impossible to distinguish. All failure cases should be confirmed parasitologically preferably by blood slide examination as in HRPII-based rapid diagnostic tests antigenemia may persist for weeks. It is important to determine treatment adherance and whether patient has vomited the therapy. Table 18.3 shows recommended therapy to be undertaken.

Failure after 14 days

It may be also result of recrudescence or new infection. Parasitological confirmation is desirable. Even if it recrudescence then first line treatment should still be effective.

Table 18.3: Recommended treatment in failure with artemisinin combination therapy (ACT)

Drug sensitivity	Recommended treatment
Failure of ACT	Quinine + Tetracycline or Doxycycline or clindamycin orally for 7 days as in Table 18.2c.

i. Treatment failure within 14 days of receiving an ACT is very unusual. It should be confirmed parasitologically by blood slide examination. It is important to determine whether patient has vomited previous treatment or did not complete a full course.

ii. Failure after 14 days of treatment can be re-treated with first line ACT.

iii. Seven days quinine regimen shows poor adherence if not observed.

References

1. Park K. Malaria. In: Park's Text Book of Preventive and Social Medicine, 17th ed. Jabalpur: Banarasidas Bhanot, 2002;192-202.
2. Directorate General of Health Services. National Vector Borne Disease Control Programme. Malaria Drug Resistance 2004. New Delhi : Ministry of Health and Family Welfare, Govt. of India 2004.
3. WHO Guidelines for the Treatment of Malaria. WHO/HTM/MAL/2006.1108.
4. White NJ. Malaria. In: Cook GC, Zumla A, eds. Manson's Tropical Diseases, 21st ed. London: WB saunders, 2003:1207-15.
5. World Health Organisation. Assessment of Therapeutic Efficacy of Antimalarial Drugs for Complicated Falciparum Malaria in Areas with Intense transmission. Geneva: World Health Organization, 1996, WHO/MAL/96.1077.
6. Directorate General of Health Services. National Vector Borne Disease Control Programme. Malaria Drug Resistance 2008. New Delhi: Ministry of Health and Family Welfare, Govt. of India 2008.
7. Directorate of National Vector Borne Disease Control Programme. Report of Meeting of an Expert Group. New Delhi: NVBDCP, 2004.
8. Arora U, Sonal GS, Dhillon GPS, Thakor HG. Emergence of drug resistance in India. *J India Med Assoc* 2008; 106:678-83.
9. Mohapatra PK, Namchomm NS, Prakash A, Bhattacharya DR, Goswami BK, Mahajan J. Therapeutic efficacy of antimalarials. In: *Plasmodium falciparum* Malaria in Indo-Myanmar Border Area of Arunachal Pradesh. *Indian J Med Res* 2003; 118:71-6.
10. WHO Guidelines for the Treatment of Malaria. WHO/HTM/MAL/2006.16-40.
11. National Drug Policy on Malaria, 2008. Director of National Vector Borne Disease Control Program. Delhi: Directorate General of Health Services, Ministry of Health and Family Welfare, 2008.

19

Management of Severe and Complicated Malaria

Ashok Kapse, Ritabrata Kundu, Nupur Ganguly

Severe and complicated malaria is a medical emergency carrying propensity for complications and mortality, however, apt diagnosis and timely treatment can prevent most of these complications.

Definition of severe falciparum malaria—One or more of the criteria written in Table 19.1 in the presence of asexual parasitemia define severe falciparum malaria.

Management of Severe Malaria in Children

Severe life threatening malaria is nearly always due to *P. falciparum*. All cases with severe manifestations are to be treated in the same line of complicated malaria with injectable antimalarials irrespective of the species.

High degree of suspicion of severe malaria is of utmost importance and any delay in initiation of treatment can be fatal. It should be treated as a medical emergency at highest level of medical facility available preferably in an intensive care setting. Confirmation of the diagnosis is preferable but one should not delay the treatment if it needs more than 1 hour[1]. Further in cases of strong clinical suspicion prompt antimalarial therapy is needed even if parasites are not found in the initial blood examination.

Severe malaria in children differs to certain extent from adults. Progression to cerebral malaria can be very rapid, but again, recovery is also rapid. Commonest complications in children are cerebral malaria, severe anemia, respiratory distress (acidosis) and hypoglycemia. Fortunately, common complications in adults like pulmonary edema and jaundice are rare in children. The definition of severe malaria was proposed by working groups convened by WHO in 1990[1] and modified in the year 2000[2] (Tables 19.1, 19.2). In case of high degree of suspicion physician should not withhold treatment even if the patients do not clearly qualify into any one of the categories.

The main objective of treatment is to prevent the patients from dying. Prevention of recrudescence, transmission or emergence of resistance and prevention of disabilities are of secondary importance. Untreated severe malaria has a mortality of 100% but with proper treatment it falls to 15–20%. As death

Table 19.1: Features of severe malaria

Severe manifestation of P. falciparum in children

Prognostic value[a]		Frequency[a]
Clinical manifestation		
+	Prostration	+++
+++	Impaired consciousness	+++
+++	Respiratory distress (acidotic breathing)	+++
+	Multiple convulsions	+++
+++	Circulatory collapse	+
+++	Pulmonary edema (radiological)	+/−
+++	Abnormal bleeding	+/−
++	Jaundice	+
+	Hemoglobinuria	+/−
Laboratory findings		
+	Severe anemia	+++
+++	Hypoglycemia	+++
+++	Acidosis	+++
+++	Hyperlactatemia	+++
+/−	Hyperparasitemia	++
++	Renal impairment	+

[a] On a scale from + to +++; +/− indicate infrequent occurrence.

due to severe malaria often occurs within hours of admission it is essential to ensure therapeutic concentration of antimalarials as soon as possible.

Effective therapy in children with severe malaria includes antimalarial chemotherapy, supportive management and management of complications. All these three interventions are equally important and to be taken care of simultaneously.

General Danger Signs of Malarial (Table 19.2)

Table 19.2: General danger signs of malaria

Danger signs of malaria:

  i. Not able to drink or breast-feed
 ii. Vomiting everything
iii. Recent history of convulsion
 iv. Lethargic or unconscious state
  v. Unable to sit or stand up

The parent/guardian should be instructed to bring the child to the doctor if the patient develops any of the danger signs during the follow up.

Antimalarial Chemotherapy of Severe and Complicated Malaria (Table 19.3)

Ideally, antimalarial drug should be given initially by intravenous infusion, which should be replaced by oral administration as soon as condition permits.

After weighing the patient antimalarials should be given according to the body weight. If parenteral injection is not possible, referral is likely to be delayed and artemisinin is not available as suppository form, consider crushed antimalarial to be given by naso-gastric tube. But it has the risk of causing vomiting and may produce inadequate drug levels in the blood.

Table 19.3: Drug and dosage of antimalarials in complicated and severe malaria

Drug	Dosage[1,4]
Quinine salt	20 mg salt/kg (loading dose) diluted in 10 ml of isotonic fluid/kg by infusion over 4 hours. Then 12 hours after the start of loading dose give a maintenance dose of 10 mg salt/kg over 2 hours. This maintenance dose should be repeated every 8 hours, calculated from beginning of previous infusion, until the patient can swallow, then quinine tablets, 10 mg salt/kg 8 hourly to complete a 7 days course of treatment (including both parenteral and oral). Tetracycline or doxycycline or clindamycin is added to quinine as soon as the patient is able to swallow and should be continued for 7 days. Tetracycline (above 8 years) or doxycycline (above 8 years) to be given for 7 days 4 mg/kg/dose 4 times daily or 3.5 mg /kg once a day respectively. Clindamycin to be given 20 mg/kg/day in 2 divided doses for 7 days. If controlled IV infusion cannot be administered, quinine salt can be given in the same dosages by IM injection in the anterior thigh (not in buttock). The dose of quinine should be divided between two sites, half the dose in each anterior thigh. If possible IM quinine should be diluted in normal saline to a concentration of 60–100 mg salt/ml. (Quinine is usually available as 300 mg salt/ml). Tetracycline or doxycycline or clindamycin should be added as above. OR
Artesunate	2.4 mg/kg IV stat dose then at 12 and 24 hours, then once a day for total 7 days. If the patient is able to swallow, daily dose can be given orally. Tetracycline or doxycycline or clindamycin is added to artesunate as soon as the patient can swallow and should be continued for 7 days. Dosage as above. OR
Artemether	3.2 mg/kg (loading dose) IM, followed by 1.6 mg/kg daily for 6 days. If the patient is able to swallow, daily dose can be given orally. Tetracycline or doxycycline or clindamycin is added to artemether as soon as the patient can swallow and should be continued for 7 days. Dosage as above.

  i. Loading dose of quinine should not be used if the patient has received quinine, quinidine or mefloquine within the preceding 12 hours. Alternatively loading dose can be administered as 7 mg salt/kg by IV infusion pump over 30 minutes, followed immediately by 10 mg salt/kg diluted in 10 ml isotonic fluid/kg by IV infusion over 4 hours.

 ii. Quinine should not be given by bolus or push injection. Infusion rate should not exceed 5 mg salt/kg/hour.

iii. If there is no clinical improvement after 48 hours of parenteral therapy the maintenance dose of quinine should be reduced by one third to one half, i.e. 5–7 mg salt/kg.

iv. Quinine should not be given subcutaneo-usly as this may cause skin necrosis.

 v. Artesunate, 60 mg per ampoule is dissolved in 0.6 ml of 5% sodium bicarbonate diluted to 3–5 ml with 5% dextrose and given immediately by IV bolus (push injection).

vi. Artemether is dispensed in 1 ml ampoule containing 80 mg of artemether in peanut oil.

According to the National Drug Policy on Malaria 2008 in all cases of severe malaria either IV quinine or parentral artemisinin derivatives are to be given irrespective of chloroquine resistance status[3].

Quinine or Artemisinin — Which One to Use?

Artemisinin are the most rapidly acting of all known antimalarial drugs, they often produce a 10,000 fold reduction of parasites per asexual cycle. They have the broadest time window of antimalarial effects from ring forms to early schizonts. Thus they can stop parasite maturation, particularly from less pathogenic circulating ring stages to more pathogenic cytoadherent stages[5].

Artemisinin also has an excellent safety profile and the cost of therapy as compared to quinine is almost similar. There are no reports of resistance to artemisinin at present but declining sensitivity to quinine has been reported from some South East Asian countries like Thailand.

One large multicentric trial from South East Asia enrolling 1461 patients (including 202 children less than 15 years old) found a significant advantage of artesunate over quinine in mortality (15% vs 22%). There was an absolute reduction in mortality of 34.7% in the artesunate group[4]. Quinine therapy was associated with hypoglycemia. The result of this and other trials suggest that artesunate is the treatment of choice in severe malaria. Quinine is also effective and should be used when artesunate is not available.

Artesunate has better pharmacokinetic properties as it can be administered intravenously thereby assuring rapid therapeutic concentration whereas artemether is absorbed erratically following intra-muscular injection which cannot be administered intravenously. There are relatively few published comparative trials of these two drugs but artesunate has a definite pharmacokinetic advantage over artemether. Simultaneous use of quinine and artemisinin is not indicated as it may be harmful and there is no added advantage.

Supportive Management

i. Rapid clinical assessment with respect to level of consciousness (use Blantyre coma scale), blood pressure, rate and depth of respiration, anemia, state of hydration and temperature.

ii. Thick and thin blood films should be sent for detection of malarial parasite. Minimal investigation should include PCV (hematocrit), blood glucose and lumbar puncture especially in cerebral malaria. If lumbar puncture is delayed proper antibiotic cover for meningitis must be given. Antibiotics may also be considered if any secondary infection is suspected, which is common in severe malaria. Start intravenous antimalarial after drawing blood.

iii. Good nursing care with proper positioning, meticulous attention to airways, eyes, mucosa and skin should be done. Appropriate fluid therapy is to be given.

iv. For unconscious child nasogastric tube is to be inserted to reduce the risk of aspiration.

v. Oxygen therapy and respiratory support should be given if necessary.

vi. In case of shock resuscitate with normal saline or Ringer's lactate by bolus infusion, avoid under or over hydration.

vii. Convulsion should be treated with diazepam.

viii. Hyperpyrexia should be treated with tepid sponging, fanning and paracetamol.

ix. Close monitoring of the vital signs preferably every 4 hours to be done till the patient is out of danger. Also maintain intake output chart and watch for hemoglobinuria.

x. Monitoring of the response to treatment is essential. Detail clinical examination with particular emphasis on hydration status, temperature, pulse, respiratory rate, blood pressure and level of consciousness is to be given. Blood smear examination every 6 to 12 hours for parasitemia for first 48 hours is needed.

xi. In case of quinine parasite count may remain unchanged or even rise in first 18–24 hours which should not be taken as an indicator of quinine resistance. However, parasite count should fall after 24 hours of quinine therapy and should disappear within 5 days[6].

xii. In case of artemisinin derivatives parasite count usually comes down within 5 to 6 hours of starting therapy. Asexual parasitemia generally disappears after 72 hours of therapy[6].

xiii. Poor prognosis is suggested by high parasite densities (above 5% RBC infected or parasite density > 250000/µl). At any parasitemia prognosis worsens if there is predominance of more mature parasite stages. If more than 20% of the parasite contain visible pigment (mature trophozoites and schizonts) the prognosis worsens. Poor prognosis is also indicated if more than 5% of the peripheral blood polymorphonuclear leukocyte contain visible malaria pigment[1].

xiv. In follow up cases add iron and folic acid.

Management of Complications of Malaria[1]

Of various complications of falciparum malaria the common and important ones in children are as follows:

a. Cerebral malaria
b. Severe anemia
c. Respiratory distress (acidosis)
d. Hypoglycemia

Cerebral malaria

Initial presentation is usually fever followed by inability to eat or drink. The progression to coma or convulsion is usually very rapid within one or two days. Convulsions may be very subtle with nystagmus, salivation or twitching of an isolated part of the body. Effort should be given to exclude other treatable causes of coma (e.g. bacterial meningitis, hypoglycemia). Patients should be given good nursing care, convulsions should be treated with diazepam/midazolam and avoid harmful adjuvant treatment like corticosteroids, mannitol, adrenaline and phenobarbitone.

Severe anemia

Children with hyperparasitemia due to acute destruction of red cells may develop severe anemia. Packed red cell transfusion should be given cautiously when PCV is 12% or less, or hemoglobin is below 4 g/dl. Transfusion should also be considered in patients with less severe anemia in the presence of respiratory distress (acidosis), impaired consciousness or hyperparasitemia (>20% of RBCs infected).

Lactic acidosis

Deep breathing with indrawing of lower chest wall without any localizing chest signs suggest lactic acidosis. It usually accompanies cerebral malaria, anemia or dehydration. Correct hypovolemia, treat anemia and prevent seizures. Monitor acid-base status, blood glucose and urea and electrolyte level.

Hypoglycemia

It is common in children below 3 years especially with hyperparasitemia or with convulsion. It also occurs in patients treated with quinine. Manifestations are similar to those of cerebral malaria so it can be easily overlooked. Monitor blood sugar every 4 to 6 hours. If facilities to monitor blood glucose are not available assume hypoglycemia in symptomatic patient and treat accordingly. Correct hypoglycemia with IV dextrose (25% dextrose 2 to 4 ml/kg by bolus) and it should be followed by slow infusion of 5% dextrose containing fluid to prevent recurrence.

Hyperpyrexia

High fever is common in children and may lead to convulsion and altered consciousness. Tepid sponging, fanning and paracetamol 15 mg/kg should be given.

Hyperparasitemia

Specially seen in nonimmune children associated with severe disease. Consider exchange transfusion/cytapheresis if greater than 20% of RBCs are parasitized.

Circulatory collapse (Algid malaria)

In case of circulatory collapse suspect Gram-negative septicemia, send blood for culture before starting antibiotics. Resuscitate with judicious use of fluids.

Spontaneous bleeding and coagulopathy (DIC)

Usually seen is nonimmune children which should be treated with vitamin K, blood or blood products as required.

References

1. World Health Organisation. Management of Severe Malaria. A Practical Hand Book, 2nd ed. Geneva: WHO, 2000.
2. World Health Organization. Control of tropical disease. Severe and complicated malaria. *Trans R Soc Trop Med Hyg* 1990;84(Suppl 2):1-65.
3. National Drug Policy on Malaria 2008: Directorate of National Vector Borne Diseases Program. Director General of Health Services, Ministry of Health and Family Welfare, 22, Shamnath Marg, New Delhi 110054.
4. World Health Organization. Guidelines for the Treatment of Malaria. Geneva: World Health Organisation 2006. WHO/HTM/MAL/2006. 1108.
5. White NJ. Protozoan infections, malaria. In : Cook GC, Zumla A, eds Manson Tropical Diseases, 21st ed. London: Saunders, 2003:1205-95.
6. Warrell DA. Treatment and prevention of malaria. In: Warrell DA, Giles HM, eds. Essential Malariology, 4th ed. London : Hodder Arnold, 2002;270-311.

20

Prevention and Control of Malaria

Jaydeep Choudhury

Despite remarkable progress in the treatment of malaria, it is still a leading cause of morbidity and mortality among children in many parts of the world including India. Approximately two billion people, roughly a third of the world's population, live in malaria-endemic areas[1]. Malaria is a leading cause of morbidity and mortality for many of these people. It imposes a substantial economic and social burden on these societies. Recent estimates indicate that there are approximately 300–500 million clinical cases and 1.5–2.7 million deaths occur every year due to malaria worldwide[2]. The indirect costs of malaria to society include poor educational performance in children, exacerbation of malnutrition and anemia, which has a negative impact on the cognitive and physical capacity of both children and adults. Malaria is responsible for up to 45 million disability-adjusted life years (DALY) annually across Africa[3].

Malaria is endemic throughout India except at elevations above 1800 meters and in some coastal areas. In India, approximately 1.1 million malaria cases were reported in 2000.

P. vivax is the commonest (60–70%) followed by P. falciparum (30–45%), P. malariae species is rarely found and P ovale is not found in India. P. falciparum is a malignant variety of malaria as 0.5 to 2% may develop complicated malaria, of which up to 50% are fatal, if timely treatment is not commenced. Almost all malaria mortality is due to P. falciparum only[2]. Urban and periurban malaria are on the increase in South Asia and in many states of Africa. Another disquieting factor is the re-emergence of malaria in areas where it had been eradicated or its increase in countries where it was nearly eradicated.

There are many obstacles to the effective implementation of the highly efficacious treatment options. Resistance of P. falciparum to chloroquine is now common in practically all malaria endemic countries in Africa. Resistance to sulfadoxcine/pyrimethamine is widespread in South-east Asia and South America. Mefloquine resistance is now common in the border areas of Thailand with Cambodia and Myanmar. Resistance of P. vivax to chloroquine has now been reported from Indonesia, Myanmar, Papua New Guinea and Vanuatu[3].

Although the total number of cases of malaria in India has remained relatively constant for the last five years, outbreaks have increased the number of malaria deaths[4]. *P. falciparum* cases have also consistently increased from 9.73% of malaria cases in 1977 to 34.5% of cases in 1995 with a peak of 43.3% in 1991[2]. The incidence and trend of malaria over the years in India is shown in Table 20.1.

Table 20.1: Incidence of malaria in India

Year	Total cases	P. falciparum	Deaths
1991	2.12 million	0.92 million	421
1992	2.13 million	0.88 million	422
1993	2.21 million	0.85 million	354
1994	2.51 million	0.99 million	122
1995	2.93 million	1.14 million	1151
1996	3.04 million	1.18 million	1010
1997	2.57 million	0.99 million	874
1998	2.09 million	0.91 million	648
2002	1.84 million	0.87 million	973
2003	1.86 million	0.85 million	1006
2004	1.91 million	0.89 million	949
2005	1.81 million	0.80 million	963
2006 (Nov.)	1.04 million	0.46 million	890

Malaria Control History in India

India started using DDT to control malaria in 1946. In 1953 all over India 70 million cases and 0.8 million deaths occurred due to malaria[2]. The National Malaria Control Program (NMCP) was launched in India in April 1953 and it was in operation for 5 years till 1958. The results of this program were highly successful in that the incidence of malaria declined sharply[5]. National Malaria Eradication Program (NMEP) was launched in 1958. The NMEP believed that it could eradicate malaria in seven to nine years. But vector resistance was detected in India for the first time in 1959 in Gujarat. Then in 1965, malaria began to re-emerge in various parts of India. 1976 witnessed the peak of malaria cases in the re-emergence period. This resurgence of malaria caused India to begin an attempt to control rather than eradicate malaria. Modified Plan of Operation (MPO) under the NMEP to control malaria was evolved and put into operation in April 1977. *Plasmodium falciparum* Containment Program (PfCP) was also launched in 1977. The PfPC aimed to contain the spread of *P. falciparum* malaria, which is the most commonly resistant and most deadly strain of malaria but *P. falciparum* cases peaked in 1991. Since then *P. falciparum* is a serious threat to many parts of India. In 1994, large scale malaria epidemics swept primarily Eastern India and Western Rajasthan.

In 1999, the Government of India decided to drop the term NMEP and renamed it as National Anti-malaria Program.

The proposal of urban malaria scheme (UMS) was sanctioned in 1971 when it was realized that urban malaria was a significant problem and if effective antilarval measures were not undertaken in urban areas, the proliferation of malaria cases from urban to rural might occur in a bigger way. In this scheme all the towns having more than 40,000 population and showing more than 2 annual parasite incidence (API) in last 3 years are to be covered. At present 131 towns and cities in 19 states and union territories are under the UMS. The National Antimalaria Drug Policy was drafted in 1982 to combat the increasing level of resistance to chloroquine detected in *P. falciparum*.

Antimalaria month is observed every year in the month of June throughout the country to enhance the level of awareness.

Recently Roll Back Malaria (RBM) initiative was started in may 1998. Though initially malaria control program was upgraded to eradication program, yet due to the practical difficulty in eradication, this roll back to control program is inevitable. This RBM initiative was announced by WHO, UNICEF and the World Bank. RBM is a global strategy to improve the health system with the goal of 50% reduction in malaria deaths by 2010[7].

The main strategies of this initiative are[8]:

i. Strengthen health system to ensure better delivery of health care at the district and community level. Prevention of and timely responses to epidemics.

ii. Ensure proper and expanded use of insecticide treated mosquito nets.

iii. Ensure adequate access to basic health care and training of health workers.

iv. Encourage the development of simpler and more effective means of administering medicines, e.g. training of village health workers and mothers on early and appropriate treatment of malaria, especially in children.

v. Encourage the development of more effective and new antimalarial drugs and vaccines.

Insecticide Policy

DDT should be the insecticide of choice for residual spray. If resistance found to DDT, malathion is the alternative choice. In case of resistance to DDT and malathion, synthetic pyrethroids is the choice[2]. Resistance to pesticides was first noted in India in 1959. As resistance to DDT increased, so did the use of alternative insecticides, which resulted in emergence of vectors resistant to those insecticides as well. The use of some of the same pesticides in agriculture could have increased the speed with which malaria-transmitting mosquitoes became resistant. Pesticides are also toxic to humans and the environment. Currently, 70% of all insecticides in India are DDT and BHC (benzene hexachloride), and their use is increasing at a rate of 6% a year in India. Both of these pesticides are persistent and accumulate in soil, water, and biological organisms, and thus were banned in the US. Due to the increasing use of DDT and BHC in India, food contamination is also expected to increase.

Malaria Control

The concept of vector control is ancient. That stagnant water and marshlands are unhealthy was known even centuries ago. Drainage and landfill to control diseases have been practised since ages. The classic description by Sir Ronald Ross, 1910 on prevention of malaria is a testimony, but even today malaria control is a complex and multidisciplinary field.

I. Vector Control Strategies

It is one of the major weapons to control malaria in endemic areas. The various methods used are shown in Table 20.2[5].

Anti-adult measures

Insecticide spray—Malathion and fenitrothion are organophosphate insecticides which are being used for malaria control following the development of vector resistance to DDT[5].

Space application—It involves application of pesticides in the form of fog or mist using special equipment. Outdoor space sprays reduce vector population quickly.

Individual protection—Personal protection by repellants, bed-nets and others.

Antilarval measures

Larvicides—Temephos confer long-lasting effect with low toxicity. It must be repeated at frequent intervals.

Source reduction—Reduction of mosquito breeding sites.

Water level management

Though this is an old method, drainage remains the most cost effective mode of vector control. Water level management to flush out

Table 20.2: Malaria vector control measures

Action	Individual protection	Community protection
Reduction of human-mosquito contact	Insecticide treated bed-nets and other personal protection	Insecticide treated bed-nets
Destruction of adult mosquito		Insecticide treated bed-nets, spraying
Destruction of larva	Peri-domestic sanitation	Larviciding of water surfaces,
Source reduction	Small-scale drainage	biological control, irrigation
Social participation	Motivation of family members	Water management, sanitation Health education, community participation

mosquito breeding areas and to provide a hostile aquatic environment for mosquito egg and larval development is an alternative to drainage. Changing water salinity or allowing organic matter pollution may also reduce vector population. But major alterations to the environment should not be undertaken without proper planning.

Personal prevention

Most anopheline mosquito remain within 2 km of their breeding sites, they cannot fly more than 4 km[9]. Many vectors bite inside houses. The chances of being bitten by a malaria-infected female anopheline mosquito can be reduced by simple measures. Most mosquitoes feed at night, sleeping indoor under insecticide treated bed-nets reduces human-vector contact. Pyrethroid insecticide (permethrin, deltamethrin) impregnated nylon nets are the best, a single impregnation of cotton or nylon mosquito net will provide protection for one year[9]. The impregnated bed-nets (IBN) can be washed and can tolerate small tears or holes without reducing the protective effects. The protective efficacy of unimpregnated bed-nets is variable. Wire-mesh screens of windows and doors are effective but expensive and may also reduce ventilation. The use of insect repellants

applied to exposed skin (diethyl toluamide) can be relative cheap and easy.

Larviciding

It includes environmental and water manipulation to prevent creation of mosquito breeding sites, use of larvivorous fish and bacterial toxins, application of chemical agents. Organophosphorus compounds such as temephos are widely used and are relatively safe to warm-blooded animals and fish[9].

II. Parasite Control Strategies

The crucial factor for disease control is case detection and proper drug treatment. All fever cases in endemic areas must be investigated for malaria. The ideal approach is diagnosis and treatment on the same day.

Chemoprophylaxis

Chemoprophylaxis recommendations vary considerably depending on risk, prevalence and drug resistance. Antimalarial prophylaxis must be taken regularly to ensure therapeutic antimalarial concentrations are maintained, drugs should be continued for 4 weeks after leaving the transmission area. The WHO recommended prophylactic drug regimens are shown in Table 20.3[10].

Table 20.3: Antimalarial chemoprophylaxis

Drug	Weight adjusted dose for children
Chloroquine-sensitive malaria	
Chloroquine and/or	5 mg base/kg weekly or 1.6 mg base/kg daily
Proguanil	3.5 mg/kg daily
Chloroquine-resistant malaria	
Mefloquine or	5 mg base/kg weekly
Doxycycline or	1.5 mg/kg daily
Primaquine or	0.5 mg base/kg daily with food
Atovaquone-proguanil	4/1.6 mg/kg daily

Chemoprophylaxis is recommended for travelers from non-endemic areas and as a short-term measure for people serving in highly endemic areas. Chemoprophylaxis should be complemented by personal protection and other methods of vector control.

Chemoprophylaxis is desirable for pregnant women living in areas where transmission is very intense and leads to parasitemias causing low birth weight and anemia or to a high risk of life-threatening malaria attacks.

i. Chloroquine and proguanil are safe during pregnancy; mefloquine is used in second and third trimester.

ii. Primaquine and artemether is contra-indicated in pregnancy.

Mass drug administration

Under revised strategy mass drug administration has been recommended in highly endemic areas with API more than 5/1000 population. Mass prophylaxis is not recommended under 5 years as it may interfere with the development of immunity, may accelerate drug resistance and increase the risk of retinopathy.

Remote Sensing (RS)

Remote sensing (RS) technology is a tool for the surveillance of habitat, densities of vector species and even prediction of the incidence of disease that must be considered as new invention in the epidemiology of malaria and vector-borne diseases[6]. Literal meaning of remote sensing is to sense any object from a distance. Such data is generated in National Remote Sensing Agency, Hyderabad, India. A feasibility study using satellite data in collaboration with the Indian Space Research Organization in and around Delhi was carried out and correlation of changes in the areas of land use features, viz. water bodies and vegetations with mosquito density was found significant in some sites.

Malaria Vaccine Approach

Malaria parasite is complex and adaptable, and it has survived for millennia. We need many tools to defeat this disease. We need tools that save lives today and those with the potential to save lives in the future. A safe, effective, and affordable malaria vaccine would close the gap left by other interventions.

A vaccine is an essential tool in stopping malaria because:

i. The fight against malaria is being waged on a variety of fronts. A vaccine would be complementary to these consorted efforts.

ii. Malaria routinely develops resistance to drugs. Mosquitoes routinely develop resistance to insecticides.

iii. Vaccines have offered a cost-effective and efficacious means of preventing disease and death against many diseases.

iv. Even a modestly efficacious malaria vaccine would protect hundreds of thousands of people from disease and death each year.

Malaria vaccine roadmap

The leading international health organizations have developed a global strategy for accelerating the development and licensing of a highly effective malaria vaccine. The plan is known as the Malaria Vaccine Technology Roadmap.

A 2007 report by the Australia-based George Institute for International Health shows that the global malaria vaccine portfolio has grown from no malaria vaccines in clinical trials in 1985 to 16 candidates in clinical development in 2006[10].

The most significant challenge that malaria vaccine scientists face is a lack of understanding of the specific immune responses associated with protection against the parasitic disease. Because the malaria parasite is so complex, scientists pursue a diversity of vaccine development approaches. Many believe that a malaria vaccine will need to encompass more than a single approach to reach a high degree of efficacy.

Types of malaria vaccines

1. *Pre-erythrocytic vaccine candidates*—The pre-erythrocytic vaccine candidates target the early stage of malaria infection, the stage at which the parasite enters or matures in an infected person's liver cells. Plasmodium sporozoites are inoculated by the infected mosquito during the blood meal before they invade the liver cells. The sporozoites then multiply within the liver cells to give rise to merozoites.

   The circumsporozoite protein (CSP) is the major surface protein of the sporozoites. In the infective stage the parasite is covered by an acidic peptide—CS protein. Specific humoral immune responses to sporozoites are stimulated by natural infection and are directed against CS protein. Immunization with irradiated sporozoites has produced protection associated with the development of high levels of polyclonal CS antibodies which has been shown to inhibit sporozoite invasion of human hepatic cells.

   The basic aim is to generate humoral immune response, once sporozoite has reached the relatively immuno-protected intracellular haven of a hepatocyte, cell-mediated immunity is called upon to contain the infection.

   These sporozoites may be the vaccine target. These vaccines would elicit an immune response that would either prevent infection or attack the infected liver cell if infection does occur. These candidates include:

   i. Recombinant or genetically engineered proteins or antigens from the surface of the parasite or from the infected liver cell.

   ii. DNA vaccines that contain the genetic information for producing the vaccine antigen in the vaccine recipient.

   iii. Live, attenuated vaccines that consist of a weakened form of the whole parasite (the sporozoite) as the vaccine's main component.

   A successful pre-erythrocytic vaccine will either kill the sporozoites before they invade hepatocyte or destroy it once they are inside the hepatocyte. This vaccine will be a *disease-preventing vaccine*. Actually these are the ideal vaccine candidates, which will result in sterile immunity.

   Liver stage antigens (LSA) are a difficult proposition as the liver stage malaria parasites are difficult to cultivate. The prospect has brightened with the recent development in molecular biology. LSA1 is the first liver stage specific antigen isolated.

2. *Blood-stage vaccine candidates*—Inside the red cell merozoites transform into trophozoites, grow and then divide finally to give dozens of merozoites, which reinvade the new red cells after bursting of the infected cells. During intracellular growth of the parasites they express some antigens on the

surface of the RBC. These merozoites and antigens on the surface of red cells (MSP1, AMA1, MSP3, GLLRP, SERA) may be the vaccine target.

Blood-stage malaria vaccine will either destroy merozoite in the short time before they invade red cells or target malarial antigens expressed on red cell surface by invading parasites. Protection offered by these vaccines will be both antibody dependent and cell-mediated immunity.

Blood-stage vaccine candidates target the malaria parasite at its most destructive stage, the rapid replication of the organism in human red blood cells. These vaccines do not aim to block all infection. These vaccines will suppress the exponential growth of dividing merozoites thereby reducing the disease manifestation. This is a *disease reduction vaccine*. They will simulate the natural immunity that is found in highly endemic zones.

Evidence suggests that people who have survived regular exposure to malaria develop natural immunity over time. The goal of a vaccine that contains antigens or proteins from the surface of the blood-stage parasite (the merozoite) would be to allow the body to develop that natural immunity with much less risk of getting ill.

3. *Transmission-blocking vaccine candidates*— Vaccines targeted against gametocyte or gametes are known as *transmission- blocking vaccines*. Some trophozoites differentiate into sexual form, male and female gameto-cytes which mature to gametes in the digestive tract of the mosquito. Antibodies produced by these vaccines against gameto-cytes will be taken up by the mosquito during its blood meal along with the gametocytes.

Within the mosquito the antigens become exposed to antibody thereby neutralizing the sexual stages. These vaccines are termed *altruistic*, since they mediate their action within the mosquito and would protect not the vaccinee, but the next person bitten.

Reduction in the transmission rate could radically alter the incidence of the disease particularly in areas of low or moderate endemicity.

Transmission-blocking vaccine candidates seek to interrupt the life cycle of the parasite by inducing antibodies that prevent the parasite from maturing in the mosquito after it takes a blood meal from a vaccinated person. These vaccines would not prevent a person from getting malaria, nor would they lessen the symptoms of disease. They would, however, limit the spread of infection by preventing mosquitoes that fed on an infected person from spreading malaria to new hosts. A successful transmission-blocking vaccine would be expected to reduce deaths and illness related to malaria in at-risk communities.

The main development approaches to malaria vaccines are the following:

i. Subunit vaccines – More than 60% of the candidate vaccines are recombinant proteins.

ii. Recombinant viral vector vaccines.

iii. Long synthetic peptides, DNA vaccines, whole parasite vaccines are the other approaches.

SPf66 vaccine

This was the first synthetic peptide human vaccine invented to prevent *P. falciparum* malaria. A total of 1257 subjects comprising vaccinated and placebo group received the three dose vaccination schedule on days 0, 30 and 180 and were followed up for 22 months. Altogether 134 *P. falciparum* malaria episodes were detected, 53 in vaccinated group and 81 in placebo group. The protective efficacy of the vaccine was 35.2%[11]. This was given up due to poor efficacy.

There is no single malaria antigen and corresponding antibody which can be targeted for a specific and effective vaccine. Of the various antigens, 5 important antigens have been tried which include CSP (circumsporozoite protein), TRAP/SSP2 (thrombospondin related adhesive protein or sporozoite surface protein 2), LSA1 (liver stage antigen 1), MSP1 (merozoite surface protein 1), and AMA1 (apical membrane antigen 1). Only CSP vaccine has shown some promising results and is set to enter phase 3 studies[12].

CSP vaccine

CSP is expressed on the surface of the sporozoites of malaria parasites in liver stage[12]. Antibodies against this antigen have been correlated with protection in natural exposure studies done in endemic areas.

RTS, S/AS02

RTS, S/AS02 is the most successful malarial vaccine so far[13]. Since 2003 it is being developed by GSK in collaboration with Program for Appropriate Technology in Health-Malaria Vaccine Initiative (PATH-MVI). It is a recombinant protein-based virus- like particle (VLP), fused to hepatitis B surface antigen (HBsAg), co-compressed in yeast with unfused HBsAg along with ASO4 adjuvant[12]. In phase IIb pediatric study done in Mozambique it showed 30% protection against first episode of malaria at 6 months which was preserved at 36% till 18 months follow-up. Efficacy was 58% against severe malaria at 6 months and 49% at 18 months[14,15]. These are the best results ever shown by any malaria vaccine so far which have also persisted at 18 months follow-up. Obviously this vaccine is ready to enter phase III[13]. Several prime-boost principles are being used for this purpose including priming with DNA encoding CSP or modified vaccinia Ankara recombinant virus (MVA)[12].

Other approaches

ME-TRAP vaccine has been developed by fusing TRAP/SSP2 with multi-epitope string of mainly CD8+ T helper epitopes from 6 pre-erythrocytic antigens. But it has not been very promising. Early results are also not very promising with LSA2 based FMP011 vaccine. Work is on with MSP1 expressed on merozoites. Other vaccines being tried include combination vaccines containing more than one malaria antigens like CSP and AMA1 or chimeric vaccine containing MSP1 and AMA1[12].

Whole organism vaccine is being developed by bioengineering technique with the help of PATH-MVI.

Chinese Malaria Vaccine

PfCP2.9 malaria vaccine: This vaccine developed by medical experts with the Shanghai No. 2 Medical College of the Chinese People's Liberation Army (PLA), is one of 20 new malaria vaccines around the world which have received funding from PATH for clinical trials[12].

Blueprint for Developing Malaria Vaccines

The Malaria Vaccine Technology Roadmap process was jointly sponsored by the Bill and Melinda Gates Foundation, the PATH Malaria Vaccine Initiative (MVI), and the Wellcome Trust. As laid out in the Malaria Vaccine Technology Roadmap, in the Roadmap Workshop, held in March 2005, in Provence, France, an interim goal is to develop and license a first-generation vaccine by 2015 that has 50% protective efficacy against severe disease and death, with protection lasting at least one year without the need for boosting. The global malaria vaccine community has laid out a blueprint for moving forward, a pathway for developing by 2025 a malaria vaccine with protective efficacy of more than 80% against clinical disease and with protection lasting for many years without a booster immunization[16,17]. Evidence suggests that the malaria vaccine community is on track, with RTS,S/AS02 to meet the 2015 mark[18].

Considering the seriousness of malaria in India, World Bank in February 2009 has announced USD 520 million for Malaria Project for India[10]. Over 100 million people in India will be provided prevention services and treatment. The scheme has been designed by the Government of India, United Nations and WHO to fight AIDS, tuberculosis and malaria. This is the largest of such projects by the international body for any country.

References

1. Guerin PJ, Olliaro P, Nosten F, *et al*. Malaria: current status of control, diagnosis, treatment, and a proposed agenda for research and development. *Lancet Infect Dis* 2002;2:564-73.

2. National Antimalaria Program. URL: www. mohfw.nic.in/reports. Accessed on 1 March 2009.

3. World Health Organization. World Health Report. Geneva: WHO: 2002.

4. Singh N, Nagpal AC, Saxena A, Singh MP. Changing scenario of malaria in central India, the replacement of *Plasmodium vivax* by *Plasmodium falciparum* (1986–2000). *Trop Med International Health* 2004;9:364-71.

5. Park K. Health programmes in India. In: Park K, ed. Park's Textbook of Preventive and Social Medicine, 19 ed. Jabalpur: Banarasidas Bhanot Publishers, 2007,346-78.

6. WHO. South East Asia. Progress Health for All, 1997-2000. New Delhi: Regional Office of SEARO, 2000.

7. Sharma VP. Re-emergence of malaria in India. *Indian J Med Res* 1996;103:26-45.

8. Mukhopadhyay M, Ghosh TK. Prevention and control of malaria. In; Ganguly N, Kundu R, Ghosh TK, eds. Common MDR Infections in Children — Typhoid, Tuberculosis, Malaria. New Delhi: CBS Publishers, 2005,208-14.

9. White NJ. Malaria. In: Cook G, Zumla A, eds. Manson's Tropical Diseases, 21st ed. London: Saunders, 2003,1205-96.

10. WHO. URL: www.who.int. Accessed on 1 March, 2009.

11. Valero MV, Amador R, Aponte JJ, *et al*. Evaluation of SPf66 malaria vaccine during a 22 month follow-up field trial in the Pacific coast of Columbia. *Vaccine* 1996;14;1466-70.

12. Epstein JE, Giersing B, Mullen G, Moorthy V, Richie TL. Malaria vaccines: Are we getting closer? Curr Opin Mol Ther 2007;9:12-24.

13. Shah NK. Malaria vaccines. Ghosh TK, ed. Vaccines at Doorstep and in Pipeline, 1st ed. Kolkata: IAP Infectious Diseases Chapter 2008, 105-9.

14. Alonso Pl, Sacarlal J, Aponte JJ, Leach A, Macete E, Milman J, *et al*. Efficacy of the RTS, S/AS02A vaccine against *Plasmodium falciparum* infection and disease in young African children: Randomised controlled trial. *Lancet* 2004;364: 1411-20.

15. Alonso Pl, Sacarlal J, Aponte JJ, *et al*. Duration of protection with RTS, S/AS02A malaria vaccine in prevention of *Plasmodium falciparum* disease in Mozambican children: Single-blind extended follow-up of a randomised controlled trial. *Lancet* 2005;366:2012-8.

16. Malkin E, Dubovsky F, Moree M. Progress Towards the Development of Malaria Vaccines. *Trends Parasitol*. 2006;22:292–5.

17. www.MalariaVaccineRoadmap.net

18. Program for Appropriate Technology in Health (PATH), Accelerating Progress Towards Malaria Vaccines. Bethesda, MD: PATH; 2007.

Section 4
Other Resistant Bacterial Infections

21

Antibacterial Resistance: Evolution, Epidemiology and Strategies for Prevention

Jaydeep Choudhury, Ashok Kapse

Antimicrobial resistance is a global pandemic. This reality is due to multiple causes and we have to share the blame too. It is imperative that antibiotic resistance is a direct consequence of antibiotic use. In spite of advocacy both continue to escalate[1].

Beginning in the 1930s, antibiotics have had a near-miraculous impact on human and animal mortality and morbidity caused by bacterial infections. But over the years they have also been exploited for other non-therapeutic uses, such as improved yields of meat from animals. The price of these dramatic benefits is that the prevalence of resistant microbes has dramatically increased to the point where, in some cases, antibiotics are no longer effective. The general trend to more widespread antibiotic resistance is relentless and, if it continues unabated, deaths from what were previously treatable infections will occur with increasing frequency. As the World Health Organization, 2004 stated unambiguously, "Today we are witnessing the emergence of drug resistance along with a decline in the discovery of new antibacterials. As a result, we are facing the possibility of a future without effective antibiotics. This would fundamentally change the way modern medicine is practised."

Evolution of Antibiotics

The history of antimicrobial therapy may be divided into 3 phases[2]:

i. *Period of empirical use*—Early days when "mouldy curd" was used in China over boils or chaulmoogra oil in leprosy in India or cinchona bark for fever.

ii. *Ehrlich's phase of dyes (1890-1935)*—Methylene blue, tryphan red, arsenicals.

iii. *Modern era ushered by Domagk in 1935*—Demonstrated the effect of Prontosil, a sulfonamide dye in pyogenic infection.

Evolution of Antimicrobial Resistance

Whenever antibiotics wage war on micro-organisms, a few of the enemy are able to survive the drug. Being living organisms, these surviving microbes want to protect themselves. Microbes are always mutating; some random mutation eventually will develop resistance against the drug.

Microbes in general are not confined by geographical, social or political boundaries. They are universal. It is quite obvious that we share a single global ecosystem in terms of antibiotic resistance too. Antibiotic resistance is a cause of great concern because detection of even a single instance of antibiotic resistance is a microcosm of a larger perspective[3].

It is obvious that the strategy to tackle a problem of such magnitude should be wide based and systematic. The whole emphasis of antibiotic policy now revolves around antibiotic resistance. Antibiotic resistance can be introduced, selected, maintained and spread in health institutions by the following six mechanisms as described by McGowan and Tenover[4].

1. Introduction of a few resistant organisms into a population where resistance previously was not present, usually by transfer from another health care system, sometimes also from the community.
2. Acquisition of resistance by a few previously susceptible strains through genetic mutation in reservoirs of high organism concentration such as an abscess.
3. Acquisition of resistance by a susceptible strain through transfer of genetic material, for example in the gut or on the skin.
4. Emergence of inducible resistance that is already present in a few strains in the bacterial population, usually from direct selection by antibiotic prescribing.
5. Selection of a small resistant subpopulation of organisms, again by antibiotic prescription.
6. Dissemination of inherently resistant organisms locally within the specific setting due to poor infection control procedures.

It is quite evident that antibiotic resistance determinants are much older than the modern era of chemotherapy. The maintenance and spread of antibiotic resistance in our health care system are by and large dependent on the unrestrained antibiotic prescribing that is prevalent.

Molecular Mechanism of Antibiotic Resistance

Antibiotic resistance refers to unresponsiveness of a microorganism to an antimicrobial agent[2]. Microbes are endowed with molecular mechanisms for resistance development.

Natural resistance

Some microbes have always been resistant to certain antimicrobial agents. They lack the metabolic process or the target site which is affected by the particular drug. This is generally a group or species specific, e.g. Gram-negative bacilli are unaffected by penicillin or *M. tuberculosis* is insensitive to tetracyclines. This type of resistance does not pose a significant clinical problem[2].

Acquired resistance

It is the development of resistance by an organism (which was sensitive before) due to the use of the antimicrobial agent over a period of time. This can happen with any microbe and it is a major clinical problem. Bacteria acquire resistance by either genetic mutation or horizontal gene transfer from other organisms[5].

Mutation—It is a stable and heritable genetic change that occurs spontaneously and randomly among microorganisms. It is not induced by antimicrobial agents. The resistant survivors may undergo separate mutations over hundreds of generations that favor maintenance of resistance. Mutation and resistance may be single step and it confers a high degree of resistance, e.g. *E. coli* and Staphylococci to rifampicin[2]. Mutation may be multistep. Here the sensitivity decreases gradually in a stepwise manner. Resistance to erythromycin, chloramphenicol is developed by many organisms in this manner[2].

Horizontal gene transfer (HGT)—Various mechanisms are conjugation, transduction and transformation. This could be by addition of plasmid or transposons.

Plasmids are circular, double-stranded unit of DNA that replicates within a cell independently of the chromosomal DNA. Plasmids carry resistant genes which could be easily transferred to other bacteria.

Transposons are short, specialized sequences of DNA that can insert into plasmids or bacterial chromosomes. Tranposons house genes for resistance determinants, some of these also contain genes for their chromosomal integration and expre-ssion.

Physiological Mechanism

Bacteria engineer varied physiological mechanisms to protect themselves from antibiotic onslaught. Majority of these mechanisms effectively decrease antibiotic efficacy. Resistant organisms can broadly be of the following 3 types:

i. *Drug tolerant*—Loss of affinity of the target biomolecule of the microorganism for a particular antimicrobial agent, e.g. certain penicillin-resistant pneumococci have altered penicillin binding proteins.

ii. *Drug destroying*—The resistant microorganism elaborates an enzyme which inactivates the drug, e.g. β-lactamases are produced by staphylococci.

iii. *Drug impermeable*—Many hydrophilic antibiotics gain access into the bacterial cell through specific channels formed by proteins called "porins", or need specific transport mechanisms. The bacteria may also acquire plasmid directed inducible energy dependent efflux proteins in their cell membrane which pump out the antibiotic.

Cross resistance: Acquisition of resistance to one antimicrobial agent conferring resistance to another antimicrobial agent, to which the organism has not been exposed, is called cross resistance. This is more commonly seen in chemically or mechanistically related drugs, e.g. resistance to one sulfonamide means resistance to all others.

Epidemiology

More than 50 years of the large-scale use of antibiotics have resulted in a number of microorganisms which have acquired resistance or multi-resistance to different antimicrobial drugs. Both Gram-negative and Gram-positive organisms have demonstrated excellent capability to undermine the effectiveness of one or more antimicrobial agents[6].

Although problems related to antibiotic resistance differ from unit to unit, hospital to hospital and country to country however, notably resistant microorganisms do not recognize boundaries between countries; hence, the epidemiology of resistance may be multinational, with some transferable determinants are prevalent worldwide. Medical literature on the transfer of resistance from city to city and country to country is widely available.

Emergence of multidrug resistance among certain strains of gram-negative bacteria such as shigella, klebsiella, enterobacter, acinetobacter, salmonella species and gram-positive organisms such as *staphylococcus, enterococcus* and *streptococcus* species is extremely troublesome. In recent years there has been a progressive increase in frequency of methicillin-resistant *Staphylococcus aureus* (MRSA), vancomycin-resistant *enterococcus* (VRE) species and extended spectrum β-lactamase (ESBL) producing *Klebsiella pneumoniae* and *Escherichia coli*[6,7].

Dynamics of Antimicrobial Resistance

According to the definition by Center for Disease Control, resistant bacteria are those judged by the infection control program, based on current state, regional or national recommendations, to be of special clinical and epidemiological significance[8].

A. *The patient*—Colonized or infected person can cause common source of outbreak. A large inoculum of infection increases the chance of pre-existing resistant organisms. Any process that lowers the drug concentration at the site of infection helps in selection of resistance and slow eradication of infection. Another major concern is the development of resistance in the normal flora, as this resistance may spread to more pathogenic flora.

B. *The organism*—Bacteria can adopt a number of ways to develop resistance to antimicrobials. One of the most remarkable traits is the genetic mechanism for resistance to antimicrobials. The various genetic mechanisms are that they can undergo chromosomal mutations, they can express latent chromosomal resistance gene or they acquire new genetic resistance material through conjugation or transduction of DNA. The information thus encoded in the genetic material enables bacteria to develop resistance through the following mechanisms:

i. Production of an enzyme that may destroy or inactivate the antibiotic.

ii. Alteration of antibiotic target site so that the antibiotic fails to attach.

iii. Prevention of antibiotic access to the target site.

Many times a single resistant bacterial strain found in a hospital may possess several of these resistant mechanisms simultaneously and this is a very complex situation. The worst scenario is the presence of an integron. It is a type of transposon, which can accommodate not only many resistant determinants (cassettes), including the *mecA* gene, but also the genes for their chromosomal integration and expression[1]. Linked resistance and resistance by active efflux of an antibiotic are other complex mechanisms of resistance.

C. *The drug*—Rational use of antibiotics is crucial. Wherever possible the pathogen and the sensitivity should be determined. Narrow spectrum antibiotics are always beneficial as they have less effect on normal flora. The antibiotic dose is also an important determinant. A higher dose which achieves higher concentration at the site of infection is less likely to cause resistance. Combination antibiotic therapy is an effective mode to tackle resistance. This has been proved effectively in the treatment of tuberculosis and HIV.

D. *The environment*—The term environment covers both institution and community. It should be distinguished whether the resistant organism originates from community or from nosocomial isolates. At the same time the isolates should be identified from body site and hospital location. The emerging resistance may be *de novo* or the result of clonal spread. In the latter, cross-infection and environmental contamination are also important. Antibiotic restriction may not be of much effect in this situation.

Surveillance for Resistant Bacterial Pathogens

It is an important role of the clinical microbiology laboratory to provide the data on bacterial isolates and antimicrobial susceptibility to guide clinicians in antibiotic therapy. Susceptibility testing data acts as the pivot for therapeutic guidance and strain typing for potential infection outbreak.

There are two components of surveillance. The first is the periodic review of minimum inhibitory concentration (MIC) or the zone diameter data for changes in resistance patterns[3]. A decrease in the mean zone diameter around antibiotic disc in susceptibility testing may be first sign of emergence of antimicrobial resistance.

The second and equally important component of surveillance is reporting of the resistance pattern to the authority.

Antibiotic resistance in hospitals

Resistant nosocomial infections are common in hospital settings. Antibiotic usage has been shown to have a critical role in the selection of antibiotic-resistant bacteria as the dominant colonizing flora as well as the nosocomial pathogens of hospitalized patients. Resistance acquisition has two mechanisms. First, antimicrobial-resistant flora may be endemic within the institution and may be transferred to the patient within the hospital setting. Second, a small population of antimicrobial-resistant bacteria that are a part of patient's endogenous flora at the time of hospitalization may emerge under the selective pressure of antibiotics and become the dominant flora.

All over the world ICU-related infections are common and often associated with resistant microorganisms.

The overall susceptibility to ciprofloxacin among aerobic gram-negative bacilli declined from 89% in 1990-1993 to 86% in 1994 and 76% in 2000. The most notable reductions in ciprofloxacin susceptibility were seen with *P. aeruginosa*. The decline in activity of ciprofloxacin correlates directly with increase in use of quinolones. Evolving problem of antimicrobial resistance in *Pseudomonas aeruginosa*, *Acinetobacter baumannii* and *K. pneumoniae* is so grave that it has led to the emergence of clinical isolates susceptible to only one class of antimicrobial agent; these isolates are termed as pandrug-resistant isolates. Pandrug-resistant strains are associated with significant treatment failures and consequent mortality[6,7].

Antibiotic resistance in community

Antibiotic resistance in the community is an emerging global problem. The normal individual flora, which is important for the maintenance of individual health, can play a critically important role in infectious diseases. Carriage of resistant bacteria such as MRSA, ESBL + enterobacteriaceae and pneumococci may result in infections.

In fact, carriage of such pathogens and infections related to them is not rare in the community. In a study performed in Saudi Arabia, fecal carriage of ESBL+ organisms was detected in 26.1% of 272 in-patients, 15.4% of 162 out-patients, and 13.1% of 426 healthy individuals. The ESBL rate of community-acquired urinary tract infections related *E. coli* strains are 7.9% in Turkey and 34.4% in India[9].

Streptococcus pneumoniae which used to be exquisitely sensitive to penicillin has acquired resistance against it; cross-resistance with other frequently used antibiotics is common among these community acquired penicillin resistant organisms. *Streptococcus pneumoniae* have important community reservoirs.

MRSA has emerged as a cause of skin infections and, less commonly, invasive infections among otherwise healthy adults and children in the community. A surveillance study was conducted simultaneously at three centers across India. A total of 13,610 test samples from various sites were obtained. Antimicrobial susceptibility testing of the isolated strains of *Staphylococcus aureus* and *Staphylococcus epidermidis* to various antimicrobial disks was carried out according to standardized disk diffusion method recommended by NCCLS. Of the total 739 cultures of *S. aureus*, 235 (32%) were found to be multiple resistant with the individual figures for resistance being 27% (Mumbai), 42.5% (Delhi) and 47% (Bengaluru). MRSA carriage was reported to be 2.6% in 500 healthy adults and 1.9% in 500 healthcare workers[10].

Development of Resistance: Clinico-epidemiological Settings

In the want of effective antibiotic policies once selected resistance rapidly grows; there are four interacting variables—patient, organism, drug and environment which need proper understanding for developing effective resistance control strategies[1].

Patient

Large inoculum of organisms as in abscess cavity potentiates the increase in pre-existent resistant mutants. Presence of foreign body which may lower antibiotic concentration at the site of infection is likely to select resistance. Immune compromised patient with slower eradication of infection may also favor resistance development.

Organism

Certain organisms are more capable of producing resistance staphylococcus, enterococcus, pseudomonas, and many other gram-negative bacilli have high potential for acquiring antibiotic resistance. Conversely antibiotic resistance has not been a problem among the atypical pulmonary pathogens, e.g. Legionella, *Mycoplasma pneumoniae*, *Chlamydia pneumoniae*. Rickettsia and spirochetal organisms also have not shown significant resistance development.

On removal of selective pressure, reversion to sensitivity may occur, although it may take longer than the initial process of resistance development, however, in certain organisms genetic compensation for the cost of resistance

may well occur, i.e. the resistant survivors can undergo separate mutations over next several generations that would favor maintenance of the resistant gene. MRSA and VRE have shown this kind of genetic compensations. Generally compensation is more likely outcome than reversion however, adaptive resistance is more likely to revert unless it is mutational.

Situation is complex where resistance evolves to multiple drugs collectively. The worst scenario is the presence of an integron, a type of transposon, which can accommodate resistant determinants for many drugs in concert. In integron coded resistance it is likely that use of any antibiotic which is represented on that integron will select evolution of resistance to all the antibiotic agents to whom the resistance determinants are coded on that particular integron. Transposons can also code for active efflux of many different classes of antibiotics (the 'sump-pump' resistance mechanism). The fluoroquinolones possess capability to activate this resistance mechanism.

Drug

Not all antibacterial drugs exert analogous resistance selection pressure. Some antibacterial drugs possess exceptional resistance development potential, while others lack this character[11]. Ceftriaxone is an excellent example of a low antibiotic resistance development potential; despite high volumes uses over a long period, it has generally remained free of significant resistance problem.

Conversely resistance against ciprofloxacin and imipenem among *Pseudomonas* was reported even during clinical trials and early after introduction in clinical use[11]. Knowledge of this particular characteristic of antibacterial agents should be one of the most vital determinants of antibiotic choice. Antibiotics with high resistance development potential should have restricted clinical uses, while antibiotics with low resistance development potential could have free clinical uses. Table 21.1 lists the antibiotics as per resistance development potential.

Table 21.1: Categorization of antibiotics as per resistance development potential[1]

AB with high resistance potential	AB with low resistance potential
Ampicillin, carbenicillin, tetracycline, ciprofloxacin, gentamicin, ceftazidime, imipenem.	Amoxycillin, piperacillin, doxycycline, ofloxacin, levofloxacin, amikacin, ceftriaxone, cefepime, meropenem.

Collateral damage

Human body is studded with lots of bacteria, according to an estimate around 5000 to 10000 different species of bacteria live in the human body, called as commensals. These bacteria constitute a significant defense mechanism of our body. When a broad spectrum antibiotic is deployed in a patient, it not only kills offending bacteria but also vastly damages commensal flora. Many of these commensals undergo mutational changes and acquire antibacterial resistance. Increasing ESBL-producing *E. coli* is a classical example of this kind of collateral damage.

Practice of using oral third-generation cephalosporins for community acquired respiratory infections and fevers is playing a huge havoc world over. Cephalosporins have a hand, not only for selecting ESBL-producing enterobacteriaceae and stably depressed mutants of inducible enterobacteriacea, but also enterococci, MRSA, *Clostridium difficile* and yeasts. Many studies have shown a reduction in the incidence, if not complete eradication of problem organisms by decreasing cephalosporin uses[1].

Inappropriate Antibiotic Therapy

Inappropriate antibiotic therapy can be defined as one or more of the following[11].

Unnecessary antibiotic prescription for viral diseases

Antibiotics are unnecessary in most of the upper respiratory infections as they are of viral etiology. It is very well known that after a short course of antibiotic like ampicillin, resistant bacteria may persist in feces for as long as three months, these resistant bugs are potentially infectious to other members of the family and community long after the cessation of therapy[9]. Physician prescribing practices in turn influence their patients' attitudes about the need for antibiotics. This creates a tremendously dangerous situation in countries where there are no controls over procuring medicines from chemist. Patients may start antibiotics by themselves in the case of fever or common cold or to overcome malaise, fatigue or pain.

Wrong choice, dose or duration of therapy

Broad spectrum antibiotic inflicts detrimental collateral damage which in turn breeds antibacterial resistance[8]. Infections should be treated with appropriate doses of narrow spectrum antibiotics and only a failed treatment should be the contemplation for upscaling the drug doses or consideration of higher antibiotic.

Ineffective initial empiric treatment of serious bacterial infection

Even at the best of the centers' pending culture sensitivity reports initial antibiotic therapy is selected empirically. A proper selection of antibiotic regimen is vitally important for patient's survival and recovery. A wrong initial choice of antibiotics invariably culminates into poor outcome.

Starting inappropriate therapy affects not only mortality but also duration of hospitalization; as inappropriate therapy is prolonged, the likelihood of resistant bacteria arising will increase, which sometimes may result in the occurrence of outbreaks. Mortality rates are higher among patients with ventilator-associated pneumonia who receive inappropriate empirical treatment[14].

Poor tissue penetration

Microbes are likely to develop resistance if exposed to low antibiotic concentrations; this is particularly true for antibiotic which has a high antibacterial resistance development potential. Antibiotic failure and resistance development is more common in body sites where achieving adequate antibiotic concentration is usually difficult. Abscess cavities, pyelonephritic kidneys, and CSF are some of the places where suboptimal antibiotic concentrations could be anticipated. Low antibiotic resistance potential and good tissue penetration should receive due considerations in making antibiotic choice in such conditions[9].

Prevention of Emergence of Resistance

The two principal goals are prevention of emergence of antibiotic resistance and control of established resistance[12]. For both these goals the approach is similar. But for obvious reason prevention of acquisition of infection is easier than curbing the established resistance.

The following strategies have to be adopted in order to reduce antimicrobial resistance and to make an antibiotic control program effective.

1. *Optimal use of all antimicrobials*—Ideally all patients should be treated with the most effective, least toxic and least costly antibiotic for the precise duration of time needed to cure or prevent an infection[3]. This is the essence of the whole strategy. Another strategy to curtail the development of antimicrobial resistance, in addition to the judicious overall use of antibiotics, is to use drugs with a narrow antimicrobial spectrum or "older" antibiotics. Several investigations suggest that some infections, such as community-acquired pneumonia and urinary tract infections, can usually be successfully treated with narrow-spectrum antibiotic agents, especially if the infections are not life-threatening[13]. New antimicrobials should be used with caution. Injudicious use of newer highly effective antibiotics like vancomycin, linezolid, meropenem should be curtailed. A common misconception is to treat all fevers with antibiotics. As a matter of fact many fevers are of viral origin. After all antibiotics are neither antipyretics nor antivirals.

2. *National protocols of common infections*—It is of utmost importance to develop national guidelines and treatment algorithms. These guidelines should be circulated among all the pediatricians and they should be asked to follow. On the other hand, the pediatricians not only get a readymade guideline for management of a particular disease but also get legal protection if they abide by a national consensus. But the authority should make it a point to update these protocols at regular intervals or whenever necessary.

Consensus-driven recommendations should be developed for the treatment of hospital-acquired and community-acquired infections. But consensus guidelines for antimicrobial therapy need to be modified at the local level (for example, according to country, city, hospital and ICU) to take into account local patterns of antimicrobial resistance. Such information may help clinicians develop more rational prescribing practices that will reduce the unnecessary administration of broad-spectrum drugs and avoid inadequate antimicrobial treatment of critically ill patients.

Locally developed guidelines, therefore, often have the best chance of being accepted by local health care providers and hence of being better implemented[18].

3. *Restriction policy*—Selective removal or control of use of specific agents or classes of agents has been employed in many hospitals[3]. But the strategy has to be determined by careful consideration of the resident flora. Here also the role of clinical microbiologist is crucial.

4. *Antibiotic cycling and scheduled antibiotic changes*—It is also known as rotation of antibiotics. A class of antibiotics or a specific antibiotic drug is withdrawn from use for a defined period and is reintroduced at a later time in an attempt to limit bacterial resistance[13]. Antibiotic class cycling has been advocated as a potential strategy for reducing the emergence of antimicrobial resistance. Antibiotic cycling cannot be used as a replacement for judicious overall antibiotic use and rigorous adherence to infection control practices as a means of controlling resistance.

5. *Combination antimicrobial therapy*—Combination antimicrobial therapy has been used successfully for *Mycobacterium tuberculosis* and has been proposed as a strategy to reduce the emergence of bacterial resistance. In addition, combination antimicrobial therapy may be more effective at producing clinical and microbiological responses. This could also help to minimize antibiotic resistance by preventing the horizontal transmission of inadequately treated antibiotic-resistant pathogens[13].

6. *Newer antibiotic research*—During 1960-69, altogether 12 new antibiotics were added to the armamentarium and during 1970-79 further 6 antibiotics were added. Since then very few new antibiotics are being discovered. According to the Infectious Diseases Society of America (IDSA), the pipeline for new antibacterial is drying up, since 1998, only 10 new antibiotics have been approved, and only two of those were truly novel, defined as having a new mechanism of action with no crossresistance with other antibiotics[19]. Resistance to antibacterial continues to increase; maybe it is time to look at older antibiotics again.

7. *Pseudoresistance*—Some antimicrobials are resistant by *in vitro* susceptibility testing but are effective *in vivo*[20].

Non-antimicrobial Prevention Strategies

The specific prevention strategies may not be effective if it is not complimented by the non-antimicrobial prevention strategies. The non-antimicrobial prevention strategies may be implemented at two levels, primary prevention program for specific infections and use of infection control practices to prevent horizontal transmission of nosocomial infection.

A. *Primary prevention program for specific infections*

   i. *Adoption of WHO strategies*—Integrated Management of Childhood Illness (IMCI), DOTS for tuberculosis, HIV/AIDS control program are some of the policies.

   ii. *Vaccination and immunoglobulins*—It is the most effective means to contain resistance. Some of the possible options are microbial surface components recognizing adhesive matrix molecules like MSCRAMM polyclonal and monoclonal antibodies, anti-lipoteichoic acid (LTA), anti-poly-N-acetyl glucosamine, C5, C8 capsular polysaccharide vaccine.

iii. Reducing length of stay in hospital and avoidance of invasive procedures.

B. *Prevention of horizontal transmission*

i. *Hand-washings*—Hand-washing is still considered the most important and effective infection control measure to prevent horizontal transmission of nosocomial pathogens[14]. Increased patient workload and decreased staffing may contribute to poor compliance of handwashing. In such cases alternate methods to soap-water hand-washing may be considered.

ii. *Gloves and gowns*—In addition to handwashing, the use of gloves and gowns has also been shown to reduce horizontal transmission of specific bacterial pathogens particularly in NICU and PICU settings.

Community Level Prevention

i. *Reduction of use of antimicrobials in livestock*—Antimicrobials normally prescribed for humans should be prohibited as growth promoters or as an alternative to high quality hygiene in animals[15]. While evidences are lacking that such addition of antibiotics to livestock feed prevents infection; there are enough data that these practices disgustingly increase antibacterial resistance[16]. Resistant bacteria developed in livestock can taint the meat or foods exposed to the animals and thereby gain into human gut[17].

ii. *Vector control*—Proper control of vectors can prevent the vector-borne diseases.

iii. *Increased availability and access to antimicrobials*—Inadequate access to appropriate antimicrobials results in improper treatment which, in turn, hastens the development of resistance. Often cost is inhibitory, which prompts premature discontinuation of antimicrobials.

iv. *Education and awareness of health workers and public*—The aim is to inculcate sense of hygiene and curb the misuse of antibiotics. Proper cleanliness goes a long way in preventing infection.

Table 21.2: Recommendations for prevention and reduction of antimicrobial resistance in hospitals[3]

Recommendation	Strength of recommendation*
Hospitals have a system for monitoring antimicrobial resistance of both community and nosocomial isolates on a monthly basis or at a frequency appropriate to the volume of isolates	A
Monitoring use of antimicrobials by hospital location or prescribing service is recommended on a monthly basis or at a frequency appropriate to the prescription volume	A
Hospitals monitor the relationship between antimicrobial use and resistance and assign responsibility through practice guidelines or other institutional policies	A
Hospitals apply contact precautions to specified patients known or suspected to be colonized or infected with epidemiologically important microorganisms that can be transmitted by direct or indirect contact	A

* Categories for strength of recommendations: A good evidence for support.

Controlling Dissemination of Resistant Bacteria in Hospitals[3]

The Society for Health care Epidemiology of America (SHEA) and Infectious Diseases Society of America (IDSA) Joint Committee on Antibiotics support the CDC "Guidelines for Isolation Precautions in Hospitals". It applies to preventing the selection and spread of resistant microorganisms. The recommendations are summarized in Table 21.2.

Antimicrobial resistance is costly in both human and financial terms[3]. Moreover, the consequences of a single case of antimicrobial resistance is far reaching. As newer antimicrobials are entering the market, it is time each and every individual should be aware and conscious in dealing with them. Although awareness of the consequences of antibiotic misuse is increasing, overprescribing remains widespread, driven largely by patient demand, time pressure on clinicians and diagnostic uncertainty[21]. It is much easier to prevent antimicrobial resistance than to treat even a single case.

References

1. Gould IM. A review of the role of antibiotic policies in the control of antibiotic resistance. *J Antimicrobial Chemother* 1999; 43: 459-465.

2. Tripathi KD. Essentials of Medical Pharmacology, 6th ed. New Delhi: Jaypee Brothers, 2008.

3. Shlaes DM, Gerding DN, John JF, *et al*. Society for Healthcare Epidemiology of America and Infectious Diseases Society of America Joint Committee on Prevention of Antimicrobial Resistance: Guidelines for the Prevention of Antimicrobial Resistance in Hospitals. *Clin Infect Dis* 1997;25:584-99.

4. McGowan JE, Tenover FC. Control of antimicrobial resistance in the health care system. *Infect Dis Clinics North Am* 1997;11:297-311.

5. Kaye SK. Pathogens resistant to antimicrobial agents: epidemiology, molecular mechanism, and clinical management. *Infect Dis Clin N Am* 2004; 467-511.

6. Hooper. *Lancet Infect Dis* 2002;2:530–38

7. Gross R. Consequences of Antibiotic Resistance. *Clin Infect Dis*:2001;33:289.

8. Garner JS. Hospital Infection Control Practices Advisory Committee, Centers for Disease Control and Prevention, Guideline for Isolation Precautions in Hospitals. *Infect Control Hosp Epidemiol* 1996;17:53-80.

9. Goossens H, Sprenger MJW. Community-acquired infections and bacterial resistance. *BMJ* 1998; 317:654-7.

10. Antibiotic surveillance. *J Postgrad Med* 1996;42: 1-3.

11. Cunha BA:Antibiotic resistance: *Med Clin Am*: 2000;84:1407-21.

12. Choudhury J. Strategies to prevent antimicrobial resistance. *Indian J Pract Ped* 2007;9:47-52.

13. Kollef MH, Fraser VJ. Antibiotic resistance in intensive care unit. *Ann Intern Med* 2001;134:298-314.

14. Goldman D, Larson E. Hand-washing and nosocomial infections (Editorial). *Lancet* 1992; 327: 120-122.

15. Jain RK. Antimicrobial resistance: can we overcome it? In: Ghosh TK ed. Infectious Diseases in Children and Newer Vaccines: Part 1, 1st ed. Ahmedabad, Kolkata: IAP Infectious Diseases Chapter Publication, 2003;113-24.

16. Bennish ML. Animals, humans, and antibiotics: implications of the veterinary use of antibiotics on human health. *Adv Pediatr Infect Dis* 1999; 14:269-90.

17. Cunha BA. Antibiotic resistance: control strategies. *Crit Care Clin* 1996;8:309.

18. Kish MA. Guide to development of practice guidelines. *Clin Infect Dis* 2001;32:851-4.

19. Spellberg B, Guidos R, Gilbert D, *et al*. The epidemic of antibiotic-resistant infections: a call to action for the medical community from the Infectious Diseases Society of America. *Clin Infect Dis* 2008; 46: 155-64.

20. Rodrigues C. Antimicrobial resistance. Shah NK, Singhal T, ed. Rational Antimicrobial Practice in Pediatrics, 1st ed. Mumbai: Indian Academy of Pediatrics, 2008, 15-22.

21. Chambers HF. General principles of antimicrobial therapy. In: Goodman and Gilman's The Pharmacological Basis of Therapeutics, 11th ed. New York: McGraw-Hill, 2006; 1095-110.

22

Microbial Drug Resistance: MRSA, VRE, ESBL, Pan Drug Resistant Organisms

Raju C Shah, Pratima Shah

The problem of microbial drug resistance is a major public health concern, due to its global dimension and alarming magnitude, although the epidemiology of resistance can exhibit remarkable geographical variability and rapid temporal evolution. The major resistance issues overall are those related to: (a) Methicillin-resistant *Staphylococcus aureus* (MRSA), (b) Vancomycin-resistant enterococci (VRE), (c) Enterobacteriaceae producing extended-spectrum beta-lactamases (ESBLs), and (d) Pan drug-resistant *Pseudomonas aeruginosa* and *Acinetobacter baumannii*.

METHICILLIN-RESISTANT STAPHYLOCOCCUS AUREUS (MRSA)

Staphylococci are very widespread bacteria. Their main representative, *Staphylococcus aureus*, is one of the most important and successful human pathogens. According to current knowledge, the Staphylococcus genus has 50 taxons with 39 various types and several subtypes.

The high mortality rate connected to the *S. aureus* strain decreased only in the forties of the last century after the first antibiotic penicillin was introduced into staphylococcal infection treatment. Sir Alexander Fleming could not have foreseen that his discovery of penicillin would also trigger global problems. Resistant and multidrug resistant bacterial strains emerged at this moment. Towards the end of 1940, hospitals in England and the USA reported that up to 50% of *S. aureus* strains registered penicillin resistance. Clinical trials have demonstrated the resistance is caused by the penicillinase enzyme (β-lactamase). It was phage typing, a brand new method that enabled identification of the *S. aureus* strain that was infectious, penicillin-resistant, and extremely invasive[1]. The strain was first described in Australia and subsequently it spread fast to America (epidemics in maternity units) and to hospitals in the UK. The strain was termed the 80/81 strain, according to its bacteriophage. Decrease in the occurrence of this strain took place in the sixties when methicillin, the first semisynthetic penicillinase fast penicillin was introduced. The staphylococci needed a mere six months to create methicillin.

Resistant Strains

In 1960, a screening of 5000 clinical isolates identified three *S. aureus* strains resistant to methicillin. All three of them had the same phenotype and came from the same hospital in the south of England. In the medical literature there emerged an abbreviation-MRSA (methicillin-resistant *Staphylococcus aureus*) while in the English literature, the term HA-MRSA (health care-associated methicillin-resistant *Staphylococcus aureus*) is used. From that time MRSA was considered to be the most important agent of hospital infections, both in adult and child patients[1].

In the second half of the sixties, MRSA strains developed that were resistant to other antibiotics and the occurrence of multidrug-resistant MRSA was reported from several Central European countries, England, Australia and India. In 1971 in Denmark, MRSA strains with a combined resistance to penicillin, streptomycin, tetracycline and occasionally to erythromycin represented 15% of all isolated *S. aureus* strains[2]. During the seventies and at the beginning of the eighties a decrease in these strains was registered (Denmark reported only 0.2% of MRSA strains). The cause was not entirely clear but probably the change of prescribing streptomycin and tetracycline, and the introduction of strict preventive measures against spreading this infectious agent played a significant role.

In the United States, approximately 60% of staphylococcal infections in the intensive care unit are now caused by MRSA, and percentages continue to rise. Outbreaks of hospital-acquired MRSA (HA-MRSA) are typically the result of clonal spread by MRSA being transferred from patient to patient, frequently using health care personnel as intermediaries. HA-MRSA strains are generally multidrug resistant[3].

In 1996, the first clinical isolate of *S. aureus* with reduced susceptibility to vancomycin was identified in Japan (vancomycin-intermediate *S. aureus*—VISA). In July 1997 the Center for Disease Control and Prevention (CDC) issued an interim recommendation regarding prevention and control of these strains. In June 2002, a strain of *S. aureus* fully resistant to vancomycin (vancomycin-resistance *S. aureus*—VRSA) was isolated from a patient in Michigan.

Genetics and the Development of Antibiotic Resistance

Resistance to methicillin and other β-lactam antibiotics is caused by the mecA gene, which is situated on the Staphylococcal Cassette Chromosome mec (SCCmec). The mecA gene encodes the 78-kDa penicillin-binding protein (PBP) 2a or PBP2'. To date, five SCCmec types (I-V) have been distinguished, and several variants of these SCCmec types have been described. All SCCmec elements carry genes for resistance to β-lactam antibiotics, as well as genes for the regulation of the expression of mecA. Additionally, SCCmec types II and III carry non-β lactam antibiotic resistance genes on integrated plasmids and a transposon[4]. The prevalence of MRSA has been found to range from 0.6% in the Netherlands to 66.8% in Japan.

The year 1993 marked the rise of a new clone of MRSA strains. These are called community-associated MRSA strains (CA-MRSA). They were isolated from indigenous Australian patients, original inhabitants of West Australia, who had no previous contact with a health care system. In the course of the last decade, information has emerged about the spread and isolation of these strains from different countries to almost all the continents of the world, in patients with no risk factor for nosocomial acquisition of MRSA. Community-associated MRSA (CA-MRSA) infections most commonly are skin and soft-tissue infections (SSTI); however, certain cases can progress to invasive tissue infections, bacteremia, and death[5].

The main characteristics of HA-MRSA and CA-MRSA strains are shown in Table 22.1.

Laboratory Diagnostics of Methicillin-Resistant *Staphylococcus aureus* (MRSA)

The National Committee for Clinical Laboratory Standards (NCCLS), now called the Clinical and Laboratory Standards Institute (CLSI), recommends the cefoxitin disk screen test, the latex agglutination test for PBP2a, or a plate containing 6 ug/ml of oxacillin in Mueller-Hinton agar supplemented with NaCl (4% w/v; 0.68 mol/l) as alternative methods of testing for MRSA[6].

Accurate detection of oxacillin/methicillin resistance can be difficult, due to the presence of two subpopulations (one susceptible and the other resistant) that may coexist within a culture of staphylococci. All the cells in a culture may carry the genetic information for resistance, but only a small number may express the resistance in vitro. This phenomenon is termed heteroresistance. Cells expressing heteroresistance grow more slowly than the oxacillin-susceptible populations and may be missed at temperatures above 35°C. For this reason, CLSI recommends incubating isolates being tested against oxacillin, methicillin, or nafcillin at 33–35°C (maximum of 35°C) for a full 24 hours before reading.

Nucleic acid amplification tests, such as the polymerase chain reaction (PCR), can be used to detect the mecA gene, which mediates oxacillin resistance in staphylococci. Staphylococcal resistance to oxacillin/methicillin occurs when an isolate carries an altered penicillin-binding protein, PBP2a, which is encoded by the mecA gene. The classic microbiological methods (microscopy, cultivation, biochemical identification) are procedures that enable identification of bacteria strains within 24–96 hours. They are not suitable for active surveillance of the MRSA strains spreading in hospitals or for rapid identification of serious bacteremia.

Prevention of the MRSA Occurrence and its Spreading

Patient screening

Occurrence of MRSA colonized patients depends on the type of the department.

In long-term care the colonization is much higher. Literature reports that 35–84% of MRSA colonized patients fail to be identified by swabs that are ordered by doctors for clinical reasons. It is recommended that swabs mainly of the anterior nares are taken; this screening should detect up to 80% of the MRSA carriers, and other swabs from additional body sites will increase the sensitivity to over 92%. Nasal carriage of S. aureus and MRSA has been identified as a risk factor for the development of infections in various settings[1]. In Illinois, USA, introduction of

Table 22.1: Characteristics of HA-MRSA and CA-MRSA strains

Characteristic	HA-MRSA	CA-MRSA
Clinical	Surgical site infections, invasive	Skin infections, "bug bites", rarely invasive, multiple, recurrent
Epidemiology	Old, health care	Young, athletes, drug users, correctional facilities and military
Antibiotic	Resistance multidrug resistant	β-lactam resistant
Molecular markers	PVL-SCCmec I-III	PVL + SCCmec IV, V

universal admission surveillance for MRSA was associated with a large reduction in MRSA disease during admission and 30 days after discharge[7].

Screening of health care workers

As published in the literature, nasal MRSA carriers among the health care workers can be MRSA sources (transfer and spreading) but they are not considered as important a reservoir as the colonized or infectious patients. The health care worker who comes into contact with colonized or infectious patients should regularly undergo screening for the MRSA strain presence.

Hand washing and hand disinfection

The risk of transferring MRSA strains is connected to temporary (transient) microflora. The amount and level of microbial types in the transient microflora of contaminated hands reflects the microbial load of the environment and the character of the executed work. Contaminated hands are considered the most frequent way of transferring MRSA strains from health care workers to patients. All prevention of transfer and spread of the MRSA strains closely depends on using disposable gloves when treating MRSA infected patients. Hands are to be washed and disinfected prior to using the gloves and also after the attendance is over. The disposable gloves are to be disposed of. After washing, disinfecting liquid soap is recommended. For hand disinfection the most suitable preparations are the alcohol-based ones. Attention is also drawn to the fact that the sensitivity of the MRSA strains to selected used biocides (e.g. chlorhexidine digluconate) has decreased. MRSA strains survive under lower concentrations than the stated minimum bactericidal concentration (MBC)[1].

Cleaning and decontamination of the environment and the equipment

The method and intensity of cleaning and decontamination of the environment predominantly depends on the type of department and on observing all the recommended procedures and on using personal protective equipment. The percentage of contaminated surfaces is reported to be between 64–74%. The most frequently contaminated objects used by the patients include hospital beds and mattresses, bedding (bed sheets), grab bars along the walls, door handles, and taps. When changing the bed sheets not only objects of a certain size but also infectious agent (MRSA) are released into the inner environment. The highest number was detected 15 minutes after this activity was executed. This shows that the MRSA strains circulate even in the inner environment. As to various devices, keyboards are always stated as first, as to the medical equipment it is mainly the sleeves on the blood pressure gauges and tourniquets used for taking blood. Contamination of stethoscope membranes by MRSA strains, and possibilities of subsequent patient-to-patient transmission must clearly lead to realizing that its regular disinfection is vital.

Conclusion

"Methicillin-resistant *Staphylococcus aureus* (MRSA)" is an important cause of nosocomial infection worldwide. Interpretation of community MRSA trends is problematical, in that the term is ill-defined, and related data are difficult to put into context. There are four relevant battlefronts, all of interest to risk assessment and prevention.

These are: an increasing pool of patients with MRSA discharged from hospitals into the community. MRSA spreading to patients in nursing and residential homes. MRSA spreading from patients and health care workers to others in community. There are often difficulties in determining whether the fourth issue, MRSA arising apparently *de novo* in the community, is in fact due to one of these other fronts. All these battlefronts are important and not yet lost. However, we must agree on definitions and design-appropriate surveillance strategies, so that we can best plan prevention and control activities to contain these emerged or emerging problems".

References

1. Matouskova I, Janout V. Current knowledge of MRSA and CMRSA. Biomed Pap Med Fac Univ Palacky Olomouc Czech Repub. 2008, 152:191-202.

2. Reinert RR, Low DE, Rossi F, Zhang X, Wattal C, Dowzicky MJ. Antimicrobial susceptibility among organisms from the Asia/Pacific Rim, Europe and Latin and North America collected as part of TEST and the in vitro activity of tigecycline.

3. Kuehnert MJ, Kruszon-Moran D, Hill HA, McQuillan G, McAllister K, Fosheim G, *et al.* Prevalence of *Staphylococcus aureus* Nasal Colonization in the United States, 2001-2002. *J Infect Dis* 2006; 193:172-9.

4. Ito T, Okuma K, Ma XX, Yuzawa H, Hiramatsu K. Insights on antibiotic resistance of *Staphylococcus aureus* from its whole genome: genomic island SCC. *Drug Resist Updat* 2003;6:41-52.

5. CDC. Department of Health and Human Services. Community-Associated MRSA information for Clinicians. Date last modified: February 3, 2005. Available from: http://www.cdc.gov.

6. CDC. Department of Health and Human Services. Laboratory Detection of Oxacillin/Methicillin-resistant *Staphylococcus aureus*. February 2, 2005. Available from: http://www.cdc.gov/ncidod/hip/Lab/FactSheet/mrsa.htm

7. Robicsek A, Beaumont JL, Paule SM, Hacek DM, Thomson RB Jr, Kaul KL, *et al.* Universal surveillance for methicillin-resistant *Staphylococcus aureus* in 3 affiliated hospitals: *Ann Intern Med* 2008;148:409-18.

VANCOMYCIN RESISTANT ENTEROCOCCI (VRE)

Enterococci with acquired resistance to vancomycin and other glycopeptides (VRE) were first found as a cause of human infections in the Europe in 1986, and very soon afterwards in the United States. Now, VRE are a worldwide challenge[1]. Although the incidence of hospitalizations with infection due to vancomycin-resistant pathogens in the United States remained stable during 2000-2003, it increased from 4.60 to 9.48 hospitalizations per 100,000 population during 2003-2006. Hospitalizations with infection due to vancomycin-resistant pathogens also increased as a proportion of all US hospitalizations, from 3.16 to 6.51 hospitalizations with VRE infection per 10,000 total hospitalizations during 2003-2006[2,3]. Clonal spread of VRE has been documented, but polyclonal outbreaks associated with antimicrobial use are also common. The relations between antibiotic use and VRE colonization are complex and related to the antienterococcal activity, biliary excretion, and antianerobic activity of the antibiotic. VRE is most often transmitted by the contaminated hands, clothing, and equipment of health care workers. Nowadays, six types of acquired vancomycin resistance in enterococci are known; however, only VanA and, to a lesser extent, VanB are widely prevalent. Various genes encode acquired vancomycin resistance and these are typically associated with mobile genetic elements which allow resistance to spread clonally and laterally.

Vancomycin resistance was seen in <5% of *E. faecalis* isolates, North America 4.6%; Europe 1.5%; Latin America 1.4%; and Asia/Pacific Rim 0%. Vancomycin resistance in *E. faecium* varied widely among regions: North America 65.6%; Latin America 46.7%; Asia/Pacific Rim 31%; and Europe 12%. In terms of country distribution, only 14 of the 29 countries submitted more than 10 *E. faecium* isolates and among these, the numbers of vancomycin-resistant isolates were small, except in the USA (n=477). The USA, Argentina and Korea had the highest percentages of vancomycin-resistant *E. faecium* (60%)[4-6].

A possible link between the use of antimicrobials in food animal husbandry and vancomycin-resistant enterococci (VRE) subsequently arose in 1994 in Europe. A number of European investigators detected vancomycin-resistant *Enterococci faecium* (VREF) in the normal flora in certain food animals, in raw meats from those animals and in sewage in Germany, Denmark and the UK. Later studies in Europe suggested that VRE were common in intensively raised food animals, especially poultry and pigs, their waste and their meats, and that carriage of VRE in some segments of the population is common[1-5].

Emergence of Antimicrobial Resistance

An important feature in the emergence of the enterococci as a cause of nosocomial infection is their increasing resistance to a wide range of antibiotics. They demonstrate both intrinsic and acquired resistance.

Intrinsic resistance—Enterococci exhibits intrinsic resistance to penicillinase-susceptible penicillin (low level), penicillinase-resistant penicillin, cephalosporin, nalidixic acid aminoglycoside and clindamycin[1]. Enterococci are resistant to most beta-lactam antibiotics because of low affinity penicillin binding proteins (PBP), which enable them to synthesize cell wall components even in the presence of modest concentration of most beta-lactam antibiotics.

Frequency of vancomycin-resistant strains among isolates of *E. faecium* is shown in Fig. 22.1.

The three types of resistance of most significance in the enterococci are high-level resistance to the aminoglycosides, ampicillin resistance caused by beta lactamase production, and glycopeptide resistance.

Acquired resistance—Acquired resistance in enterococci can occur either via mutations in existing DNA or through the acquisition of new DNA. High-level resistance (MIC 2000 µg/ml) is usually due to the transferable plasmid mediated production of aminoglycoside-inactivating enzymes[5,7].

Vancomycin resistance—From the perspective of *E. faecium* antimicrobial resistance, there is an association between ampicillin and vancomycin resistance. Ampicillin resistant *E. faecium* isolates are most often detected before vancomycin resistance is detected. Together, the genetic linkage in *E. faecium* between ampicillin, PBP-5, and vancomycin and clinical studies that have shown prior beta-lactam use as a leading predisposing factor suggest that antimicrobial agents such as cephalosporins contribute to the emergence of vancomycin-resistant *E. faecium*.

Phenotypic classification—Six glycopeptide resistance types, van A, van B, van C, van D, van E, and van G, have been described in enterococci[7]; they can usually be distinguished on the basis of the level, inducibility, and transferability of resistance to vancomycin and teicoplanin, although they are most specifically distinguished by their associated genes (Table 22.2)[7]. The first two types are the most clinically relevant. Two of these (van A and van B) are mediated by newly acquired gene clusters not previously found in enterococci. van A and van B resistance phenotypes were described primarily in *E. faecalis* and *E. faecium*, van A-resistant strains possess inducible, high-level resistance to vancomycin (MICs >64 µg/ml) and teicoplanin (MICs >16 µg/ml).

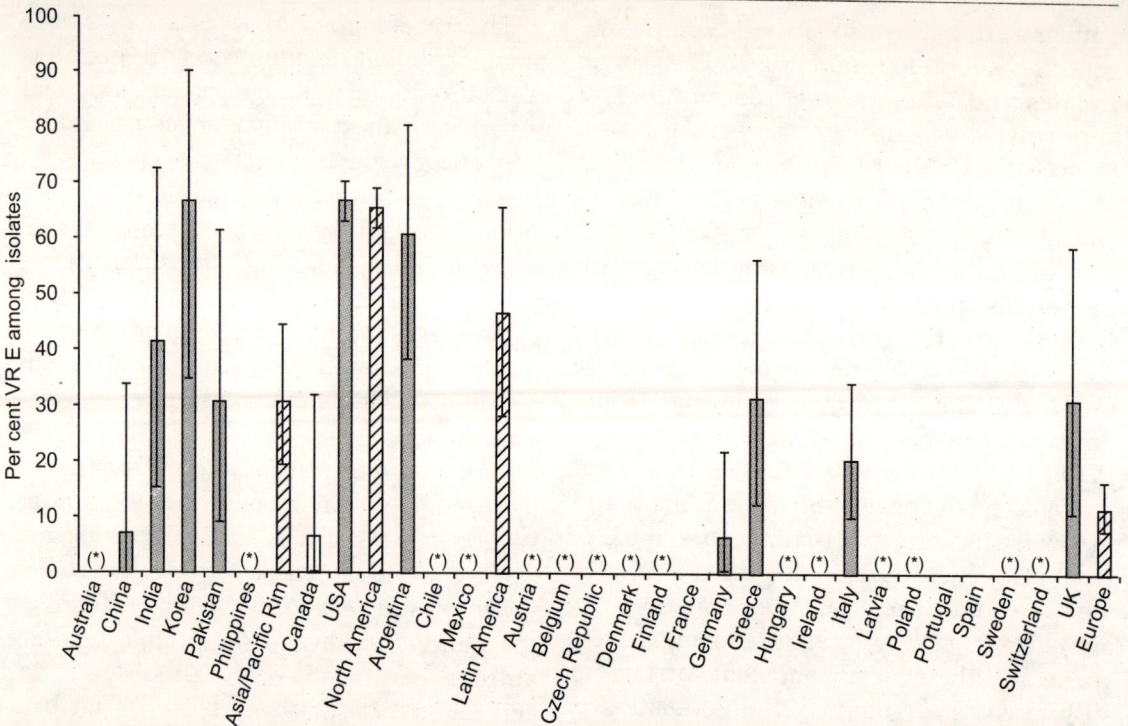

Fig. 22.1: Frequency of vancomycin-resistant strains among isolates of *E. faecium* (January 2004-August 2006), by country submitting >10 isolates (with 95% confidence intervals). *Indicates data not shown as country submitting,10 *E. faecium* isolates. Data for Singapore, Brazil and the Netherlands are not presented as these countries did not submit *E. faecium* isolates to test during the study period[6]

The genes associated with high level vancomycin resistance in enterococci, van A, van B, and van D, encode a ligase responsible for the synthesis of the depsipeptide D-alanyl-D-lactate which is incorporated into a pentapeptide peptidoglycan cell wall precursor (which terminates in D-alanyl-D-lactate) to which vanconycin binds poorly. In contrast, in vancomycin-susceptible cells, vancomycin complexes with the D-alanyl-D-alanine termini of normal pentapeptide peptidoglycan cell wall precursor thereby inhibiting cell wall synthesis.

Van A-type phenotypic glycopeptide resistance has traditionally been characterized by acquired inducible resistance to both vancomycin and teicoplanin, although there can be variability in the phenotype. Van A

resistance is mediated by Tn1546 or closely related elements. Tn1546 consists of 10,851 base pairs and encodes nine polypeptides that can be assigned to different functional groups: Transposition functions, regulation of glyco-peptide resistance genes (van R and van S), synthesis of depsipeptide D-alanyl-D-lactate which, when incorporated into the penta-peptide peptidoglycan precursor, form a pentapeptide precursor to which neither vancomycin nor teicoplanin will bind (van H and van A), and hydrolysis of precursors of normal peptidoglycan (van X and van Y). Van Y and van Z are accessory peptides not required for resistance. Genetic heterogeneity has been described in the van A gene clusters of VRE, and the van A gene cluster has been found on the chromosome as well as plasmids.

Table 22.2: Resistance to Glycopeptides in Entercoci

Phenotype	Genotype MIC (ug/ml)	Vancomycin MIC (ug/ml)	Teicoplanin	Expression	Tranfer	Species
Van A	Van A	64–>1000	16–512	Iinducible	+	E. faecium E. faecalis E. avium E. gallinarum E. durans E. mundtii E. casseliflavus E. raffinosus E. hirae
Van B	Van B	4–1000	0.25–2	Inducible	+	E. faecium E. faecalis E. gallinarum E. durans
Van C	Van C–1	2–32	0.12–2	Constitutive Inducible	–	E. gallinarum
Van C	Van C–2	2–32	0.12–2	Constitutive	–	E. casseliflavus
Van C	Van C–3	2–32	0.12–2	Constitutive	–	E. flavescens
Van D	Van D	16–256	2–64	Constitutive	–	E. faecium E. faecalis E. raffinosus
Van E	Van E	16	0.5	Inducible	–	E. faecalis
Van G	Van G	16	0.5	Inducible	–	E. faecalis

Van B-type glycopeptide resistance is characterized by acquired inducible resistance to various concentrations of vancomycin but not to teicoplanin. The van B gene cluster, as described in *Enterococcus faecalis* V583, has homology to the van A gene cluster, it consists of genes encoding polypeptides assigned to regulation of glycopeptide resistance genes (van RB and van SB), synthesis of the depsipeptide D-alanyl-lactate (van HB and van B), and hydrolysis of precursors of normal peptidoglycan (van XB and YB). Several groups have identified sequence variability in van B amongst different enterococcal isolates.

Van C-type glycopeptide resistance is characterized by low-level vancomycin resistance but teicoplanin susceptibility is an intrinsic property of *Enterococcus gallinarum* and *Enterococcus casseliflavus* flavescens. Pentapeptide peptigoglycan precursors in isolates with Van C vancomycin resistance terminate in D-alanyl-D-serine rather than in D-alanyl-D-alanine

High-level vancomycin resistace has been described in *Staphylococous aureus*, as a result of transfer of vancomycin resistance- associated genes from *Enterococcus faecalis*. Van A has been found in vancomycin-resistant clinical isolates of *Oerskovia turbata*, *Arcanobacterium haemolyticum*, and *Bacillus circulans*, and Van B in glycopeptide-resistant isolates of *Streptococcus bovis* and *Streptococcus gallolytiticus* and anaerobic bacteria present in human feces.

Gene clusters similar to van HAX and van BBXB have been identified in several soil dwelling glycopeptide-producing members of the glycopeptide producing (and glycopeptide resistant) actinomycete, *Streptomyces coelicolor*. It has been shown that Paenibacillus popilliae contains van F encoding a putative D-alanine: D-lactate ligase, Van F as part of the van R, S, Y, Z, H, FX, cluster similar in structure to the enterococcal van A and vab B clusters . It is also found a short sequence of DNA with homology to the enterococcal Tn1546 transposase gene within the glycopeptide resistance cluster of several strains of *P. popilliae* possibly representing a "footprint" of a Tn1546-like element that was necessary for an intermediate combinational step in the molecular evolution of the *P. popilliae* glycopeptide resistance cluster[5,7].

Vancomycin-dependent enterococci—An interesting phenomenon that has developed in some strains of van A- and van B-type VRE is that of vancomycin dependence. These enterococci are not just resistant to vancomycin but require it for growth. A likely explanation for this phenomenon is that these enterococci turn-off their normal production of D-Ala-D-Ala and then can grow only if a substitute dipeptide like structure is made. With most van A- and vanB-type enterococci, this occurs only in the presence of vancomycin, which induces the synthesis of associated dehydrogenase (van H) and ligase (van A or van B) that make D-Ala-D-Lac. The reason for the cell turning-off the synthesis of D-Ala-D-Ala is that as long as vancomycin is present, D-Ala-D-Ala is not necessary for cell wall synthesis by VRE. Indeed, it is being destroyed by the action of van X. Once the vancomycin is removed, D-Ala-D-Lac is no longer synthesized, and without either D-Ala-D-Ala or D-Ala-D-Lac, the cell cannot continue to grow or replicate. Reversion to vancomycin independence has been observed[5-7].

Over the past few years, linezolid resistance has emerged in vancomycin-resistant enterococci. Herrera *et al.* reported nosocomial transmission of linezolid-resistant vancomycin-resistant entercococci. In almost all clinical studies, linezolid resistance has been associated with a G2576T mutation gene (in the absence of G2576T mutation) associated with linozolide resistance in *E. faecium*. Bonora *et al.* reported several linezolid-resistant vancomycin-resistant enterococcal isolates from intensive care unit patients that belonged to different clones. Bae *et al* reported the first clinical isolate of linezolid and vancomycin-resistant *Enterococcus faecium* in Korea; the minimum inhibitory concentration of linezolid was proportional to the number or copies of the G2576U mutation. Daptomycin resistance in vancomycin-enterococci is also being reported.

Risk Factors

Earlier studies in US revealed that most patients with VRE were in ICUs[2]. However, VRE is now being seen with increasing frequency among patients with chronic renal failure, cancer, organ transplant recipients and patients who experience prolonged hospitalization. They tend to occur in more debilitated or seriously ill hospitalized patients. Risk factors include longer duration of hospitalization, longer duration of stay in ICU, gastrointestinal colonization with VRE (it may precede infection in many patients but all colonized patients do not get infected), previous antimicrobial therapy (especially with multiple antibiotics), severity of illness, exposure to contaminated medical equipment, proximity to a previously known VRE patient, exposure to a nurse who has assigned on the same shift to another known patient, hematological malignancy/bone marrow transplantation, parenteral/oral vancomycin and receipt of third-generation cephalosporins and drugs with activity against anaerobes. Vancomycin most probably predisposes patients to colonization and infection with VRE by inhibiting the growth of the normal Gram-positive bowel flora and by providing selective advantage for VRE that may be present in small numbers in the individuals bowel[5].

Prevention and Control

It has been demonstrated that enterococci, including VRE, can be spread by direct patient-to-patient contact or indirectly via transient carriage on the hands of personnel, contaminated environmental surfaces or patient care equipment.

In response to the dramatic increase in vancomycin resistance in enterococci, the CDC Hospital Infection Control Practices Advisory Committee (HICPAC) has made the following recommendations[5]:

i. *Prudent use of vancomycin*—Encouraging the appropriate use of oral and parenteral vancomycin is an important component of HICPAC recommendations.

Other measures include formulary policies discouraging the use of third-generation cephalosporins and agents most likely to cause *C. difficile* colitis.

ii. *Education of hospital staff*—Continuous education programs for health care workers should include information about the epidemiology of VRE and the potential impact of this pathogen on the cost and outcome of patient care.

iii. *Effective use of the microbiology laboratory*— Early detection of patients colonized or infected with VRE is an essential component of any hospital program designed to prevent nosocomial transmission of VRE.

There are at present eight available susceptibility test methods (agar dilution, disk diffusion, E-test, agar screen plate, Vitek GPS-TA and GPS-101, MicroScan overnight and rapid panels). Enterococci may also be tested for vancomycin resistance by using PCR assays designed to detect the genes responsible for glycopeptide resistance in these organisms. Surveillance cultures for VRE are time consuming and expensive for the laboratory to perform.

iv. *Implementation of infection control measures*— Including the use of gloves and gowns and isolation or cohorting of patients, as appropriate to specific conditions.

Treatment

Treatment is difficult due to resistance and because of the fact that it is necessary to use specialized techniques to demonstrate their true susceptibility in clinical laboratory.

A number of new approaches to the treatment of VRE infections including beta lactam-beta lactamase, beta lactam-glycopeptide, Lactamase inhibitor and beta lactam-fluoroquinolone combinations have been explored in experimental animal models[67]. Each approach has its limitations and the treatment is at best, experimental. Dalfopristin-quinupristin (RP 59,500), a streptogramin antibiotic, is the first antibiotic approved for the treatment of patients with serious or life-threatening infections associated with vancomycin-resistant *E. faecium* bacteremia. Amongst all the other agents, it is the oxazolidinones, a new class of synthetic antibiotics, which have a good antienterococcal activity[2,7].

Conclusion

The occurrence of VRE is a persisting clinical problem in all geographic areas and continues to be exacerbated by clonal dissemination within the health care facility leading to limited therapeutic options. Only a comprehensive program (consisting of active surveillance, isolation of colonized/infected patients, strict adherence to proper infection control practices and antimicrobial stewardship) can limit the spread of these organisms. In addition to monitoring the compliance with traditional infection control measures, new strategies that merit consideration include pre-emptive isolation of patients in high-risk units and molecular techniques for the detection of VRE.

References

1. Werner G, Coque TM, Hammerum AM, *et al.* Emergence and spread of Vancomycin resistance among Enterococci in Europe. *Euro Surveill* 2008; 13: 47-20.

2. Ramsey AM, Zilberberg MD. Secular trends of hospitalization with vancomycin-resistant enterococcus infection in the United States, 2000-2006. *Infect Control Hosp Epidemiol* 2009;30:184-6.

3. Rice LB. Antimicrobial resistance in gram-positive bacteria. *Am J Infect Control.* 2006:34(5 Suppl 1):S64-73.

4. Zhu W, Clark NC, McDougal LK, Hageman J, McDonald LC, Patel JB. Vancomycin-resistant *Staphylococcus aureus* associated with Inc18-like van A plasmids in Michigan. *Antimicrob Agents Chemother* 2008;52:452-7.

5. Chlebicki M P, Kurup A. Vancomycin-resistant Enterococcus - A Review From a Singapore Perspective. *Ann Acad Med Singapore* 2008;37:861-9.

6. Reinert RR, Low DE, Rossi F, Zhang X, Wattal C, Dowzicky MJ. Antimicrobial susceptibility among organisms from the Asia/Pacific Rim, Europe and Latin and North America collected as part of TEST and the in vitro activity of tigecycline

7. Werner G, Strommenger B, Witte W. Acquired vancomycin resistance in clinically relevant pathogens. *Future Microbiol.* 2008;3:547-62.

EXTENDED-SPECTRUM BETA LACTAMASE (ESBL) ORGANISMS

Extended-spectrum β-lactamases (ESBLs) are extremely broad spectrum β-lactamase enzymes found in a variety of enterobacteriaceae ESBL organisms. They are among the fastest growing problems in the area of infectious diseases and have become global invaders of virtually all hospitals where serious infections are treated. These β-lactamases can be produced by a variety of Enterobacteriaceae; however, the most common ESBL-producing organisms are *Klebsiella pneumoniae*, other Klebsiella sp (i.e. *K. oxytoca*), and *Escherichia coli*. With the ability to produce highly effective β-lactamase enzymes, these organisms are resistant to all β-lactam antibiotics except cephamycins (cefoxitin, cefotetan) and carbapenems. In addition, ESBL-producing organisms are frequently resistant to many other classes of antibiotics, including aminoglycosides and fluoroquinolones. Hence, a more appropriate name would be "multidrug resistant organisms"[1].

The introduction of the third-generation cephalosporins into clinical practice in the early 1980s was heralded as a major breakthrough in the fight against β -lactamase-mediated bacterial resistance to antibiotics[2]. These cephalosporins had been developed in response to the increased prevalence of β-lactamases in certain organisms (for example, ampicillin hydrolyzing TEM-1 and SHV-1 β-lactamases in *Escherichia coli* and *Klebsiella pneumoniae*) and the spread of these β-lactamases into new hosts (for example, *Hemophilus influenzae* and *Neisseria gonorrheae*). Not only were the third- generation cephalosporins effective against most β-lactamase-producing organisms but they had the major advantage of lessened nephrotoxic effects compared to aminoglycosides and polymyxins.

The first report of plasmid-encoded β-lactamases capable of hydrolyzing the extended-spectrum cephalosporins was published in 1983[3]. The gene encoding the β-lactamase showed a mutation of a single nucelotide compared to the gene encoding SHV-1. Other β-lactamases were soon discovered which were closely related to TEM-1 and TEM-2, but which had the ability to confer resistance to the extended-spectrum cephalosporins. Hence, these new β-lactamases were coined extended-spectrum β-lactamases (ESBLs). In the first substantial review of ESBLs in 1989, it was noted by Philippon, Labia, and Jacoby that the ESBLs represented the first example in which β-lactamase-mediated resistance to β-lactam antibiotics resulted from fundamental changes in the substrate spectra of the enzymes[4].

The occurrence of ESBL producers among *K. pneumoniae* isolates collected over 3 years was highest in Latin America (44%), compared with Asia/Pacific Rim (22.4%), North America (7.5%) and Europe (13.3%) (Fig. 22.2). By country, the highest ESBL rates occurred in India (72%) and Mexico (71.4%). Also notable were the rates in the other Latin American countries (37.8% to 55.3%), Greece (43.1%) and Poland (37.5%). No ESBL-producing isolates were reported in Austria, Czech Republic, Denmark, Finland, Ireland, Switzerland and the Netherlands[5].

Against all *K. pneumoniae* collected, imipenem was the most active antimicrobial, with >99% susceptibility in each region. This was followed by tigecycline (>94% of isolates susceptible in each region). Imipenem and tigecycline were also the most active agents

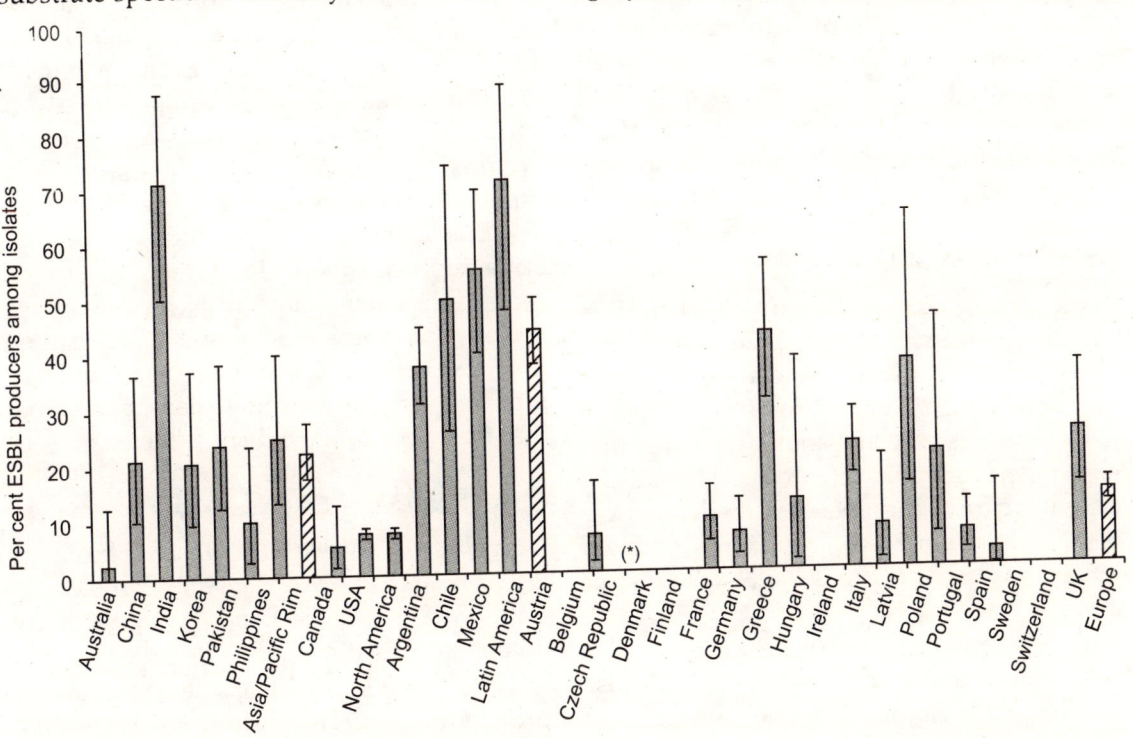

Fig. 22.2: Frequency of ESBL producers among *K. pneumoniae* isolates (January 2004-August 2006), by country submitting >10 isolates (with 95% confidence intervals). *Indicates data not shown as country submitting <10 *K. pneumoniae* isolates (Reinert *et al*)[5]

against the subpopulation of ESBL-producing *K. pneumoniae*. The susceptibility rates for β-lactams and levofloxacin varied widely among the regions and were markedly lower in Latin America than the other regions in the cases of amoxicillin/clavulanate and piperacillin/tazobactam[5]. Figure 22.2 shows frequency of ESBL procedures among *K. pneumoniae* oneumoniae (January 2004-August 2005).

ESBL production among *E. coli* was variable among the regions; Asia/Pacific Rim and Latin America had the highest rates (12.0% and 13.5%, respectively) and North America had the lowest rate (2.2%). In Europe, 7.6% of *E. coli* were ESBL producers. *E. coli* isolates showed 100% susceptibility to tigecycline and imipenem and >90% susceptibility to piperacillin/tazobactam and amikacin in the four regions. Overall, antimicrobial susceptibility was comparable in the four regions. However, the MIC90 values varied widely for ceftriaxone (0.25 to >128 mg/l) and cefepime (<0.5–32 mg/l). Ampicillin, amoxicillin/clavulanic acid and levofloxacin showed poor activity against *E. coli*[5].

Definition of ESBLs

There is no consensus of the precise definition of ESBLs. A commonly used working definition is that the ESBLs are β-lactamases capable of conferring bacterial resistance to the penicillins, first, second, and third-generation cephalosporins, and aztreonam (but not the cephamycins or carbapenems) by hydrolysis of these antibiotics, and which are inhibited by β-lactamase inhibitors such as clavulanic acid[4].

ESBLs are plasmid-encoded enzymes that belong to a limited number of beta-lactamase families, with various members appearing in geographically distinct clusters. Initially, the TEM and SHV families of ESBLs predominated in the United States beginning in the mid- to late-1980s, with occasional reports of ESBLs from the OXA beta-lactamase family a few years later. However, as the newly described CTX-M family of beta lactamases emerged in the mid-1990s in Germany and South America, these enzymes began to displace the "traditional" ESBLs from many geographic areas. Today the CTX-M family of enzymes has become the dominant ESBL in most of the world, and TEM ESBLs are now rarely, or never, reported from many countries. For some unexplained reason, however, the SHV and TEM families remain the ESBLs in the United States, with little reporting of CTX-M enzymes.

Epidemiological surveys of ESBLs production demonstrate higher levels of these enzymes in klebsiella sp. in contrast to *E. coli*. These enzymes have also appeared in almost all other Enterobacteriaceae, but at lower prevalence. Detection of theses enzymes in all the Enterobacteriaceae, and reporting of cephalosporin susceptibilities in these organisms, remains a controversial topic, especially in pathogens other than Klebsiella and *E. coli*. Pharmacodynamic properties and epidemiological considerations are often at odds with each other, and clinical microbiology laboratories struggle to determine how low cephalosporin resistance should be reported in hospitals that may have clonal outbreaks of ESBL-producing bacteria.

Classification of ESBLs

β-Lactamases are commonly classified according to two general schemes: The Ambler molecular classification and the Bush-Jacoby-Medeiros functional classification[4].

The Ambler scheme classifies β-lactamases into four classes according to the protein homology of enzymes. β-lactamases of class A, C, and D are serine β-lactamase and class B enzymes are metallo-β-lactamases. The

Bush-Jacoby-Medeiros functional scheme is based on functional properties of enzymes, i.e. the substrate and inhibitor profiles. The term 'extended-spectrum β-lactamases' was originally applied to the TEM and SHV derivatives that can hydrolyze oxyimino-cephalosporins, and these enzymes were classified as group 2be with the Bush-Jacoby-Medeiros functional scheme. The 2be designation consists of '2b'denoting that the enzyme is derived from a 2b enzyme (e.g. SHV–1, TEM–1, and TEM–2) and 'e' represen-ting the extended spectrum of activity. The definition of extended spectrum of activity is to have a hydrolytic activity against oxyimino-cephalosporins or aztreonam at more than 10% of that against benzyl penicillin to be the enzymes that cannot hydrolyze cephamycins or carbapenems efficiently and are inhibited by β-lactamase inhibitors such as clavulunate. TEM-ESBLs and SHV-ESBLs belong to class A in the Ambler scheme. In last few years discovery of several novel enzymes have blurred the original definition of ESBLs.

Typical class C enzymes can confer resistance to oxyimino-cephalosporins if they are hyperproduced as a consequence of mutational derepression or are expressed constitutively on plasmid. Class C enzymes are resistant to the inhibition by β-lactamase inhibitors and are not deemed a member of ESBLs. Recently, AmpC mutants with increased hydrolytic activity against cefepime and cefpirome (extended-spectrum cephalosporinases) have been reported. Although it has been determined that such mutants were mainly located on bacterial chromosome, two plasmid-mediated extended-spectrum cephalosporinases, CMY-19 and CMY-10, have been reported. Some specialists may insist on regarding such enzymes as ESBLs because of their wide spectrum of activity.

In recent years class A β-lactamases that can hydrolyze carbapenems have been reported (e.g. KPC, NMC/IMI, and SME). Most of these enzymes also hydrolyze oxyimino-cephalosporins. From the clinical point of view, it is not practical to categorize these enzymes as ESBLs because carbapenems are regarded as the drug of choice for ESBL-producing organisms. GES enzymes pose a more difficult problem on this matter. GES-1 possesses hydrolytic activity similar to the classic class A ESBLs, is inhibited by β-lactamase inhibitors, and is generally classified into ESBL. The total number of ESBLs now characterized exceeds 200. These are detailed on the authorative website on the nomenclature of ESBLs hosted by George Jacoby and Karen Bush. (http://www.lahey. org/ studies/webt.htm).

The current beta-lactamase classifications have reached a high level of complexity, making them less accessible to clinicians, infection control professionals, hospital management and politicians. From the clinical perspective, a revised comprehensible nomenclature scheme is, therefore, needed. The term extended-spectrum beta-lactamases (ESBLs) has reached a broader audience over time, but is currently restricted to functional class 2be/ molecular class A, clavulanic acid inhibited enzymes with activity against extended-spectrum cephalosporins. The proposed new classification expands the definition of ESBL to other clinically important acquired beta-lactamases with activity against extended-spectrum cephalosporins and/or carbapenems[6]. The classical class A ESBLs have been designated ESBLA in this classification, whereas plasmid-mediated AmpC and OXA-ESBLs are classed as miscellaneous ESBLs (ESBLM). Lastly, the carbapenemases have been designated ESBLCARBA, ESBLs with hydrolytic activity against carbapenems. It is believed that this simplified classification may encourage new groups of health care professionals to engage in the effort to prevent the spread of acquired β-lactamases.

Mechanism of Resistance

The ESBL enzymes are plasmid-mediated enzymes capable of hydrolyzing and inactivating a wide variety of β-lactams, including third-generation cephalosporins, penicillins, and aztreonam. These enzymes are the result of mutations of TEM1, TEM2 and SHV1, all of which are β-lactamase enzymes commonly found in the Enterobacteriaceae family. Normally TEM1, TEM2, and SHV1 enzymes confer high-level resistance to early penicillins and low-level resistance to first-generation cephalosporins[4]. The widespread use of third-generation cephalosporins and aztreonam is believed to be the major cause of the mutations in these enzymes that have led to the emergence of ESBLs[1,7].

A distinction must be made between AmpC β-lactamases and ESBL enzymes. The AmpC β-lactamases are encoded by genes located on chromosomes, are often inducible, and are commonly found in Enterobacter sp, Citrobacter freundii, Morganella morganii, *Serratia marcescens*, and *Pseudomonas aeruginosa*[8]. Since genes encoding these enzymes are located on chromosomes, they are not easily transferable to other bacterial species. Resistance patterns associated with AmpC β-lactamase enzymes are strikingly similar to those of ESBLs; however, AmpC β-lactamases are only weakly inhibited by β-lactamase inhibitors and usually confer resistance to cephamycins. In contrast, ESBLs are generally well inhibited by β-lactamase inhibitors and usually retain sensitivity to the cephamycins. The ESBLs are encoded by genes located on plasmids, resulting in easy transfer to other bacterial species. Table 22.3 shows type of plasmid-mediated ESBL.

Diversity of ESBL Types

SHV

The SHV-type ESBLs may be more frequently found in clinical isolates than any other type of ESBLs. SHV refers to sulfhydryl variable. This designation was made because it was thought that the inhibition of SHV activity by p-chloromercuribenzoate was substrate-related, and was variable according to the substrate used for the assay. SHV-type ESBLs have been detected in a wide range of Enterobacteriaceae and outbreaks of SHV-producing *Pseudomonas aeruginosa* and Acinetobacter spp. have now been reported[7].

TEM

The TEM-type ESBLs are derivatives of TEM-1 and TEM-2[7]. TEM-1 was first reported in 1965 from an *Escherichia coli* isolate from a patient in Athens, Greece, named Temoneira (hence the designation TEM). In 1987 *Klebsiella pneumoniae* isolates detected in France as early as 1984 were found to harbor a novel plasmid-mediated β-lactamase coined CTX-1. The enzyme was originally named CTX-1 because of its enhanced activity against cefotaxime. The enzyme, now termed TEM-3, differed from TEM-2 by two amino acid substitutions. The first TEM-type ESBL is now called TEM-12. Well over 100 TEM-type β-lactamases have been described, of which the majority are ESBLs. Their isoelectric points range from 5.2 to 6.5. However, interesting mutants of TEM β-lactamases are being recovered that maintain the ability to hydrolyze third-generation cephalosporins but which also demonstrate inhibitor resistance. These are referred to as complex mutants of TEM (CMT-1 to 4). A unique TEM-derived enzyme, TEM-AQ, has been found in Italy. This enzyme has an amino acid deletion not seen in other TEM enzymes plus several amino acid substitutions.

CTX-M and Toho β-lactamases[2]

The name CTX reflects the potent hydrolytic activity of these β-lactamases against cefotaxime. Organisms producing CTX-M-

Table 22.3: Type of plasmid-mediated extended-spectrum β-lactamase enzymes[4]

Type	Classification	Preferred substrates	β-lactamase Inhibitors	Location
TEM and SHV	Bush: Class 2be Ambler: Class A	Oxyiminocephalosporins and other β-Lactams except cephamycin and carbapenems	Susceptible	Worldwide
Inhibitor-resistant TEMs	Bush: Class 2br Ambler: Class A	Penicillins	Resistant	Worldwide
PER	Bush: Class 2be Ambler: Class D	Oxyiminocephalosporins and other β-lactams except cephamycin and carbapenems	Susceptible	Turkey, South America
OXA	Bush: Class 2d Ambler: Class D	Oxyiminocephalosporins, cephamycin, and other β-Lactams except carbapenems	Resistant	Turkey
Plasmid-mediated AmpC	Bush: Class 1 Ambler: Class C	Oxyiminocephalosporins, cephamycin, and other β-Lactams except carbapenems	Resistant	Worldwide
Plasmid-mediated carbapenemases	Bush: Class 3 Ambler: Class B	All β-Lactams, including carbapenems	Resistant	Japan, Singapore, Italy; not yet reported in the U.S.

type β-lactamases typically have cefotaxime MICs in the resistant range (>64 μg/ml), while ceftazidime MICs are usually in the apparently susceptible range (2 to 8 μg/ml). However, some CTX-M-type ESBLs may actually hydrolyze ceftazidime and confer resistance to this cephalosporin (MICs as high as 256 μg/ml). Aztreonam MICs are variable. CTX-M-type β-lactamases hydrolyze cefepime with high efficiency, and cefepime MICs are higher than observed in bacteria producing other ESBL types. Tazobactam exhibits an almost 10-fold greater inhibitory activity than clavulanic acid against CTX-M-type β-lactamases.

Toho-1 and Toho-2 are β-lactamases related structurally to CTX-M-type β-lactamases. (Toho refers to the Toho University School of Medicine Omori Hospital in Tokyo, where a child was hospitalized who was infected with Toho-1 β-lactamase-producing *Escherichia coli.*) Like most CTX-M-type β-lactamases, the hydrolytic activity of the Toho-1 and Toho-2 enzymes is more potent against cefotaxime than ceftazidime. The number of CTX-M-type ESBLs is rapidly expanding. Given the widespread findings of CTX-M-type ESBLs in China and India, it could be speculated that CTX-M-type ESBLs are now actually the most frequent ESBL type worldwide.

OXA

The OXA-type β-lactamases are so named because of their oxacillin-hydrolyzing abilities. These β-lactamases (group 2d) are characterized by hydrolysis rates for cloxacillin and oxacillin greater than 50% that for benzylpenicillin. Most OXA-type β-lactamases do not hydrolyze the extended-spectrum cephalosporins to a significant degree and are not regarded as ESBLs. However, OXA-10 hydrolyzes (weakly) cefotaxime, ceftriaxone, and aztreonam, giving most organisms reduced susceptibility to these antibiotics. Unfortunately there are very few epidemiologic data on the geographical spread of OXA-type ESBLs[6].

GES

GES-1 was initially described in a *K. pneumoniae* isolate from a neonatal patient just transferred to France from French Guiana. GES-1 has hydrolytic activity against penicillins and extended-spectrum cephalosporins, but not against cephamycins or carbapenems, and is inhibited by β-lactamase inhibitors. These enzymatic properties resemble those of other class A ESBLs; thus, GES-1 was recognized as a member of ESBLs. GES-2 is only weakly inhibited by β-lactamase inhibitors. GES-4, which has a Gly170Ser substitution compared with GES-3, is also capable of hydrolyzing carbapenems and weakly inhibited by β-lactamase inhibitors. Furthermore, GES-4 extends its hydrolytic activity towards cephamycins[6].

PER

The PER-type ESBLs share only around 25 to 27% homology with known TEM- and SHV-type ESBLs. PER-1 β-lactamase efficiently hydrolyze penicillins and cephalosporins and are susceptible to clavulanic acid inhibition. Worryingly, a *Pseudomonas aeruginosa* strain producing both PER-1 and the carbapenemase VIM-2 has been detected in Italy. The co-existence of these enzymes renders an organism resistant to virtually all β-lactam antibiotics[2].

VEB-1, BES-1, and other ESBLs

A variety of other β-lactamases which are plasmid-mediated or integron-associated class A enzymes have been recently discovered. They are not simple point mutant derivatives of any known β-lactamases. They are remarkable for their geographic diversity. Novel chromosomally encoded ESBLs have also been described. VEB-1 has greatest homology with PER-1 and PER-2 (38%). It confers high-level resistance to ceftazidime, cefotaxime, and aztreonam, which is reversed by clavulanic acid. The gene encoding VEB-1 was found to be plasmid mediated; such plasmids also confer resistance to non-β-lactam antibiotics. The patient from whom the β-lactamase was originally described was a Vietnamese infant hospitalized in France hance the name[2].

TLA, SFO, and IBC are other examples of non-TEM, non-SHV ESBLs and have been found in a wide range of geographic locations.

Risk Factors for Colonization and Infection with ESBL Producers

Numerous studies have used a case-control design with which to assess risk factors for colonization and infection with ESBL-producing organisms. Analysis of the results of these studies yields a plethora of conflicting results, likely due to the differences in study populations, selection of cases, selection of controls, and sample size[1,9]. Nevertheless, some generalizations can be made. Patients at high risk for developing colonization or infection with ESBL-producing organisms are often seriously ill patients with prolonged hospital stays and in whom invasive medical devices are present (urinary catheters, endotracheal tubes, central venous lines) for a prolonged duration. The median length of hospital stay prior to isolation of an ESBL producer has ranged from 11 to 67 days, depending on the study. In addition to those already mentioned, a myriad of other risk factors have been found in individual studies. All these risk factors are summarized in Table 22.4[1].

Table 22.4: Risk factors associated with ESBL colonization and infection

Prolonged hospitalization	Gut colonization
Prolonged ICU stay	Indwelling catheter
Long-term care facility residency	Gastrostomy or jejunostomy tube
Exposure to ceftazidime or aztreonam	Ventilator dependence
Exposure to amino-glycoside	Age <12 wks
Exposure to any antibiotic	Low birth weight
Number of antibiotics received	Nasogastric tube
Emergency abdominal surgery	Severity of illness

Detection of ESBLs in Clinical Laboratories

Detection of organisms harboring ESBLs provides clinicians with helpful information. Treatment of infections caused by ESBL-producing organisms with extended-spectrum cephalosporins or aztreonam may result in treatment failure even when the causative organisms appear to be susceptible to these antimicrobial agents by routine susceptibility testing. In addition, patients colonized or infected with ESBL-producing organism should be placed under contact precautions to avoid hospital transmission. These benefits warrant the detection of ESBL-producing organisms in clinical laboratories[7]. On the other hand, revision of cephalosporin breakpoints has been achieved by the European Committee on Antimicrobial Susceptibility Testing (EUCAST) and is under way by the Clinical and Laboratory Standards Institute (CLSI) for better prediction of clinical

outcome by MIC values[10]. It is still controversial whether this revision might allow clinical laboratories to dispense with ESBL detection. Since the 1980s, several phenotypic tests for detection of ESBL-producing organisms have been developed. All methods utilize the characteristics of ESBLs, conferring a reduced susceptibility to extended-spectrum cephalosporins and inhibition by clavulanate. Detection of ESBL production by organisms with inducible chromosomal AmpC β-lactamase is difficult using these methods because AmpC β-lactamase resists inhibition by clavulanate. In addition, clavulanate may act as an inducer of chromosomal AmpC β-lactamases of these organisms. The CLSI recommends screening of *E. coli*, *K. pneumoniae*, and *Klebsiella oxytoca* (and *Proteus mirabilis*, if clinically relevant such as bacteremic isolates) for potential production of ESBL. The CLSI method for ESBL detection consists of the initial screen test and the phenotypic confirmatory test.

Treatment and outcome of Infections with ESBL-producing Organisms

Given the ability of ESBL-producing organisms to hydrolyze many β-lactam antibiotics, it is not surprising that antibiotic choice for infections with such organisms is seriously reduced. Furthermore, however, the plasmids bearing the genes encoding ESBLs frequently also carry genes encoding resistance to aminoglycosides and trimethioprim/sulfamethoxazole. There have been increasing reports of plasmid-encoded decrease in susceptibility to quinolones, frequently in association with plasmid-mediated cephalosporin resistance. Third-generation cephalosporins are poor choices for the treatment of serious infections due to ESBL-producing organisms. Failure rates are high when MICs of the cephalosporins are elevated (for example, 4 or 8 µg/ml) but still within the susceptible range.

Stochastic modeling suggests that cefepime at 2 g every 12 h may have a high probability of achieving pharmacokinetic/pharmaco-dynamic targets which have previously been correlated with clinical success. However, published clinical experience with the use of cefepime for the treatment of ESBL-producing organisms has been quite limited. In a randomized trial of cefepime versus imipenem for nosocomial pneumonia, clinical response for infections with ESBL-producing organisms was seen in 100% patients treated with imipenem but only 69% patients treated with cefepime. In common with other extended-spectrum cephalosporins, MICs for cefepime rise substantially when the ino-culums of infecting organisms rise. Cefepime resistance may be more frequent in strains which produce the CTX-M type ESBLs. Cefepime should not be used as first-line therapy against ESBL-producing organisms; if it is used (for example, against organisms with a cefepime MIC of <2 μg/ml), it should be used in high dosage (at least 2 g twice a day). In vitro synergy may be achievable between cefepime and amikacin[2].

β-lactam/β-lactamase inhibitor combina-tions are subject to rising MICs as inoculum rises. Additionally, it is well known that ESBL-producing organisms may continue to harbor parent enyzmes (for example, SHV-1 or TEM-1). Hyperproduction of these non-ESBL-producing β-lactamases or the combination of β-lactamase production and porin loss can also lead to a reduction in activity of β-lactamase inhibitors. Stochastic modeling suggests that some dosing regimens of piperacillin-tazobactam may not have a high probability of achieving pharmacokinetic/pharmacodynamic targets which have pre-viously been correlated with clinical success.

Carbapenems should be regarded as the drugs of choice for serious infections with ESBL-producing organisms[11,12]. The basis for this statement is not just the almost uniform susceptibility in vitro of these compounds but also increasingly extensive clinical experience. There is no evidence that combination therapy with a carbapenem and antibiotics of other classes is superior to use of a carbapenem alone. Carbapenem resistant, ESBL-producing isolates remain exceedingly rare. Neither ESBLs nor plasmid-mediated AmpC β-lactamases are capable of hydrolyzing carba-penems to any great degree.

Carbapenem-Resistant *Klebsiella pneumoniae* Isolates

In studies which have investigated clinical isolates of *Klebsiella pneumoniae* exhibiting carbapenem resistance, the combination of porin loss and β-lactamase production has resulted in carbapenem resistance[13]. The relevant β-lactamases have included previous-ly characterized ESBLs (SHV-2) and AmpC-type enzymes (ACT-1 and CMY-4).

A second documented mechanism for carbapenem resistance is the presence of a β-lactamase capable of hydrolysis of carba-penems. Worryingly, such carbapene-mases have been found to be plasmid-mediated[2]. This is a great concern given the propensity for klebsiellae to host plasmids. Two types of carbapenemases have thus far been detected. The first are Bush-Jacoby-Medeiros group 3 enzymes. These metallo-enzymes were originally found in *Klebsiella pneumoniae* isolates in Japan in 1994. This IMP-1 enzyme has now been found in a *Klebsiella pneumoniae* isolate in Singapore, where a combination with porin loss contributed to high-level carbapenem resistance. A recent report from Taiwan has described a *Klebsiella pneumoniae* isolate with a novel IMP-type carbapenemase (IMP-7), which was encoded on a plasmid also harboring genes encoding TEM-1 and the ESBL SHV-12. Several other examples of IMP and VIM metalloenzyme producing klebsiellae have been reported.

The second carbapenemase detected in *Klebsiella pneumoniae* was the novel Bush-Jacoby-Medeiros group 2f β-lactamase, coined KPC-1. The amino acid sequence of this β-lactamase showed 45% homology to the Sme-1 carbapenemase of *Serratia marcescens*. Although the strain also harbored an ESBL, SHV-29, the carbapenemase was also responsible for resistance to extended-spectrum cephalosporins and aztreonam. Related carbapenemases, KPC-2 and KPC-3, have also been reported, especially from New York City .

Prevention

Institutions with endemic ESBL-producing organisms need to determine whether there is a high rate of cephalosporin use, especially third-generation cephalosporins. Several studies have shown that by limiting the use of these agents, alone or in combination with infection control measures, the frequency of ESBL isolates can be reduced substantially. During 1993 and 1994, the frequency of ceftazidime-resistant *K. pneumoniae* increased from 6 to 28% at the Cleveland Department of Veterans Affairs Medical Center. In February 1994, piperacillin-tazobactam was added to the formulary, and educational programs encouraged its use over ceftazidime for empiric treatment of nosocomial infections. This formulary change resulted in a significant decrease in ceftazidime use and a concomitant decrease in the percentage of ceftazidime-resistant isolates. No significant rise in the rate of resistance to piperacillin-tazobactam was seen among clinical isolates of *K. pneumoniae*[1].

A study published in 1998 evaluated the effect of restricting all cephalosporin use (parenteral and oral) to control ceftazidime-resistant Klebsiella isolates. The only indications for cephalosporin administration without an infectious disease by physician's approval were pediatric infections, meningitis, spontaneous bacterial peritonitis, and surgical prophylaxis. These controls resulted in an 80% reduction in cephalosporin use hospital wide and a 44% decline in the number of ceftazidime-resistant Klebsiella isolates. However, a significant increase in imipenem use (140%) during the study was accompanied by a 69% increase in imipenem-resistant *P. aeruginosa* and emergence of imipenem-resistant Acinetobacter sp.

With this congruence of data, it is clear that limiting the use of cephalosporins, especially third-generation cephalosporins, is an effective way to reduce the frequency of ESBLs[14]. The dramatic decline in resistance rates was seen within a short period of time. Appropriate alternatives for third-generation cephalosporins are β-lactams-β-lactamase inhibitors, especially piperacillin-tazobactam, since a number of studies indicate no significant rise in the rate of resistance to these agents among clinical isolates of *K. pneumoniae* despite increased use. Table 22.5 shows recommended treatment for infections with ESBL-producing organisms.

Conclusions

The ESBL-producing organisms are a breed of multidrug-resistant pathogens that are increasing rapidly and becoming a major problem in the area of infectious diseases. High rates of third-generation cephalosporin use have been implicated as a major cause of this problem. Problems associated with ESBLs include multidrug resistance, difficulty in detection and treatment, and increased mortality. Of all available antimicrobial agents, carbapenems are the most active and reliable treatment options for infections caused by ESBL isolates. However, overuse of carbapenems may lead to resistance of other

Table 22.5: Recommended treatment for infections with ESBL-producing organisms[2]

Infection type	Therapy of choice	Second-line therapy
Urinary tract infection	Amoxicillin/clavualante	Quinolone (a)
Bacteremia	Carbapenem	Quinolone (a)
Hospital-acquired pneumonia	Carbapenem	Quinolone (a)
Intra-abdominal infection	Carbapenem	Qinolone (a) (plus metronidazole)
Meningitis	Meropenem	Intrathecal polymyxin B

a If the organism is quinolone susceptible

gram-negative organisms. Therefore, restricting the use of third-generation cephalosporins, along with implementation of infection control measures, are the most effective means of controlling and decreasing the spread of ESBL isolates.

References

1. Surakit Nathisuwan, Pharm.D., David S. Burgess, Pharm.D., and James S. Lewis II, Pharm.D. Extended-Spectrum β-Lactamases: Epidemiology, Detection, and Treatment *Pharmacotherapy* 2001; 21(8):920-928.

2. David L. Paterson and Robert A. Bonomo. Extended Spectrum Lactamases: a Clinical Update, Clin. Microbiol. Rev. 2005; Vol. 18, No. 4, 657-686.

3. Knothe H, Shah P, Kromery V, Antal M, and Mitsuhashi S. Transferable resistance to cefotaxime, cefoxitin, cefamandole and cefuroxime in clinical isolates of *Klebsiella pneumoniae* and *Serratia marcescens*. *Infection* 1983; 11:315-17.

4. Bush K, Jacoby GA, Medeiros AA. A functional classification scheme for β-Lactamases and its correlation with molecular structure. *Antimicrob Agents Chemother* 1995;39:1211-33.

5. Ralf Rene Reinert, Donald E. Low, Fla´via Rossi, Xiaojiang Zhang, Chand Wattal and Michael J. Dowzicky. Antimicrobial susceptibility among organisms from the Asia/Pacific Rim, Europe and Latin and North America collected as part of TEST and the in vitro activity of tigecycline. *J Antimicro Chemother*; 2007; 60:1018-29.

6. Giske CG, Sundsfjord AS, Kahlmeter G, Woodford N, Nordmann P, Paterson DL, Cantón R, Walsh TR. Redefining extended-spectrum beta-lactamases: balancing science and clinical need. *J Antimicrob Chemother*. 2009;63(1):1-4.

7. Sohei Harada, M.D.1,2, Yoshikazu Ishii, M.D.1, and Keizo Yamaguchi, M.D.1. Extended-spectrum β-lactamases: Implications for the Clinical Laboratory and Therapy. *Korean J Lab Med* 2008;28:401-12.

8. Wiener J, Quinn JP, Bradford PA, *et al.* Multiple antibiotic-resistant Klebsiella and *Escherichia coli* in nursing homes. *JAMA* 1999;281,517-23.

9. Asensio A, Oliver A, Gonzalez-Diego P, *et al.* Outbreak of a multiresistant *Klebsiella pneumoniae* strain in an intensive care unit: antibiotic use as risk factor for colonization and infection. *Clin Infect Dis* 2000;30:55-60.

10. Taneja N and Sharma M. ESBLs detection in clinical microbiology: why & how? *Indian J Med Res* 2008;127:297-300.

11. Kang CI, Kim SH, Park WB, Lee KD, Kim HD, Kim EC, Oh MD, and Choe KW. Bloodstream infections due to extended-spectrum beta-lactamase-producing *Escherichia coli* and Klebsiella pneumoniae: risk factors for mortality and treatment outcome, with special emphasis on antimicrobial therapy. *Antimicrob. Agents Chemother* 2004; 48:4574-81.

12. Paterson DL, KOWC, Von Gottberg A, *et al* Antibiotic therapy for *Klebsiella Pneumoniae* bacteremia: implications of production of extended-spectrum beta-lactamases. *Clin. Infect. Dis.* 2004;39:31-37.

13. Luzzaro F, Docquier JD, Colinon C, *et al.* Emergence in *Klebsiella pneumoniae* and Enterobacter cloacae clinical isolates of the VIM-4 metallobeta-lactamase encoded by a conjugative plasmid. *Antimicrob Agents Chemother.* 2004;48:648-50.

14. Rahal JJ, Urban C, Horn D, *et al*. Class restriction of cephalosporin use to control total cephalosporin resistance in nosocomial Klebsiella. *JAMA* 1998;280:1233-7.

PAN DRUG RESISTANT ORGANISMS

In Singapore a number of isolates have been found which appear susceptible to ceftriaxone and aztreonam at the dilutions performed during routine testing[1]. However, these isolates readily develop mutants at higher inoculums which constitutively hyper-produce the β-lactamase, giving rise to a >30-fold increase in minimal inhibitory concentration (MIC). This may be clinically relevant to infection at sites with poor antimicrobial penetration and high bacterial cell densities. The use of cephalosporins to treat infections with bacteria known to produce AmpC β-lactamases (Enterobacter sp., Serratia sp. C freundii, P. vulgaris, Providencia spp. M. morganii, and now pAmpC-producing E. coli and K. pneumoniae) is prone to failure regardless of the in-vitro susceptibility result and alternative antimicrobials (possibly a carbapenem or fluoroquinolone) should be preferred. Second, because they are weak carbapenemases, hyperproduction of pAmpC in association with porin loss may even lead to carbapenem resistance. Forty per cent of 20 carbapenem-resistant K. pneumoniae isolated in SGH between 2004 and 2006 were positive for blaDHA. Such isolates are sporadic but have been increasing in recent years[2].

Carbapenemases

ESBLs and pAmpCs are able to hydrolyze ESCs, but remain susceptible to carbapenem antibiotics. The carbapenems have consequently become the treatment of last resort. The metallo-β-lactamases (MBLs) are able to hydrolyze even the carbapenems but until recently were only found in the chromosomes of relatively uncommon and less pathogenic gram-negative bacilli like *Stenotrophomonas maltophilia* and *Elizabethkingia meningoseptica* (formerly *Flavobacterium meningosepticum*).

The first transferable MBL IMP-1 was found on plasmids in *Pseudomonas aeruginosa* in Japan in 1988. The first description of IMP-1 outside Japan was in a *K. pneumoniae* strain isolated from a hematology patient in SGH, Singapore in 1996[3]. When the blaIMP-1 gene was transferred by conjugation to an *E. coli* recipient, the transconjugant showed an 8-fold rise in imipenem MIC from 0.25 mg/L to 2 mg/l. This was much lower than the imipenem MIC of the original *K. pneumoniae* isolate (>128 mg/l). However, on repeated subculture, the *K. pneumoniae* isolates become imipenem susceptible again (4 mg/l). Further investigation showed that a porin that was not expressed in the resistant isolate was now being expressed. Taken together, these two findings imply that Enterobacteriaceae that carry MBL genes may appear carbapenem susceptible, while still retaining the potential for developing full-blown carbapenem resistance. The anticipated spread of MBLs in *K. pneumoniae* does not seem to have materialized as carbapenem resistance in this species in Singapore seems to be largely due to pAmpC .

Carbapenem resistance is more common in *P. aeruginosa* than in the enterobacteriaceae. As early as 1991, 10% of *P. aeruginosa* were resistant to imipenem. Because blaIMP-1 had been found in *P. aeruginosa* in Japan, it was logical to see if these genes could also be found in this species in Singapore. blaIMP-1 and another acquired MBL gene blaVIM-6 have also been found in multiresistant *Pseudomonas putida* and *Pseudomonas fluorescens*. While these are relatively nonpathogenic, they may serve as reservoirs of resistance genes which may eventually be transferred to more pathogenic bacteria[2].

Another group of significant multiresistant gram-negative bacilli in the local context are the Acinetobacter sp. Multidrug-resistant Acinetobacter emerged as important pathogens in Singapore from November 1990 onwards, with a strain that was resistant to all antibiotics (including amikacin, ampicillin-sulbactam, ceftriaxone, ceftazidime, gentamicin, netilmicin, perfloxacine, ciprofloxacin, minocycline, imipenem) except polymyxin B. In 1992, two strains were reported as being resistant to even polymixin B. In 1991, 6% of 165 Acinetobacter sp. isolated in NUH, Singapore, were resistant to imipenem. This had increased to 12.9% of 70 isolates by 1993 to 1994[3].

The first transferable carbapenemase to be described in Acinetobacter sp., OXA-23 (then called ARI-1) was found in an isolate in Scotland in 1985. An Acinetobacter sp. from Singapore isolated in 1995 to 1997 was found to have a related oxacillinase, OXA-27, that shares 99% amino acid similarity to OXA-23. Brown *et al.* described 2 new OXA-51-type β-lactamases (OXA-66 and OXA 69) in Acinetobacter baumannii collected from KKWCH between 1996 and 2000. We now know that there are 4 distantly-related families of OXA carbapenemases found in Acineto-bacter spp. OXA-23-type, OXA-24-type, and OXA-58-type are transferable, whereas OXA-51-type appears to be specific to *A. baumannii*. These are even more remotely related to the non-carbapenem hydrolysing oxacillinases like OXA-1[4,5].

All *A. baumannii* that showed carbapenemase activity contained blaOXA-51-type and blaOXA-23 genes. There was a great diversity of blaOXA-51-type genes. Many were blaOXA-66 and blaOXA-69 as had been described by Brown but in addition there was blaOXA-64 and the novel blaOXA-88,

blaOXA-91, and blaOXA-95. Since blaOXA-51-type genes are now thought to be intrinsic to A. baumannii, it was not surprising to also find them (blaOXA-93, blaOXA-94) in isolates which were susceptible to imipenem[4,5]. The problem with multiresistant Acinetobacter species is compounded by their ability to rapidly develop resistance to new antimicrobials. Tigecycline is one of the few recently developed novel antimicrobials with activity against gram negative bacilli.

In19 PDR- *Pseudomonas aerugionosa* strains in China, the resistance mechanism of PDR-PA to cephalosporins, beta-lactam/beta-lactamase inhibitor, carbapenem, fluoroquinolones, and aminoglycosides are due to production of VEB-3-ESBL, aac (3) II, and ant (3") I aminoglycoside modifying enzyme, mutations of DNA gyrase gyrA and topoisomerase parC gene, OprD2 protein deficiencies, and efflux pump overexpression were found[3].

Quinolone Resistance in Enterobacteriaceae

While attention tends to focus on β-lactam resistance, quinolone resistance is also increasing to become a significant problem Hirataka noted in the 1998-2002 SENTRY study that ciprofloxacin coresistance (46%) in ESBL-producing Klebsiella sp. in Singapore (TTSH) was high compared to most other countries[14]. During a recent survey of local hospitals in the public sector, we found that 42% of Klebsiella sp. were ciprofloxacin resistant[5].

References

1. Koh TH, Wang GC, Sng LH. IMP-1 and a novel metallo-beta-lactamase, VIM-6, in fluorescent pseudomonads isolated in Singapore. *Antimicrob Agents Chemother* 2004;48:2334-6.
2. Kouda S, Kuwahara R, Ohara M, Shigeta M, Fujiwara T, Komatsuzawa H, *et al.* First isolation

of bla(IMP-7) in a *Pseudomonas aeruginosa* in Japan. *J Infect Chemother.* 2007;13:276-7.

3. Koh T H. Gram-negative resistance in Singapore: A historical perspective. *Ann Acad Med Singapore* 2008;37:847-54.

4. Walther-Rasmussen J, Høiby N. OXA-type carbapenemases. *J Antimicrob Chemother* 2006;57: 373-83.

5. European Antimicrobial Resistance Surveillance System. Available at: http://www.rivm.nl/earss/database.

6. Robicsek A, Jacoby GA, Hooper DC. The worldwide emergence of plasmid-mediated quinolone resistance. *Lancet Infect Dis* 2006;6:629-40.

Index

TYPHOID